PRAISE FOR *SACRED MEDICINE*

"*Sacred Medicine* is a must-read for anyone who respects the importance of conventional medicine and also wants to dive in to the transformative possibilities of emotional and spiritual healing. Dr. Rankin's healthy dose of skepticism and careful eye for safety make her the perfect guide to introduce the reader to a wide array of healing theories and practices."

Kelly A. Turner, PhD

New York Times bestselling author of *Radical Hope* and *Radical Remission*

"*Sacred Medicine* delivers on the promise of its title, and more. As a well-ness advocate who believes that there is no separation between healing and justice, I was delighted to read every one of Lissa Rankin's words. She has managed to honor both the sacred and the science while illuminating the truth that the two are inextricably linked. Themes of curiosity, compassion, and justice artfully weave throughout the pages in a way that compels the reader to see community as a foundational element of healing. I am so grateful for this expansive, intentional, and incredibly well-researched and well-experienced text on medicine. Brava!"

Rebekah Borucki

mother, author, publisher, advocate

"*Sacred Medicine* takes you on an exciting tour of nontraditional approaches to healing through the eyes of a traditionally trained physician who also carries the heart of a spiritually evolved guide. Ancient and modern healing practices are submitted to the rigors of rational, scientific thought and tapped for their inherent utility and sacred wisdom. Ultimately, you will be the beneficiary of this unique exploration as you navigate your own way through your culture's confusion about healing and spiritual development."

Donna Eden and David Feinstein, PhD

coauthors of *Energy Medicine*

"This is the wisest, most thorough analysis of the mysteries of healing to appear in years. As a physician/healer, Lissa Rankin approaches this subject with scientific thoroughness, but also with the respect and tenderness it requires. This book will be enormously valuable for anyone in the helping professions and for anyone who needs healing—and who doesn't?"

Larry Dossey, MD
author of *One Mind*

"This is *the* book we've all been waiting for—the one that helps us harness the power to heal ourselves while also acknowledging a sacred truth: we often need each other too. Take this book and hold it close to your heart, for there is no better guide than Lissa Rankin for the journey. Through this book, she helps us surrender to the mystery of healing while also supporting us fully in finding the medicine we each deserve."

Amy B. Scher
bestselling author of *This Is How I Save My Life*

"As an integrative medicine physician who constantly navigates this confusing world of science (which I love with my whole heart, but it is limited in its scope) and the vital but murky waters of spirit, faith, energy, *qi*, *prana*, and a host of healing modalities, I deeply respect the journey that this book took Lissa Rankin on personally and professionally. And to navigate these waters within a societal structure that is inherently sexist, racist, professional-ist (not a word, but should be), and infinitely inequitable is a monumental challenge. Dr. Rankin is an admirable warrior in this realm, calling out the shadow and trauma in ourselves and in the fallible humans who can sometimes also be talented and effective healers. In *Sacred Medicine*, she puts the tools of transformation into our hands and gently leads us to the experiences that can unlock healing."

Rachel Carlton Abrams, MD, MHS, ABOIM

"Once in a rare while, one happens upon a writer who is capable of linking worlds and healing the soul. Dr. Rankin is, on one hand, a highly trained physician devoted to evidence and all that the unblinking rational mind can tell us. And on the other hand, she is an explorer who walks into the deeper, less-mapped mysteries of healing where only the prostrate soul can pass. She examines, she pokes, she asks for evidence, she asks what works, she questions herself, and she slowly moves us ahead. It's about the physical, yes, but also about healing the deeper developmental and acute traumas. It's about the science, yes, but also about opening one's heart and knowing how to protect that which is most beautiful and essential. It's about healing the individual, yes, but also about healing the communities and culture. Read this book with attention to the particularities of your own spectacular, wild, and utterly unique life. This is a deeper medicine."

Jeffrey D. Rediger, MD, MDiv
author of *Cured*

"My father was a physician/researcher who wouldn't have believed much of what is contained in this book. Yet he taught me to follow the data, even if it takes you far outside your paradigm. Lissa Rankin is uniquely positioned to lead us on a journey far outside the paradigm of conventional medicine. She is a well-trained physician who appreciates Western medicine and became intrigued by stories of other kinds of healing. She keeps her skeptical part close by as she opens her mind enough to explore the territory of miracle cures and alternative treatments. As she engagingly describes this journey, interspersed with vulnerable self-disclosure and amazing stories, I found myself opening to possibilities I had dismissed. I'm so grateful for the in-person and academic research she includes, as well as for her beginner's mind approach. You will be fascinated by her journey and grateful to her for bringing you along. This book is a big step forward in bridging the gap between traditional and alternative healing!"

Richard Schwartz, PhD
developer of the Internal Family Systems model
of psychotherapy and author of *No Bad Parts*

"Dr. Lissa Rankin takes the reader by the hand on a multidimensional quest for healing and personal transformation through stories, ponderings, and wisdom gleaned from her own life's journey. A bold and stimulating book."

Beverly Rubik, PhD

"*Sacred Medicine* is a gift for our times. Through the wit, wisdom, and candor we have come to know and love from Dr. Lissa Rankin, we discover and uncover the mysteries of healing across the globe—picking up priceless gems from visits to sacred sites, energy healers, dancers, shamans, and trauma therapists along the way. Throughout the adventure, Lissa provides practical steps that allow us to take in the joy of healing with Spirit while practicing wise, trauma-informed discernment. If you're looking to open your heart, soul, and mind to the powerful adventure of healing and personal growth, please take *Sacred Medicine* as a trusted guide along with you in your journey."

Shamini Jain, PhD
founder and CEO of the Consciousness and Healing
Initiative and author of *Healing Ourselves*

"Modern medicine can be highly effective in treating some illnesses, but it can't cure everything. If you or someone you love has a medical issue where doctors shrug and give up, *Sacred Medicine* is the book for you. Dr. Lissa Rankin writes in an engaging, encouraging, and empathic manner, and her survey of 'whole health' approaches to healing is accurate, timely, and authoritative. Bravo!"

Dean Radin, PhD
chief scientist at the Institute of Noetic Sciences and author of *Real Magic*

"I strongly recommend *Sacred Medicine*. There is so much wisdom and information in this book for healing professionals of all kinds, as well as for those struggling with health problems. Dr. Rankin integrates a strong Western scientific basis with an openness to methods of healing that are non-Western and nontraditional. She addresses the paradoxes of healing, writing with nuance about the intersection of science with spirituality, medicine, energy healing, cutting-edge trauma treatments, and making informed medical decisions that are grounded in research and critical thinking and while in touch with emotional, somatic, and intuitive intelligence. This book is an important addition to the broad field of healing."

Laurence Heller, PhD
founder of the NeuroAffective Relational Model (NARM)
and coauthor of *Healing Developmental Trauma*

"*Sacred Medicine* is an account of Dr. Lissa Rankin's valuable and moving ten-year adventure in the science and art of healing, complete with a powerful smorgasbord of methods to try and healers to learn about. Whether she's writing about healing with energy, going on retreat at Lourdes, sampling the arts as forms of healing, describing scientific research on healing, or experiencing potent, emerging therapies, Lissa's evocative prose, deep insight, and wonderful storytelling make for an absorbing and valuable read. Be ready to try it all."

Asha Clinton, PhD

"In this age when dogmatism dominates discussion and people seek out only the like-minded in order to reinforce their beliefs, along comes a breath of fresh air in Dr. Lissa Rankin! Traditionally trained in Western medicine and a fan of its impressive accomplishments, Lissa nonetheless dives deep into a dizzying array of alternative and complementary approaches to healing. She takes us on a rollicking ride into worlds of healing, not just as a critical thinker (which she surely is) but also as someone unafraid to experience her subject firsthand with open eyes, an open heart, and an unquenchable sense of adventure.

Join Lissa on this adventure and, regardless of your starting point, you will have your beliefs and ideas challenged as she continuously challenges her own thinking. This book is not for those who want to remain safe in their own dogmatic silos. How refreshingly delightful!"

William F. Bengston, PhD
president of the Society for Scientific Exploration

"In a time of increasing polarity and othering, we find ourselves, our society, and our planet growing sicker than ever. *Sacred Medicine* is a bridge to real wholeness and healing, an embrace of the paradox, and an integration of both the conventional and the natural, the spiritual and the scientific. This book is a comprehensive and generous gift, not only for those who are seeking healing but also for those who are the healers, doctors, and practitioners who nobly set out to help humanity—but have found it hard to make peace and healing within the fields they inhabit."

Kelly Noonan Gores
writer/director/producer of the documentary *HEAL*

"Lissa Rankin's eye-opening new book offers a binary prescription: make use of both science *and* spirituality, conventional *and* unconventional medicine, in the great work of healing. With a passionate, compassionate, and humble heart, she will help expand your definition—and conception—of what's within your power when it comes to your own healing journey."

Gregg Levoy
author of *Callings* and *Vital Signs*

SACRED
MEDICINE

Also by Lissa Rankin

Encaustic Art: The Complete Guide to Creating Fine Art with Wax

*What's Up Down There? Questions You'd Only Ask
Your Gynecologist If She Was Your Best Friend*

Mind Over Medicine: Scientific Proof That You Can Heal Yourself

*The Fear Cure: Cultivating Courage as Medicine
for the Body, Mind, and Soul*

*The Anatomy of a Calling: A Doctor's Journey from the Head
to the Heart and a Prescription for Finding Your Life's Purpose*

The Daily Flame: 365 Love Letters from Your Inner Pilot Light

LISSA RANKIN, MD

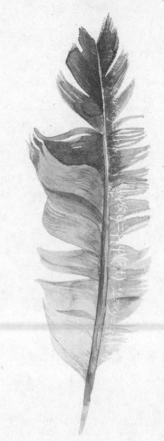

SACRED MEDICINE

A Doctor's Quest to Unravel the Mysteries of Healing

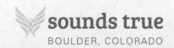

sounds true

BOULDER, COLORADO

Published 2022

Book design Linsey Dodaro

The wood used to produce this book is from Forest
Stewardship Council (FSC) certified forests, recycled materials,
or controlled wood.

Printed in the United States of America

BK06160

Library of Congress Cataloging-in-Publication Data

Names: Rankin, Lissa, 1969-
Title: Sacred medicine : a doctor's quest to unravel the mysteries of healing / Lissa Rankin.
Description: Boulder : Sounds True, 2022. | Includes bibliographical references and index.
Identifiers: LCCN 2021027932 (print) | LCCN 2021027933 (ebook) | ISBN
    9781683647423 (hardcover) | ISBN 9781683647430 (ebook)
Subjects: LCSH: Mental healing. | Mind and body therapies. | Spiritual healing.
Classification: LCC RZ400 .R153 2022 (print) | LCC RZ400 (ebook) | DDC
    615.8/528–dc23
LC record available at https://lccn.loc.gov/2021027932
LC ebook record available at https://lccn.loc.gov/2021027933

10 9 8 7 6 5 4 3 2 1

To Rachel Naomi Remen, MD,
who taught me the difference between healing and
curing and helped me and countless others to heal

Contents

Foreword

n this brave and ambitious volume, Dr. Lissa Rankin set herself a double task. First, to reconcile within herself two parts: the Western-trained, linear thinking, evidence informed and scientifically inclined physician and her own open-hearted, spiritually alive and emotionally ardent self that feels confined within the barriers erected by the former. The latter part, intrigued by the mysteries of healing, calls her to move beyond strict definitions of illness and cure embraced by mainstream medicine and to trust anecdote, story, intuition, and the witness of her own senses. The second task taken on in this work is to bring together age-old tradition, human experience, the wisdom of Indigenous masters, modern forms of healing, such as energy medicine, and deeply intuitive and scientifically well thought out mind-body approaches without, at the same time, denigrating or dismissing the marvelous and truly miraculous achievements of modern medicine.

As an appreciative reader of this book and a Western-educated physician myself, I can well relate to my colleague Lissa's challenge. Not long after I began my own decades of clinical practice within the mainstream medical system, I, too, could not help noticing its limitations and found myself constrained by its ideological narrow-mindedness, notably its failure to see the whole person in his/her/their full humanity with a whole range of physiological, emotional, social, and spiritual attributes and needs, each inseparable from the others. This blindness, as Dr. Rankin shows, extends even to ignoring the well-documented science that has for decades now rendered obsolete any notion of mind/body separation. The result is a reductionist perspective dominated by biology and focused only on our ability to act on the physiology of the body. None of this invalidates the triumphs of scientific medicine, but it helps explain its failures when confronted by chronic conditions of body and mind. Both as a traumatized and suffering person and as a highly trained specialist, Lissa had to envision, stumble toward, struggle to identify, seek, and forge her own path, not only to her personal healing but also to becoming a healer herself. As she clearly articulates, healing may or may not correlate with cure. The latter is not always possible, she acknowledges; the former is always a vibrant potentiality.

If there is a foe Lissa identifies in *Sacred Medicine*, it is dogmatism of any kind: both a dogmatism that would reflexively mistrust medical science but also the too prevalent narrow dogmatism of mainstream medicine that looks down its nose at approaches outside its ken. *Sacred Medicine* is, therefore, a book of inclusion. It does not prescribe nor preach nor prose-lytize: it illustrates, informs, and illuminates. It asks more questions than it answers, and it invites the reader's engagement with these questions to allow the voice within us all to come to the conclusions that suit us, each for ourselves—just as the author intends.

This book is a journey conducted by an informed, inquisitive, and keenly intelligent guide who insists on experiencing—or at least visiting—realms her medical education could not even conceive of, but which humans have explored for eons and continue to. Her path takes her deeply into herself but also to points scattered across the globe from Bali to Latin America, from scientific laboratories to shamanic ceremonies, from encounters with medical intuitives to the latest Western psychother-apeutic modalities. True to her rigorous training, Lissa always wants evidence when available. She does not spare the reader the perhaps discouraging news that various cherished "alternative" approaches are less than solidly established in verifiable fact. Although she hazards some very educated guesses, she does not claim to explain why certain spiritual experiences may, at times, yield seemingly miraculous results in terms of both cure and healing. But her essential point is that suf-fering, even if it cannot always be cured, can always be carried with grace—and even with gratitude. Her personal access to that healing realization has been hard won and, one senses, continues to demand ongoing work. As for all of us.

Filled with telling anecdotes, vivid descriptions, irreverent humor, fearless self-revelation, judiciously used and meticulous research, and personal histories, this book is both a journal of individual transformation and a guide for the reader into worlds that main-stream medical practice dare not stray. By means of guidelines and specific exercises at the end of each section, the reader is invited to deepen their experience of the methods and modalities uncovered by Lissa's eclectic and questing mind.

If there is one rule Lissa Rankin seems to insist on, it is only this: Follow neither her nor anyone else unthinkingly. Open yourself to considering pathways toward healing that may seem strange or even culturally alien but be your own decision maker. To paraphrase Shakespeare, there is much more in this world than the usual medical ideology dreams of. Respect science *and* hold your mind alive to possibilities that may lie outside its narrowly drawn borders. Whichever path you take, whether conventional or complementary or some combination of both, your decision-making capacity will be enhanced by the rich explorations Lissa has here under-taken on our behalf.

Gabor Maté, MD
author of *When the Body Says No: Exploring the Stress-Disease Connection*

Prologue

MY UNEXPECTED
HEALING JOURNEY

The sun rose over the mountains as I hiked to the Muir Beach over look, where the Pacific Ocean was serene after many days of high winds. Although the world around me was calm, my inner land-scape was turbulent. My beloved seventy-one-year-old mother had just received a stage-four cancer diagnosis and dismal prognosis. She wanted palliative chemotherapy and hospice, a decision our family respected, although we were frightened and sad.

Although I knew radical remissions were possible, most of the mi-raculous healing stories I'd heard began with patients taking extreme measures to assert their will to live. And although I held glimmers of hope that my mother might be cured by effortless grace, because she accepted her death as inevitable, I figured hers would be a self-fulfilling prophecy. Still, I was unsure how to survive without her. She was my best friend, my most intimate relationship. I'd always assumed I would wither away when she died, but now I had a daughter—a reason to continue after Mom crossed the threshold of human incar-nation. I had no idea how I could handle losing my mother, but as I watched the sun rise, I recited a prayer I learned from spiritual teacher Tosha Silver: "Divine Beloved, change me into someone who can sur-vive helping my mother die."

When I'd finished, I noticed two young men at the overlook, enjoying the ocean view, beaming. One of them yanked on the leash of his dog, and it slobbered on the grass, lying down to take a nap.

We were chatting about the best places to hike when I moved closer to the dog, *and it struck me like a snake*! None of us saw it coming. The dog had been docile and obedient, his leash slack, resting by his owner's side, until he lunged toward me, locking onto my inner thigh, inches from my crotch and cell layers from my femoral artery. He clenched my flesh in the vise of his teeth and shook my leg like he was trying to pull a wing off a chicken. The three of us were paralyzed as the gravity of the situation kicked in. *This animal could kill me.*

The men screamed. They pulled on the leash with all their might and managed to extricate the dog from my leg. Looking down at my black yoga pants, wet with blood, I realized I'd been mauled.

I heard the terror-stricken dog owner cry, "What do I do? Call 911?"

Most people in that situation would and should call 911 or rush to the ER. Because I am a doctor and knew enough to make that choice for myself, I chose not to go to the hospital. The next day, after seeking an outpatient plastic surgery consultation and being told I'd have to wait at least six weeks and undergo multiple procedures, I declined surgery, although the surgeon warned me the wound wouldn't close without skin grafts.

Four months later, I was dancing and hiking, the gash in my leg fully healed.

I can't take full credit for that outcome, and my fortune was a mark of many unearned privileges, including access to good conventional medicine, expert healers, and all the Sacred Medicine tools I share in this book. Although I wouldn't expect everyone to replicate my good health outcome, my journey inspired me to write what I hope is a clinically relevant book that shows, without exaggerations or sweeping promises, what is within your power to know, practice, and accomplish so you can rest assured that you've done what you can to ease the kinds of suffering Sacred Medicine might help you relieve.

To navigate and get the best results, you'll need to know how to make wise decisions about which conventional medicine and/or complementary and alternative interventions suit you best. You'll need to take a firm stand, even if health-care providers and loved ones pressure you, such as my mother, boyfriend, and surgeon thinking I was crazy to let my dog-bite wound try to close without surgery. You'll want to consider the *objective* aspects of healing—the evidence-based science, statistics, and measurable elements of optimal recovery. But you won't want to neglect the impossible-to-measure but equally important *subjective* aspects—such as the consciousness of your health-care providers; the impact of your consciousness on the repair of your body; and the roles that love, spiritual development, community interconnection, intention, nutrition, movement, creativity, meditation, prayer, feeling your emotions, and healing trauma might have in your recovery.

The best outcomes usually result from a carefully titrated brew of many healing interventions, guided by a recipe only you will know. This isn't to suggest you won't want science, experts, and experience informing your choices. To close my wound nonsurgically, I worked with a wound-care physician who was also a longtime meditator and a restorative presence. She knew I'd declined surgery and supported me with cutting-edge interventions, although she recognized that my choice was risky and was scared along with me. I also sought treatment from an energy healer and a Native American medicine man, applied nutritional interventions to help my body produce collagen, took immune-boosting supplements to prevent infection, and got an energy psychologist involved to help clear the trauma and avoid PTSD symptoms or a dog phobia. I avoided working with health-care providers who weren't willing to cooperate and hold my best interests at heart. I consider the ragged scar on my inner thigh a testament to my struggle but also a reminder of my resilience.

What guided me even more than my medical knowledge was the God inside me, who helps me organize my life and make wise decisions and whom I call my Inner Pilot Light. You have one inside of you too. We all do. The tools in this book will help you strengthen that bond between you and your inner healer so you won't feel adrift on your journey. You'll need that wisdom to make your body miracle prone.

INTRODUCTION

We are all likely to get sick or injured at some point in our lives, as are those we love. None of us are superhuman, so our frailty will catch up to us one day. Even if you're someone who eats a perfect diet, works out every day, avoids bad habits, follows doctor's orders, masters self-care, gulps down a dozen supplements, and meditates daily, there is no permanent immunity to guarantee you disease- and disability-free longevity. Although the body is brilliantly designed to heal itself, it can also break down, and our fragile psyches and souls might endure dark nights for reasons entirely outside our control.

Sometimes we get sick in ways easy to cure. When we do, we would be wise to use whatever medicine works, thanking our lucky stars that a cure exists. Even curable illness can humble us, stripping us of our hubris and shattering our illusions of invincibility. Such temporary setbacks might give us a taste of frailty and humility, but that brush with vulnerability rarely sticks. We bounce back and carry on with business as usual.

Not so when we get leveled by a difficult-to-cure health condition that hits the limit of conventional medicine's mighty powers and leaves doctors flummoxed and patients desperate. When this happens, you might feel cast aside, adding insult to injury. Some doctors don't cope well with feeling powerless to cure disease. Unwittingly, they might withdraw from patients when their suffering eludes cure, telling them there's nothing more that can be done and leaning away at the moment they need someone who leans in. Feeling abandoned, disbelieved, isolated, scorned, or viewed as weak might feel even worse than whatever made you ill to begin with.

To stay present, openhearted, and empathetic with someone suffering in ways you can't relieve is no small task for those trained to "fix" people. Some are gifted in this way; some aren't, not because they're not good people but because it makes them feel uncomfortably powerless and vulnerable when, because of their own wounds, they might fancy themselves the opposite. They don't realize that connection heals, whereas pulling away hurts.

For most of us, being chronically or life-threateningly ill or disabled elicits painful vulnerability. As with sucking air over a toothache, we tend to cringe not only because being sick can hurt but also because we feel scared, impotent, helpless, and even damaged. This can evoke shame, as if it's a sign of weakness, or even worse, of moral or spiritual inferiority. We might go into our darkest places, catastrophizing and imagining that the suffering will never end, or if it does, it might end only in death.

This all-too-common situation can thrust you somewhere few would willingly go, down into the landscape of soul, where we encounter loss, fear, disappointment, loneliness, hopelessness, despair, grief, nakedness, and mortality. To those living in a culture that loves ascending, rising up, staying positive, practicing optimism, and revering strength, *down* can be a dirty word. But from the point of view of the soul, down is *holy ground.* When our health outcomes are uncertain, when we've tried what we can to get better and nothing is working, this holy ground can be a portal to healing. Whether we walk through that sacred doorway is a choice that every individual has the right to make because all are entitled to their own journeys. Whether you step into that opportunity, the portal to healing beckons those ready to cross that threshold.

Perhaps you are ready, or maybe you stand at the threshold, wondering. This book gives you ways to approach that threshold, whether you choose to tiptoe across or cannonball into the deep end.

Many books about health focus on offering hope. They tell you rare but inspiring (and difficult to prove) miracle stories. Yes, grounded hope is good medicine for combating despair. Hope can give you a boost that lifts you over a hump when you can't bear to walk even one more step uphill. Indeed, this is a book about hope because some patients who feel hopeless do get better when they're finally provided the right treatment. I'll be offering you some of these medicines, which your doctor was most likely not trained to include in your Prescription for Health, and it's possible you'll find the relief you've been praying for.

But there are no guarantees. Some suffering cannot be relieved; it can only be borne. In the face of such suffering, there might be no hope. There might be only love to help us avoid bearing our burdens alone.

Although we can do nothing but offer our compassion to those whose suffering cannot be relieved, as a physician, my heart breaks when I see patients suffer needlessly because no doctor told them there might be other options after conventional medicine hits its limits. Over the course of a decade, I set out to discover *what else* might ease suffering if you reach the point when the doctor says, "We've done all we can." For those who have eluded diagnosis or been saddled with a disease that has no known cure, are there medicines that might pick up where conventional medicine leaves off? Might there be tools in the world's medicine bag that serve as adjuncts to, or perhaps even replacements for, some conventional medical treatments with dire side effects and without the promise of a cure?

I had a hunch I had not been given the whole picture in my medical training, so I set out to find hope to offer you, dear reader. However, I want to do more than get your hopes up. I seek to offer you opportunities for healing. What does it mean to heal? By definition, it means *to become whole.* This is the work of the soul, this reclamation of wholeness, which often means venturing not only up into the light, so valorized in our culture, but also down into the holy ground of darkness, bringing the two together into something larger than the sum of their parts. As Rachel Naomi Remen—my spiritual mentor and author of *Kitchen Table Wisdom*—taught me, healing is different than curing. You can be healed without being cured, and you can be cured without being healed. But when healing happens, a cure is sometimes a welcome side effect. Even when it's not, healing makes you whole, and wholeness might just be the raison d'être of human existence.

WHOLENESS IN MEDICINE

Unfortunately, many who claim to promote health fail to realize the importance of wholeness in medicine, focusing unilaterally on the cure while neglecting the value of healing, which impoverishes everyone involved. Narrowing in on the quest for a cure while neglecting the healing process fractures human wholeness and can cause harm, even if the cure happens. Yet this dismembered approach is built into conventional medicine.

By fragmenting the human body, mind, spirit, and energy field into parts siloed into various disciplines by academia, medicine suffers from this reductionism. The body is reduced to the biology department and medical school; the mind to psychology and neuroscience in college and psychiatry and neurology in medical school; the spirit to the religion department and the divinity school. The human energy field is reduced to the physics or biology department. And forget about the heart! Aside from the cardiology department, the heart doesn't even receive a place in academia, except maybe in the literature department.

This fragmented approach to medicine goes all the way back to the mind-body dualism of Descartes in the sixteenth century. The split between spirituality and science goes even further back. But what if, instead of separating these aspects of healing into silos, we healed the rifts, housing them together in a medicine of wholeness?

Although the advent of integrative, functional, naturopathic, and osteopathic medicine is changing this picture, it's still true that few mainstream allopathic doctors prescribe anything but conventional medicine to patients. Nutritional medicine, herbs, and supplements aren't usually on an MD's radar, much less medicines from other cultures, such as Traditional Chinese Medicine (TCM), Ayurvedic or Tibetan medicine, Indigenous healing and shamanism, or spiritual medicines, such as energy healing or faith healing.

As a conventionally trained physician who has spent more than a decade trying to figure out *what else* helps us heal beyond what they taught me in medical school, I now realize that, although medical reductionism comprises either/or polarizations (conventional medicine *or* natural medicine, doctors and drugs *or* spiritual healing), healing is full of both/and paradoxes (conventional medicine *and* natural/spiritual healing).

Perhaps you, dear reader, have approached your own health care in black or white. Maybe you've always thought optimal health comes only from following your doctor's orders—but now you're struggling with a physical or mental health issue your doctor can't seem to solve. Perhaps you've gone the other route, avoiding doctors, drugs, and surgeries altogether and always relying only on natural approaches—yet now you're wrestling with something your naturopath, chiropractor, and acupuncturist can't seem to cure.

As a doctor who took a sacred vow to lean in and devote my life to doing whatever I can to ease the suffering of others, my heart breaks when I see people suffering needlessly because they only know about or are only willing to use the kind of medicine authorized by whatever side of the conventional medicine/complementary and alternative medicine (CAM) divide they find themselves. It can be disheartening to see how much the conventional medicine camp and the CAM camp demonize and diminish each other. Some doctors are skeptical of CAM methods, dismissing them as "unscientific," mouthing off about how it's all snake oil, and treating the people who practice or seek these treatments with derision and contempt. On the other side, some CAM providers or people who use them fall into an "antimedicine" camp, avoiding doctors at all costs; holding reality-denying, antiscience beliefs; feeling betrayed by conventional medicine; and fearing the legitimate damage it can cause. The problem is that when we polarize into camps, we miss out on symptom-relieving or even curative treatments that might be on the other side of the divide. Then people needlessly suffer and die. Why do we do this? Because far too many people stubbornly care more about being *right* than being *healed*.

This is not a book about who's right and who's not; it's a book about healing. When healing happens, you might even find you don't care so much about which camp is right. You care about easing suffering—using *whatever works*.

BRIDGING THE CAMPS

My life path has situated me smack dab in the middle of these two polarities. I am a doctor who loves science and is in awe of what modern medicine can do. I trained at fancy universities, such as Duke and Northwestern, and was fully indoctrinated and stubbornly dogmatic in my adherence to the conventional medicine camp as a result of both my academic training and my physician father. But my worldview shattered by the time I was thirty-six. I wound up leaving my job at the hospital not only because I became disillusioned and "morally injured" by the limitations of conventional medicine and the US health-care system but also because, by the time I was thirty-three, I was a patient taking seven drugs for a variety of health conditions my doctors couldn't seem to cure, and I was afraid I might not live to forty.

In 2007, after becoming a mother, losing my father to cancer, getting fed up with life in the hospital, and feeling hopeless about my medical issues and suicidal to boot, I quit my job as an OB/GYN and embarked upon a journey to discover *what else* helps us heal. I stepped out of the silo of what I was taught in medical school. This took me down a path of exploration beyond conventional medicine—mind-body medicine; psychoneuroimmunology; natural, integrative, and functional medicine; bioidentical hormones; supplements; acupuncture; Qigong; food as medicine; yoga; meditation; all kinds of spirituality; Indigenous healing; energy medicine; dance; creativity; and, ultimately, trauma therapy as it relates to curing illness.

Unlike some doctors who leave medicine and rebel against their training, turning their backs on what they learned and entrenching themselves in the CAM camp, I never lost my respect for the life-saving aspects of conventional medicine. Even though I had my eyes wide open to the limitations and potential dangers of my profession, and I no longer believed it was the *only* medicine in the medicine bag, I neither turned my back on it nor joined the other camp.

By the time I was fifty-two, I had spent fourteen years studying and practicing conventional medicine and another fourteen years studying and practicing everything else along the health, wellness, psychology, yoga, and spirituality gamut. I found just as much shadow in that world as I did in the world of conventional medicine, if not more. You might say I've been a doe-eyed devotee of both camps, but I've also been disillusioned by both. I'm sort of a unicorn but also a bit of an unusual expert in both camps. I know from direct experience that both offer gems and garbage. Both can wow us with miracles or horrify us with malpractice, ethics breaches, criminal acts of fraud and corruption, and even violent crimes, such as rape. This makes me incapable of idealistically lauding either camp as the panacea that will cure all that ails you or unilaterally demonizing, disavowing, or blaming either camp. In other words, there's light and shadow in all medicines, and your job, dear reader, is to educate yourself, practice discernment, and make wise choices about which tools from the world's medicine bag will serve you best. This book will help you learn how.

I started perceiving medicine not as black or white but as the kind of both/ and you might experience if you've ever looked at one of those Gestalt images. You know the black-and-white image that looks like either two black facial silhouettes gazing toward each other or a white vase? Depending on how you alter your perception, you can see the two faces or you can see the white vase, but it's practically impossible to see both images simultaneously. You can almost hear the two camps of medicine arguing.

"It's two black faces, asshole!"

"No, you idiot, can't you see? It's so *obviously* a white vase!"

Both are right, and both are wrong—because both have an incomplete view of the whole picture.

Some people approach medicine the same way. But make no mistake about it: Limiting how you approach health care to one camp or the other could prevent you from having the best possible health outcome, and as I said, it would be heartbreaking if you continued to suffer needlessly. As someone standing on the bridge between camps, I can see both the two faces and the white vase—and I'm here to help you expand your perception too. Especially if you or someone you love is wrestling with a mental or physical illness your conventional or CAM providers have not been able to help you cure, *this book is for you.*

I'll tell you a story about the health-care providers I teach in the training program I founded almost a decade ago—the Whole Health Medicine Institute (WHMI). I started WHMI as a kind of Medical School 2.0. In the beginning, it was for medical doctors only, to teach physicians everything I was learning about the camp of healing we didn't hear about in medical school. But so many healers with letters after their names got insulted! By making the program exclusively for MDs and DOs, we inadvertently triggered a long-festering wound among the naturopaths, chiropractors, acupuncturists, therapists, energy healers, nurses and nurse practitioners, midwives, and physician assistants. Our exclusion criteria needled all their inferiority complexes born of a hierarchy in modern culture that tends to put doctors at the top and undermine the value of what all other health-care providers offer. Not wanting to exclude anyone genuinely interested in Whole Health, we decided to allow anyone who wanted to learn this material to enroll as a student. To avoid setting up an internal hierarchy, we didn't even put any letters at the ends of names on student nametags. We decided to be the "camp of no camps," a bridge between them that recognizes and honors *all* medicines. We figured that everyone was equal and had something of value to offer, and we were all here to learn, heal, love, and accept each other and to humble ourselves before the mystery of healing.

A curious thing kept happening. All our students were healers of some sort, but many were also patients struggling with illnesses and disabilities and longing for relief. Doctors with mystery illnesses conventional medicine hadn't been able to diagnose or cure enrolled. So did chiropractors with back pain chiropractic medicine hadn't helped. Energy healers who avoided doctors like the plague got illnesses energy medicine couldn't cure, and TCM doctors found their herbs and acupuncture needles failing to relieve their symptoms. So, in search of a cure—and in close proximity to healers from other camps because they were all students in the same school—many wound up having to venture into what they often considered an enemy camp.

Voilà! A curious percentage of them had unexpectedly good health outcomes that felt like miracles after their own camp had failed to offer relief. This was both a surprise and a wound to their egos. As it turns out, crossing the bridge from one camp to the other—and humbly walking back and forth across that bridge as needed, guided by a symphony of intelligences you can learn to cultivate within yourself—seems to make some people miracle prone. And that is what I wish for you, dear reader, not as a false promise but as a prayer that you might find relief, and that if you can't, your suffering might be carried on the wings of compassion.

In order to make yourself miracle prone, you'll need to let go of seeing your health care in black or white and bridge the camps with a more paradoxical way of getting your health-care needs met. How? By embracing what I call the *paradoxes of healing*. I'll unpack these paradoxes throughout the book, but to show you how much you might need to stretch beyond black-and-white binaries, I'll introduce you to some key paradoxes.

THE PARADOXES OF HEALING

- You can heal yourself *and* you can't do it alone.

- Conventional medicine can save lives *and* conventional medicine is the third highest cause of death in the United States.[1]

- Keep an open mind *and* don't be so open your brains fall out.

- Be clear in your intention to heal *and* surrender attachment to outcomes.

- Trust your intuition *and* follow the science and apply critical thinking.

- Believe in magic and miracles *and* avoid indulging in magical thinking and denial.

- Be proactive about taking back your power *and* go with the flow.

- Your disease is not your fault, *and* your healing journey *is* your responsibility.

- Stay hopeful *and* be realistic.

- Lead with your heart *and* use your head.

- Be guided by germ theory *and* terrain theory.

- Your thoughts *influence* reality, *and* your thoughts cannot *control* reality.

- We are one, *and* we are separate.

- Maximize self-help *and* be willing to ask for help and rely on others.

- Seek pain relief *and* feel your pain.

- Fear can cause disease *and* repressing or ignoring fear can kill you.

- We are not our bodies, our emotions, or our identities, *and* we are all those things.

- Identifying with your ego can limit your growth and lead to illness, *and* the only way to grow beyond the ego is to stop demonizing it—befriend it, love it, heal it, and integrate it.

- Follow spiritual guidance *and* never be too
  certain that you've got a direct line to God.

Take some time with each of these paradoxes, dear reader. Notice if you feel resistance, relief, or perhaps just curiosity. Whatever arises, welcome it. As you'll learn, welcoming your direct experience and allowing yourself to feel it will be a theme in this book, so you might as well start now. While we're talking about feelings, if you're reading this, I assume you're either struggling with the symptoms of a chronic mental or physical illness you haven't been able to kick (or maybe it has even eluded diagnosis); you've been diagnosed with an "incurable" illness, and you're desperate for that proclamation to be untrue; you're supporting a loved one who is suffering; or you're a health-care provider who wants to make sure you're up to date on all possible avenues of treatment for your patients or clients. If any of this is true, then I'll begin by saying I'm sorry if what you're going through is hard. I'm sorry if the camp of medicine you genuinely believed could cure you, your loved ones, or your patients has failed you. I'm sorry if you're in pain or scared or feeling helpless, hopeless, defeated, ashamed, or exhausted from trying to get better. I've felt all those ways, too, and I mean it when I say it's my intention to hold you and your tender feelings with great care as we navigate this journey. If I mess that up, I'm sorry about that too. As you'll see, this is not an easy journey we are about to embark upon. But I hope you will sense through my words that you journey in good company, not just with me but also with everyone else who reads this book, with everyone who has ever suffered illness, and with all people who have devoted themselves to healing themselves or others. This is the human experience, and you are not alone.

EMBRACING THE MYSTERY

The good news is that although our bodies, psyches, and spirits are vulnerable, fragile, sensitive, and prone to imperfect functioning, we are also marvelous creations with healing abilities and resilient capacities not fully understood by doctors, CAM providers, scientists, psychologists, theologians, or philosophers. There are mysteries we have yet to solve, like why some people have "spontaneous" remissions from "incurable" diseases such as stage-four cancer or human immunodeficiency virus (HIV) infection and others don't, something radical remission researchers have studied ad nauseum without answering definitively. Other mysteries, such as the placebo effect, could not be solved even by a multidisciplinary team of geniuses who convened for a conference at Harvard in the 1990s to try to figure it out, as detailed in Anne Harrington's book *The Placebo Effect*.

Over the years, as I became particularly curious about the mystery of various forms of spiritual healing, shamanism, and energy medicine, which I came to call Sacred Medicine, I started asking questions: "What is it? Does it work? Is there any proof that it's effective? If so, what is the mechanism? What diseases does it work best for, if at all? How might we use it clinically alongside other medicines to relieve suffering in the vulnerable? How can we make wise, ethical, sound choices about its usefulness as part of the world's medicine bag?" I set out to answer some of these questions, knowing my quest might be futile, because many had journeyed before me, and nobody I'd met had found the holy grail that held the secrets of healing.

What we do know is that we make cancer cells every day, and our bodies mostly keep us cancer-free. We're exposed to infectious diseases all the time, and unless it's a novel virus our immune systems have never encountered before, such as the coronavirus that caused the recent pandemic, we rarely catch those infections. Cutting-edge science even shows us that blocked coronary arteries can sometimes unblock themselves. What happens to inhibit this natural self-healing process, allowing heart attacks to flatten us, cancers to take hold, autoimmune diseases to settle in, or infections such as Lyme disease or Covid-19 to disable us?

Sure, we can engage in healthy behaviors so the body is less likely to get sick in the first place, but what else can sick people do to jump-start healing when the body's natural abilities have broken down? And what can we make of all the alleged miracle cures floating around the internet? Are any of them real or replicable? Might we learn something from those stories that could help you, dear reader, become more miracle prone?

The *Oxford English Dictionary* defines a miracle as "a surprising and welcome event that is not explicable by natural or scientific laws and is therefore considered to be the work of a divine agency." While I was doing research for my book *Mind Over Medicine: Scientific Proof You Can Heal Yourself*, I bumped into a lot of stories of healings that fit this dictionary definition. At first, puffed up by my scientific certainty, I felt fairly comfortable with my conclusion that these stories I was hearing could be written off as

unscientific exaggerations or at least demystified and explained physiologically. No need to entertain the idea that something magical or supernatural
or even divine was happening. I thought I could explain it all with hard
science. But after publishing that book in 2013, I kept meeting people
whose stories didn't fit the neat, tidy scientific explanation I promoted in it,
so I revised it in 2020 to bring it up to date with what I'd learned.

I also questioned whether sharing those rare miracle stories actually
helped sick people. If you or someone you love is struggling with a chronic or life-threatening illness, those stories might elicit a frustrated eye roll
or cause you to wonder whether you're doing something wrong or are
not worthy or special enough to be granted your own miracle. I wasn't
sure if collecting more of those rare stories and getting people's hopes up
was helpful, but I also didn't want to leave any stone unturned that might
help suffering people experience relief or assist dying people to live a few
more years worth living.

The truth is that seemingly miraculous stories of healing are far out-
numbered by heartbreaking stories of innocent children and adults who
did everything they could to try to get their miracle, yet stayed sick or
died seemingly before their time. I wound up asking every spiritual healer
I met how they wrestled with the question: "What story do you tell yourself about why innocent people suffer?" None of their answers satisfied
me, but I didn't have a better one. I wondered whether much of spirituality is an attempt to answer that unanswerable question because we find
this mystery unbearable. Can we not cope with feeling that out of control
or concluding, "I don't know"?

As a mystic with an intimate, lifelong relationship to the Divine, I was
willing to accept that maybe some people are granted mystery cures as
an act of God, something humans can't control and have no business
messing with. But as a skeptical physician who respects the objectivi-
ty of science, who retired from clinical practice to research and write
about radical remission, I wanted to see if I could discover the "whys" and
"hows" of people who exceeded expectations.

I want to make it explicitly clear that it is not my intention to suggest
that people who are sick, injured, or suffering brought it upon themselves
or aren't good enough at creating the conditions for healing. The global
Covid pandemic showed us that some people—including world-famous
doctors—in wellness communities, the yoga world, alternative medicine,
mind-body healing, and spirituality circles hold the belief that "keeping

your vibe high," eating a "pristine" diet, meditating hard enough, saying enough positive affirmations, holding the thought form that you'll never get sick, or cleaning up your "terrain" will make you immune to disease. This dangerous delusion spread by many online wellness influencers who became entangled in "conspirituality" was responsible for countless unnecessary deaths and a lot of shaming of those who did get sick or died of Covid.[2] That is the *opposite* of healing.

We'd be wise to be honest and humble about how much power we really have to cure illness, regardless of which camp we might lean toward. Although I've seen more than my share of treatment failures by doctors full of hubris, I've seen just as many or more treatment failures by equally arrogant energy healers, faith healers, shamans, herbalists, and fad-diet promoters. Contrary to widespread belief, not only genetic predisposition, hindered access to good medical care, poor nutrition, bad habits such as smoking, exposure to environmental toxins and infectious diseases, and lack of exercise make people sick. It's also not simply whether you see the best doctors at the most stellar university hospitals, meditate regularly, drink your green juice, perfect your downward dog, load yourself up with supplements, and eat only organic food that can lead to healing.

In 2020, it became clear that so many of our kindred human beings wind up sick because of conditions utterly beyond their control—the traumas of poverty, systemic racism, relentless oppression, patriarchal cultural norms, or ongoing personal or institutional abuse, along with the brutal aftermath of enslavement, colonization, land theft, unethical wars, and environmental degradation. Massive traumas such as these affect not only mental but also physical health. The coronavirus pandemic made it glaringly obvious that health is not just an individual issue but a collective one.

I do believe we have *some* power over whether we experience an optimal health outcome. I also believe life doesn't always cooperate with giving us what we want, and our attempts to control all aspects of our lives usually fail. Although some people believe we can "manifest" our miracles, it's also true that we might not be as powerful as we think to change the countless factors that influence why some people get their greatest longings fulfilled and others don't. As Black antiracism activist Rachel Cargle posted on her Instagram, "Maybe you manifested it. Maybe it's white privilege."[3]

Whether we're talking about good health, financial abundance, the fulfillment of creative or career ambitions, or finding a soul-mate, the conversation about whether we can heal ourselves, control our reality, and get whatever we want with the power of our positive thinking or spiritual power is not complete without considering the impacts of opportunity, access, financial inequity, and social injustice as they relate to race, gender identity, sexual orientation, and the consequences of massive collective traumas.

With all those disclaimers, this book distills down to one overriding question: *What is within your power to ease your suffering and make yourself miracle prone?* Recovery programs often say the Serenity Prayer: "God, grant me the serenity to accept the things I cannot change, the courage to change the things I can, and the wisdom to know the difference." This book seeks to help you do all three. It also invites us to help each other carry together—in community—the burdens of suffering we can neither change nor accept.

CAN WE DEMYSTIFY HEALING?

I had no idea a decade ago that my attempt to answer these questions would lead me to the *paqos* in the Andes in Peru; the backyards of healers in Bali; Indigenous medicine men and women in the United States, Canada, Colombia, Africa, and Australia; kahunas in Hawaii; Qigong healers from China; researchers and renegade scientists pursuing the thankless task of validating things not seen; mystics in caves, monasteries, and ashrams; swamis, gurus, and pastors from many religions; and a variety of energy healers and faith healers from around the globe. I would be led to sacred sites reputed to be places of healing, participate in group healings facilitated by huge circles of meditators, anointed with oil, smudged with sage, poked with sticks, baptized with water, chanted over, strewn with coca leaves, surrounded by bones, and touched with healing hands. I would dance, make art, chant, pray, meditate, and meet many of my inner children, alongside spirit guides and demons. I would go "bliss hunting" and feel ecstatic. I would study trauma healing and cry, grieve, rage, scream, and shake. I would be frightened, threatened, and psychically attacked by dark energies I didn't even believe in. I would feel exploited and grow disillusioned, despairing, and downtrodden. I would love, be loved, and feel the most extreme gratitude. My quest would take me on the wildest adventures of my life, and I would sob when it was finally over because it was the hardest thing I'd ever done. I was both awakened and wounded by the journey.

I was not sick or in need of physical healing at the time I embarked upon this journey, having already experienced my own radical remission from a whole host of medical conditions that got me off the seven drugs I was taking when I left the hospital. This was meant to be more of an intellectual exploration, a kind of "globe-trotting grad school" for everything they never taught me in medical school, which I intended to bring back as my sacred offering to those suffering as I once did. What I did not anticipate was that, in the course of doing this research, I would have the opportunity to apply what I was learning as I dealt with an acute medical crisis and became a patient myself.

WHAT ARE YOUR WHOLE HEALTH INTELLIGENCES?

Although there are heartbreaking disparities in access to affordable conventional medicine, a dearth of doctors who can be good allies, and expensive alternative medicine practitioners and trauma therapists who don't take insurance, we all have equal access to the same powerful inner tools, no matter the difference in our outer circumstances. An essential element of my healing success—and yours—is what I call the four Whole Health Intelligences:

1. Mental
2. Intuitive
3. Emotional
4. Somatic

There might be other intelligences included among these, such as creative or erotic intelligence, and they can all be accessed to guide our healing, but our intelligences work best when they flow together. To create the conditions to make your body miracle prone, you'll need to connect with all four. When we synchronize and harmonize them, we wind up in the flow state that creative types and athletes describe. It's also the state that can predispose you to unexpectedly good health outcomes. Because healing is, by definition, a return to wholeness, accessing your Whole Health Intelligences must be a foundational part of any healing journey.

Assess Your Whole Health Intelligences

Take a personal inventory of the relative strengths and weaknesses of how you work with your four Whole Health Intelligences. Without judgment or self-criticism, get curious and be honest. On a scale of zero to ten, zero being "no access" and ten being "highly attuned," rate yourself in each of the four Whole Health Intelligences.

Mental Intelligence
Am I . . .
> a critical thinker?
> most comfortable making decisions based on accurate
>   information?
> trusting in science?
> curious, tending to process things mentally?
> skeptical of phenomena I can't explain logically?
> able to distinguish between facts, propaganda, and
>   manipulation?
> discerning?
> someone who gets lost in my head?

Intuitive Intelligence
Do I . . .
> get spontaneous, ultimately helpful information flashes?
> distinguish between "thinking things up" and intuition
>   that "drops in"?
> get feedback from others about how intuitive I am?
> know things I couldn't possibly know rationally in ways
>   later verified?
> have precognitive dreams or visions?
> access multidimensional realms others don't seem to visit,
>   or see/hear/sense beings invisible to others?

Emotional Intelligence

Can I . . .

read and feel other people's emotions accurately?

attune to my own feelings?

establish boundaries between other people's feelings and mine?

respond to what I read in other people with empathy without their emotions making me pull away, try to fix them, or flood me with their feelings?

avoid either repressing emotions or exploding with them?

care about the suffering of others (and myself) and feel motivated to help ease suffering?

feel my heart open and respond to this heart opening with my courage and sacred activism in the face of injustice?

Somatic Intelligence

Am I . . .

aware of my physical sensations on a regular basis?

attuned to "gut" feelings?

grounded, firmly planted on earth (as opposed to being flighty, uncoordinated, or ungrounded)?

able to read subtle body signals or symptoms before they become big ones?

able to ask my body questions and interpret my body's "yes" or "no" with some confidence?

able to titrate what my body and nervous system can handle without pushing myself to the point of injury or getting flooded or overwhelmed somatically?

THE WHOLE HEALTH MODEL OF HEALING

The work of integrating the Whole Health Intelligences requires developing an orchestra conductor within you who arranges and harmonizes the intelligences. In a mind-dominated, patriarchal culture, we tend to give mental intelligence more weight than it deserves, overshadowing the wisdom of more ancient feminine intelligences—intuition, body, and emotions. By contrast, in New Age spiritual circles and certain wellness communities, over-reliance on intuition can cause people to ignore the critical thinking necessary to distinguish fact from fiction, intuition from wishful thinking, and science from conspiracy. In an unbalanced psyche, we tend to fragment, and one intelligence might overpower and dominate the others, causing us to be lopsided. However, when we gather information from all our intelligences, without overlooking any (especially the oft-maligned and neglected intelligence of "negative" emotions), we make healthy, balanced decisions.

In *Mind Over Medicine,* I offer healing tools scientifically proven to optimize a patient's chance for radical remission when everything else has failed to cure disease. I collected these health-inducing interventions into one wellness model I call the Whole Health Cairn. I won't get into the details—you can read about them in *Mind Over Medicine*—but as a quick review, a cairn is a stack of balanced stones like the ones you see adorning beaches or marking hiking trails, graves, or sacred landmarks. In the Whole Health Cairn, each stone represents an element of wellness and is contained in a Healing Bubble of love, pleasure, gratitude, and service, all balanced upon the primary stone—our Inner Pilot Light. If any stone in the Whole Health Cairn is unbalanced or unaligned with the Inner Pilot Light, the entire structure is at risk of collapsing.

While treating patients and training doctors, I incorporated the Whole Health Cairn into a process I call the Six Steps to Healing Yourself. These steps help identify areas in your life that might be causing stress in the nervous system and making it difficult for the body's natural self-healing mechanisms to operate effectively. None of these steps alone is typically adequate for optimal results, but when some patients, upon whom conventional medicine has given up, combine them, they report better-than-expected results.

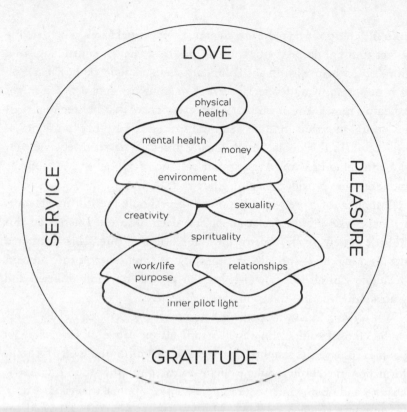

SIX STEPS TO HEALING YOURSELF

1. Believe that healing is possible.
2. Connect and surrender to your Inner Pilot Light, letting your innermost knowing guide your healing journey.
3. Surround yourself with healing support.
4. Diagnose the root cause of your illness.
5. Treat your fears and resistance.
6. Write the Prescription for Health for yourself.

This process of self-inquiry culminates in writing your Prescription, informed by the four Whole Health Intelligences. When you use your Whole Health Intelligences to guide these six steps, you'll discover that the Prescription might mean surgery, chemotherapy, or improving your diet. You might seek professional treatment for unhealed trauma or end a toxic relationship. Perhaps you will change your career to help you fulfill your life's purpose, be more honest about your sexual needs, sing the song as yet unsung, deepen your spiritual practice, change your living situation, or get help with financial limitations that might be healable even if it means applying for social services or disability support. You might take up a movement practice or other experiences that bolster your mental health and spark healing neurotransmitters and other hormones of self-repair. In this book, I'll offer many potential Sacred Medicine components to add to your Prescription because they might not be on the radar of other providers helping guide your journey.

Our ancestors surely relied upon all four Whole Health Intelligences to make wise life, health, and societal decisions, and I activated this holistic system in the face of my traumatic dog bite. This integrated decision-making, especially in times of crisis, relies upon the interconnectedness of all things and helps you protect not only yourself and your family but also the good of the collective.

When I've worked with patients, finding balance between the ten stones in the Whole Health Cairn was often difficult and sometimes triggering for people. To have the stamina, courage, and dedication necessary for transformation, the Healing Bubble offered a cushion to the grounded lifestyle changes and healing interventions necessary for optimal results. Love heals because we can do hard things with great love; service helps avoid the tendency to become self-absorbed and fosters gratitude, one of the most healing emotions; and pleasure makes everything more delightful.

Not every patient experiences every aspect of the Healing Bubble equally. Those who tend toward unbalanced hedonism might need less pleasure and more service. Others who tend toward martyrdom and excessive caretaking need less service and more pleasure. Those who use gratitude practices to deny what isn't working in their lives might need more self-love so they can quit pretending to be grateful for an abusive relationship or other hardship. Although the stones in the Whole Health Cairn are solid, evidence-based, scientifically verifiable aspects of good health and longevity, the ingredients in the Healing Bubble have to be customized—a dash of gratitude, two helpings of love, one part service, a pinch of pleasure. Perhaps this is what Sacred Medicine is—an elixir to create the conditions for healing.

The Whole Health Cairn was a sensible starting point for my healing journey after the dog-bite injury and for many of the patients I worked with over the years. However, although I had myriad testimonials from the hundreds of thousands of people who read *Mind Over Medicine* and from the doctors I trained to work with these methods, something was missing. It's like I'd catch a whiff of what I was after, but just as the smell of jasmine might waft through an open window, an ineffable aspect of healing was hard to capture. My Sacred Medicine journey became a way to bottle up aspects of healing that were elusive and difficult for science to capture, explain, and prove. It was subjective and more numinous than anything I wrote about in *Mind Over Medicine,* which focused on evidence-based science—the objective, measurable aspects of healing written up in medical journals.

IN SEARCH OF THE HOLY GRAIL

I initially set out with the hopes of helping you and those you care about relieve the suffering within your power to ease. I didn't know at the time I would wind up saving myself. As Rachel Naomi Remen, MD, once told me, "Sometimes the soul will grab you by whatever handle is sticking out. When the soul is in charge, very often, we do the right thing for the wrong reasons."

I look back at my grandiose fantasies of who I was when I first embarked upon this Sacred Medicine quest more than a decade ago, and I feel tender amusement that I had the chutzpah to even try to hack healing, as if radical remissions were Nancy Drew mysteries that just needed a smart enough girl detective to solve them. I will disappoint you from the beginning with a spoiler alert, dear reader, and confess that this book does not end with the triumphant news that I have cracked the code of miraculous healing that will stave off illness, disability, and death for everyone forever. I did not discover the secret to immortality, the cure for cancer, or a guaranteed way to live to be more than a hundred with no disease or disability until you die peacefully in your sleep.

I did, however, discover another kind of holy grail, something unexpected and full of wonder, a game changer that even now, as I write this, renders me misty eyed, bursting with awe, and overflowing with gratitude. I won't spoil this surprise for you but rather will let you discover it for yourself. I promise that if you can make it through the rough patches you might experience on your journey through this book, the treasure will be worth any hiccups along the way.

Although other kinds of medicine are valuable and worthy of including in your Prescription, this book focuses on a narrow niche of what might help relieve your suffering when nothing else has worked. Specifically, the healing tools I offer in this book address the subjective approaches science doesn't yet know how to measure—subtle energies, love, community, consciousness, connection to the earth, ritual, creativity, intuition, movement practices, meditation, relationship to the Divine, what helps life force flow, and what plugs up the leaks so we stop hemorrhaging it in the first place. Because some people mistake the term *Sacred Medicine* with plant medicine, be clear that for a variety of reasons, I did not include in the scope of my study the many psychedelics and plant medicines increasingly used for healing. This is not to diminish the value of such medicines any more than it is to negate the value of evidence-based conventional medicine and more objective aspects of healing. But I did not experiment with such medicines. Nor did I research the many nutritional medicines, herbs, supplements, or anything that required crystals, potions, gadgets, or gizmos to activate your life force. My intention was to focus on what could help you *self-heal* with only the facilitation of others who hold sacred space and support your healing process.

I caution you to avoid comparing your journey to mine in the chapters that follow because the distribution of all medicines is not equal or fair on this planet. All suffering that can be treated deserves relief, not just that of the privileged but of all beings. As I reflect on my own healing journey, I'm uncomfortably aware of my privilege. Most people do not have the choice to globe-trot, work with the world's best healers, eat from the most organic gardens, or hire the best trauma therapists. Perhaps one day every patient struggling with illness, injury, or trauma can access this Whole Health care—inside or outside a hospital setting—in a way that is accessible, equitable, and affordable. That hasn't happened yet, but through my work with Heal at Last, a nonprofit we are developing to bring cutting-edge healing modalities and trauma therapies to people who would not otherwise be able to afford or access them, I'm actively working to democratize Sacred Medicine and make it available to anyone emotionally and spiritually ready to apply it, regardless of socioeconomic status, race, gender identity, sexual orientation, political affiliation, or religion. Until my vision becomes a reality, my prayer is that this book will be a democratizing bridge, guiding you through easy-to-learn self-help practices that can be implemented at no cost. Because most people are unable to take time from their life, travel around the world to sacred sites, or work directly with the world's expert healers, I did it for you. Like a treasure hunter on a quest, I've brought back what I learned to share as my offering to those who might benefit.

Keep in mind that self-help only takes us so far. Most healing comes from safe, unconditionally loving, healing relationships with those who care for us when we are weakened, vulnerable, and in need of help. Self-help tools won't replace healing touch, having someone generously listen when you're hurting, and the presence of someone—or even better, a community of someones—who hold a healing frequency of love. If you intend to use these self-help tools without healers, therapists, and other skillful facilitators, please gather your inner circle to help you heal. If you're typically the caregiver, stretch yourself to ask the people resourced to support you to envelope you in a Healing Bubble so you know you don't have to do this alone. Rugged individualism may be an American value, but even John Wayne needed help when he got stomach cancer. Nobody who has an optimal health outcome arrives there alone, so please, even if it makes you uncomfortable, let yourself receive.

HOW TO USE THIS BOOK

Each chapter will offer you invitations to play with a variety of Sacred Medicine practices. Some might resonate with you. Some might not. My recommendation is that you approach these with childlike wonder, like a kid in the Sacred Medicine candy store. Be curious. Try out what feels like it's meant for you. Toss anything that sounds like nonsense. And trust your inner guidance to know what's right for your unique journey. Remember, one person's medicine might be another's poison. You will be concocting your own alchemical recipe for healing. I'm only offering you ingredients with which you might brew your own healing potion.

Although there's some overlap in how these elements work, as a general rule, Sacred Medicine practices you'll learn in part one are intended to lift you up, fill you with life force, and serve as a kind of "energy transfusion" in case your life force is a bit anemic because of whatever is causing you to suffer. Practices in part two are mostly meant to keep you safe from harm because there can be pitfalls in the Sacred Medicine realm, just as you'd be wise to tread carefully in conventional medicine and be a savvy, empowered patient who knows how to milk an imperfect system for its healing nectar. Practices in part three are intended to unblock the areas where life force might be draining or stuck so you don't keep leaking life force and getting anemic. It works best if you marry practices in part one with practices in part three so you're simultaneously filling your tank and preventing leaks, all while using what you learn in part two to practice healthy discernment and protect yourself from harm.

This journey won't always be easy, but I'll do my best to make it as gentle as possible. In general, part one practices are relatively easy to engage, and part three practices can be more difficult. You'd do well to toggle between the two, titrating based on your comfort, tolerance, and stamina and taking breaks when needed.

This is where you have the opportunity to return to one of the paradoxes of healing. You begin by casting your vote to relieve any suffering you haven't known how to release so far. If you're up for the challenge, you start by putting the full weight of your focus, dedication, commitment, attention, intention, discipline, courage, and self-care behind your desire to get well. You declare a vow to the Universe that announces, "I'm a *yes* to healing, and I'll do *whatever* is within my power to demonstrate my commitment, even if it's uncomfortable." You double down, claim your will to actualize the highest potential of what is available to you, and fill out your ballot. In the cocreation process, your vote, and your commitment matter—*a lot*.

Then you take that ballot, and you put it in the cosmic drop box, handing over the burden of your intense desire to get well and surrendering any attachment to outcomes to whatever higher power or force of love resonates with you, whether that's God, your Higher Self, or something in nature you trust, such as a redwood tree or your favorite lake. This act of humility, trust, intimacy, and reconnection with whatever you might call the Divine helps you loosen your grip on trying to control an uncontrollable process, restoring spiritual connection, and allowing your nervous system to relax, thereby activating healing.

With your vote cast and your ballot surrendered, you are now free to begin your journey. If it feels right to you, you might want to cross over this metaphorical threshold with a gesture of your commitment that feels authentic to you. Whether you cross this threshold physically, anchoring it with some ritual or movement practice, or whether you do so in your mind's eye or inside your own heart, you can trust that your vow to commit to your healing process has begun, and your choice has been witnessed by whatever organizing intelligence or force of love feels natural to you.

Just remember, dear reader—you are loved. You are safe. *You are not alone.* I hope you can tune into the resonance of every individual who will ever read this book. Although the journey might be harder for some than for others for reasons that are no one's fault, *we are all in this together.* I hope you feel our connection in this global circle of healing as we expand to embrace each other beyond the borders of our separateness. You are witnessed by a million angels, spirit guides, ancestors, and all the other people who ever read this book who are together, cheerleading you on, waving pom-poms, and saying, "Let this one finally be free."

Part One

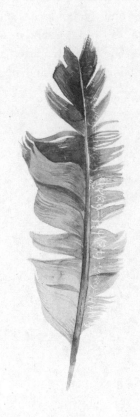

HEALING
TRANSFUSIONS

f you're on a healing journey, it's safe to assume you're experiencing a challenge or emotional or physical pain or you are stuck. Healthy life force, or what some healers call *chi* or *prana,* results when energy and information flow. When this occurs, you feel radiantly alive, your body is more capable of healing itself, and synchronicities become commonplace. You connect with your purpose and intuition, and experience a direct intimacy with all life forms. Your emotions are fluid, your mind is clear, your soul is awake, and your body tends to feel good.

Flow states are the result of energy and information in motion; however, when life force gets stuck and contracted in the body, we tend to feel depleted, sick, depressed, anxious, or numb like a vessel leaking life force. When the flow is blocked or congested, no matter how much you fill yourself with nutritious food, supplements, sleep, positivity, and other uplifting behavior, life force seems to drain away, turning the simplest efforts into Herculean tasks. Especially if illness, loss, trauma, or another crisis comes as a shock, it can bring you to your knees, making it difficult to stand.

The Sacred Medicine practices in part one are intended to restore the flow of life force, to lift you up. Although you might get this boost from a healer, it doesn't have to come from another person. It could come from a holy place or the love of a group that offers radiant healing vibes. You might find yourself raised up by earth herself through a profound encounter with nature. It might arise from a mystical experience in contemplative prayer or meditation or awaken from ritual, dance, singing, or creative expression.

I offer this medicine to strengthen, comfort, inspire, and revitalize you enough to get you back on your feet. For some, these practices are the destination, fostering self-healing and leading to enduring cures. For others, they serve to fortify, alleviate symptoms, and provide energy, but the journey might not be over.

Chapter 1

GROUP HEALING
AS MEDICINE

n 1858 in the small town of Lourdes, in the foothills of the Pyrenees in France, a fourteen-year-old peasant girl, Bernadette Soubirous, announced she'd been visited by the Virgin Mary. Over the next five months, the Virgin appeared to Bernadette eighteen times at the Grotto of Massabielle, along the Gave de Pau River. Dressed in white with a blue sash, the apparition who came to be called Our Lady of Lourdes gave Bernadette a Divine order: "Construct a chapel at the site of the visitations; offer a place for prayer, penance, and reparation with God for all who visit." She instructed Bernadette to uncover a miraculous spring that would heal people and invited her to drink and bathe in its healing waters.

Crowds of skeptical townspeople watched Bernadette squat inside the grotto and scrape away earth until water emerged. She drank until her face was covered with mud, and the bystanders assumed she'd lost her mind until a spring arose in the grotto, filling the hole Bernadette had dug with her hands. Awestruck, the observers filled containers with the water and took them home. To this day, the spring continues to flow with what's considered holy water. Pilgrims from around the world come to drink and bathe at Lourdes and touch the walls of the grotto where the Virgin appeared to Bernadette.

The first miracle is said to have happened four days after Bernadette dug up the spring. A thirty-nine-year-old woman, Catherine Latapie, from a nearby town had injured her hand after a fall, leaving two fingers paralyzed, bent toward her palm. Neither a believer nor Catholic, Catherine had paid no mind to the excited stories about Bernadette's visitations. Yet, inexplicably, in the middle of the night, burdened by the heavy belly of a third-trimester pregnancy, Catherine found herself grabbing her children and traveling to Lourdes, where Bernadette met her at dawn. They entered the grotto together and knelt in prayer. Catherine dipped her hand in the spring, and her fingers spontaneously reverted to normal, regaining all function. Later that day she delivered her third child, who became a priest.

In the years that followed, so many miraculous cures were reported that in 1883 the Catholic Church and the medical establishment developed a process to ensure no false miracles were proclaimed. Only those deemed supernatural in origin and not the result of "hysteria" were considered. In other words, an attempt was made to rule out what would come to be called the *placebo effect* to prove evidence of Divine intervention.

Lourdes is not the only place people go to receive healing from water. As reported in the *Washington Post*, many thousands of sick people line up daily to take away a can or two of the now-famous miracle "light water" from Jesus Chahin's well in Tlacote, Mexico, said to have cured everything from acquired immune deficiency syndrome (AIDS) to high cholesterol.[1] So many people reported unexplainable healings from a spring in a cave in Nordenau, Germany, that it caught the attention of the scientific community, which acknowledged the water's healing properties, naming it the Nordenau phenomenon.[2]

THE SKEPTIC ON A MYSTICAL JOURNEY

To explore interventions that tend to make people miracle prone, I knew I'd have to visit at least one sacred site reputed to cause miracles because people all over the globe often resort to pilgrimages to special places and say prayers for miracles after conventional medicine has failed them. Pilgrimages to sacred sites of healing far predate seeking what modern society thinks of as medicine. Indigenous cultures have been practicing pilgrimages to sacred sites in search of healing for millennia. In ancient Greece, healing temples were dedicated to Asclepius, the first doctor-demigod in Greek mythology, said to have the power to raise the dead. Pilgrims flocked to these temples in search of physical and spiritual healing. Those in the Greek Orthodox tradition make pilgrimages to churches dedicated to the healing saints Cosmas and Damian, hoping to receive divinely inspired dreams and cures. Muslim pilgrims visit Mecca, the birthplace of the prophet Mohammed, and the shrines of saints. Protestants visit Jerusalem and make pilgrimages to the holy sites of Jesus Christ's life and death. Along with Lourdes, Catholics visit the Black Madonna at the Basilica of Our Lady of Guadalupe, apply "healing dirt" at the Santuario de Chimayo in New Mexico, or walk the *camino* (road) to Santiago de Compostela. Hindus make their journeys to the waters of the Ganges River, the holy mountain caves of Amarnath in Kashmir, and the great Indian temples. Buddhists visit Bodh Gaya, where the Buddha is said to have attained enlightenment under the Bodhi tree. Pagans journey to Stonehenge or Glastonbury. Modern Indigenous people still undertake vision quests and pilgrimages to holy sites and vortices such as Machu Picchu in Peru, Uluru in Australia, and various mountain peaks, seeking connection to the spirit world. Some pilgrims report having dreams and visions that cured them, waking up healed after falling asleep sick at these places. Others are said to be cured on the spot.

Countless people who heard my talks, took my courses, or read *Mind Over Medicine* shared their stories of miraculous cures as a result of pilgrimages to sacred sites, ashrams, and retreat centers presided over by mystics and gurus. For example, Will was nine years old when diagnosed with a golf-ball-sized, stage-two astrocytoma, an inoperable brain tumor. His father was a cardiologist, a believer in conventional medicine. However, both parents were unsatisfied with the grim prognosis the conventional doctors made for their son. They researched countless alternative modalities, and Will wound up spending two years at a famous pilgrimage site in Brazil. Fifteen years later, Will graduated from college, free of his tumor.

Then there's Allison, who made her pilgrimage to Sedona, convinced by New Age claims that the "energy vortexes" of the red rock formations could cure her lupus. After a year of countless healing interventions, her doctor declared her cured, which he hadn't believed was possible. Or Daksha, who had been devoted to her Indian guru for twenty years when she got cancer, visited the ashram of his lineage in India, and returned cancer-free. Then there's the guy who made his pilgrimage to Burning Man with the desire to heal from heartbreak, only to fracture his foot, have the break confirmed by

X-ray, and wind up healed by the "energy" of the festival, resulting in such complete closure of the fracture that he kept dancing.

Initially I was skeptical about these claims. Puffed up by my scientific certainty, I felt comfortable with my conclusion that these stories could be demystified in the same physiological way I explained the placebo effect in *Mind Over Medicine*. I hypothesized that the nervous system reverts to the self-healing parasympathetic mode when people gather to visit a sacred site and engage in the rituals such pilgrimages often include. People dress a certain way, sit in prayer or meditation together, eat a purifying diet, listen to relaxing music, drink holy water, ingest herbs, and receive the nurturing care of whoever might be ministering to the sick at a pilgrimage site—a priest, guru, or healer in a position of authority the people believe might have the power to heal them.

Going on a pilgrimage, leaving behind the stressors of everyday life, spending time with like-minded pilgrims, and being among believers who trust in the power of the sacred site to cure them: the perfect setup for the body to physiologically heal itself with what researchers call *mega-placebo*. No need to entertain the idea that something magical, supernatural, or divine was happening. But before writing it off as scientifically plausible and easy to demystify, I wanted to check out one of these sacred sites myself.

MY SOJOURN IN LOURDES

Although I long ago left the church of my youth—incensed by the homophobia, racism, and misogyny—I was raised Christian, so I decided to join the six million pilgrims who visit Lourdes each year. The skeptical scientist in me suspected I'd debunk anything more miraculous than the brilliantly designed self-healing human body, which, given the right conditions, is certainly miracle prone. However, the scientist in me was weary when I went to Lourdes. The dog-bite gash on my leg had been closed and pain-free for about eight months, but it had caused a stressful and scary journey that required prayer and meditation to keep my nervous system calm. My mother had passed away six months earlier from cancer after being unwilling to attempt any of my own *Mind Over Medicine* teachings or the Sacred Medicine I had so wanted her to try but knew she had the right to decline. I was still grieving hard and experiencing frequent and sometimes confusing visitations from her, which she had promised me she would do if contacting me from the other side was within her power.

Although I can often be more of an analytical intellectual, tipping toward mental intelligence, feeling certain and in control of my reality, this time in my life was tender and pregnant with mystery. After years of being the strong Lissa, who ministers to the sick and suffering, I was now the vulnerable one, still in recovery from injury, trauma, and loss. Maybe because my analytical parts were exhausted from trying to control my increasingly uncertain and disorienting world, I'd let go of my quest for certainty, which left me floating, open, and admittedly ungrounded. Perhaps because I'd loosened my grip on the reins of my life, signs and synchronicity showed up to guide me. Rather than directing events, I allowed myself to be carried.

My skeptical scientist part went along for the ride, but the seeker in me was dominant and open to awe. If an angel had fallen from the sky and offered to take a selfie with me, I would have pulled out my camera. As I traveled to Lourdes, I was ready to believe anything was possible.

As my best friend, Diane, and I drove from Bordeaux in our tiny European rental car, we saw a black cloud forming over the Pyrenees in the direction we were headed. "That looks like a tornado sky you'd see in the Midwest," I said. As I spoke, the heavens opened and hail crashed down. It sounded like the roof of the car was about to collapse. Diane, who was driving, careened through deep water into someone's backyard. We parked under an awning to prevent our windshield from shattering.

Somewhat protected, we burst into giggles. Of course, something like this would happen to us! We hadn't summited treacherous mountains or fasted or slayed dragons, so we figured it wouldn't be a real, honest-to-God pilgrimage unless we experienced some adversity. When the hail let up, the clouds parted and revealed one of those spotlights of luminous light my mother always called a "God beam." It was pointing toward Lourdes.

Although there have been more than 7,000 cases of miraculous cures reported by pilgrims who traveled to Lourdes in search of a miracle, only those documented by a medical team and approved by the bishop qualify as supernatural events. In 2013, the sixty-ninth miracle was proclaimed for Danila Castelli from Italy. The most recent Lourdes miracle as of this writing was pronounced in 2018 by Bishop Jacques Benoit-Gonnin of Beauvais, who deemed the recovery of Sister Bernadette Moriau, a long-debilitated nun, the seventieth. After four operations on her spinal column, one foot remained permanently twisted. The sister had been dependent on morphine, leg braces, and a wheelchair. After her miracle, she heard a voice say, "Take off your braces," and she hiked five kilometers a few days later—without morphine!

By the time Diane and I arrived at our hotel, the hail had subsided to a drizzle. We stumbled around the grounds in the damp and hushed silence. Crossing the bridge over the Gave de Pau River, I sought shelter from more rain in one of the many covered pavilions where people light candles in honor of loved ones. I bought a glass candle decorated with the image of the Virgin Mary dressed in white with a blue sash. Although I was raised Methodist, I knew that my mother would have liked having a candle lit for her at Lourdes.

THE HOLY GROTTO

That afternoon, Diane and I attended a gathering of people listening to mass outside the Grotto of Massabielle, where Bernadette reportedly received the eighteen visitations. We didn't understand much because it was spoken in Latin. A group of attendants in blue raincoats held umbrellas over the line of mostly elderly people in blue wheelchairs. These attendants were the "angels of Lourdes," volunteers who came from all over the world as part of their spiritual practice to meet the thousands of pilgrims arriving at the local train station each day. The angel volunteers helped the pilgrims get to their hotels; pushed their wheelchairs to the grotto; assisted as they bathed in the holy waters of Lourdes; and attended the nightly sunset processional, when thousands of pilgrims and volunteers walk at a snail's pace through the square in front of the cathedral, where a priest holds mass and offers a blessing for the sick who have come seeking healing.

After the mass, those in wheelchairs are first to enter the sacred grotto, a dark, wet-walled cave with stones rubbed smooth as obsidian by pilgrims. A small waterfall streams into a pool behind a cordoned area strewn with bouquets of flowers, photographs, and handwritten notes people leave as offerings to the holy place. An offering is different than a gift. It's an act of devotion, something that feels like a sacrifice, humbly given to a deity, aspect of nature, or any object of your devotion—as a prayer and expression of gratitude. An offering is not necessarily received; there is the offer, and if you're lucky, your offering will be received by the being to whom you are offering it. Having your offering received is a blessing, an act of grace, and an acknowledgment of your devotion.

I marveled at how every faith tradition includes offerings, and it struck me that the offering tradition of the Protestant church of my childhood had been flattened from the beautiful flowers, handwritten letters, statues, and crystals of Lourdes to five-dollar bills collected in fake gold offering plates by ushers. I'd never felt moved by that, but I was affected as I watched people fall to their knees in tears and lay bouquets of roses at the feet of the statue of the Virgin Mary glowing in ethereal candlelight and presiding over the grotto.

Even so, my first trip through the grotto felt mechanical. I stood in line with Diane in silence and touched the stone walls. I placed my offering at the holy spring. I said my prayers, but overall, I was underwhelmed.

THE LOURDES PROCESSIONAL

That night, however, someone asked us if we were going to the processional. We had seen hundreds of people in raincoats with umbrellas rushing through the crowded tourist shops, buying small candles perched on plastic handles, but we hadn't known why. By the time we arrived in the main square in front of the cathedral, thousands of people were lined up alongside the rushing river, whose roar was louder than the church bells. A statue of Our Lady of Lourdes was lit from inside, adorned with flowers, and carried on the shoulders of four men in rain gear. Behind them, hundreds of angel volunteers pushed the sick pilgrims in wheelchairs covered in blue bonnets, like baby buggies. Those who needed healing but could walk lined up behind the wheelchairs, and those there to participate in the group healing of others followed last.

The sunset cast a mysterious glow on the scene, amplifying the flickering light of thousands of candles. The music swelled, and the processional began. It took about an hour for the massive crowd to move around the square like a giant serpent, slithering like a singular being, until the snake coiled right before the cathedral, everyone lined up, bonneted wheelchairs in front, before the priest, who led mass in Latin.

To get a better view of the snaking crowd, Diane and I stood on a balcony of the cathedral overlooking the square. From our vantage point, Lourdes looked otherworldly. I felt like an outsider; I attended the processional not as someone in need of physical healing, not as a Catholic, and not as someone who had come to be a healing presence. I had embarked on the experience with an anthropologist's curiosity and a scientist's detachment. But, to my surprise, the experience drew me in on an emotional level, and I found myself engulfed. The sky was growing dark, making everyone's candles shine brighter. I caught the far-off eye of a frail old woman in one of the bonneted wheelchairs. Her gaze was soft and surrendered, her eyes alight with tears that reflected the flame of the candle she held. I felt penetrated and overcome. It was as though the God in me was admiring and beholding the God in her, and she was beholding me too. She seemed peaceful, glowing. Had she come to Lourdes not with a prayer for a miracle but with the intention to die well? It would be a wonderful place to pass, like this, during a mass at sunset. You could follow the light and make a graceful exit.

I felt the organ music reverberate as awe swept through me, my heart opening to all beings in that square—to their pain and longing; to their grief and loss; to their love of God and each other; to their fear, faith, and doubt. For the duration of the processional, I felt as if "I" were a single cell in a great body. My mind slowed, and the chatter disappeared, replaced by a pulsing in my chest slower and stronger than my heartbeat. I later learned to interpret this sensation as my own somatic signal that the group field has unified, and the individuals have synced into brain, heart, and energetic coherence.

At the time, I wasn't thinking about brainwaves or heart-rate variability. The skeptic had gone offline, and instead of analyzing the experience, I was flooded with a surge of gratitude. I felt thankful to be alive, to be with Diane, to be part of this collective weaving through the streets, feeling less existentially alone than I had in a while. I felt my mother in the ether, and her presence made me wonder. If I'd brought her here in her wheelchair and pushed her through the processional, was there any chance she might have been Lourdes's seventy-first miracle—or was that just a grieving daughter's wishful thinking?

After dinner, Diane and I wandered through the shrine. I felt drawn to the grotto that had failed to move me on my first tour. It was empty except for one man on his knees in prayer. This time, a deep silence pulled me in. Without the distractions of the rain, loudspeaker, and crowds, I could imagine young Bernadette, astonished by the appearance of an apparition who would give her such impossible instructions. What made her capable of pulling off having such a grand cathedral built? Courage, sincerity, rapture, unwavering faith, or maybe even a wounded girl's inflation, grandiosity, and exaggerated confidence? Whatever the impulse, Lourdes was second only to Paris as the most popular destination in France.

As I sat in silence, I tuned in to the emotions of the pilgrims who had visited the shrine for the past century and a half, laying their burdens down. I felt their pain, fear, grief, trust, relief, gratitude, and devotion to God. I felt the disappointment of those who arrived sick and went home still sick. I felt the ecstasy of those rare individuals granted miracles and the hope of those who bowed before such a possibility for themselves or their loved ones.

When I opened my eyes, Diane and I were alone. We knelt at the holy spring, listening to the babble of the running water as I lay a small rose quartz crystal on the altar. When I stood at the feet of Our Lady of Lourdes, in the flickering light of the candelabra, I realized that, if nothing else, Lourdes made me *feel*. Later, when I was in a more rational frame of mind, I speculated about whether all this emotional movement might be healing unto itself. In a culture allergic to feelings, perhaps this gateway to the emotional intelligence those on a healing journey need to access explains the countless unofficial miracles reported by pilgrims to Lourdes.

Or maybe not.

Part of me hoped I'd never unravel the mysteries of such miracles or succeed in dissecting them scientifically. I certainly no longer felt inclined to write them off as a mega-placebo. Now, I don't know how to explain what does or does not happen at Lourdes. I remain profoundly humbled, grateful that places like Lourdes exist, where we can let go of our understandable craving for control and cast our burdens onto something more powerful than our small minds, opening our hearts to the possibility of Something Larger than our limited selves helping us heal.

THE SACRED WATERS

The next day, Diane and I rose early to join the pilgrims who wanted to be immersed in the holy spring water. We lined up on hard wooden pews in front of the royal-blue-and-white-striped curtains as women dressed in white button-down shirts and blue smocks with burgundy kerchiefs around their necks hustled us through the process. Some people lay on stretchers covered in blue-and-white bedsheets. Others were in the bonneted wheel-chairs pushed by angel volunteers.

As I waited my turn for immersion in the holy water, I prayed for the others who came here for healing but also for myself. The impact of losing my mother still ricocheted in me like an out-of-control wasp, stinging without warning. My mother and I'd been so enmeshed, so fused without clear boundaries, so intimate but not in a healthy way. Sometimes I couldn't tell where I ended and she began, so I never let myself imagine her death. I'd carried a secret, lifelong fantasy that I would die on the same day she did, because I couldn't bear the idea of living without her. I was willing to die young if it meant I wouldn't have to survive a day without her in it.

I started therapy soon after she died, realizing I needed to break my unhealthy attachment, to individuate decades after I should have done so if I'd been raised right. But it felt like an impossible wish that a Lourdes miracle might heal. In case she could hear me, I prayed, "Please, Mom, if you love me, let me go." I could feel a tugging sensation at my belly button, like she didn't want to let me go. I figured maybe Divine intervention could finally cut the cord.

When it was my turn to be bathed, I was ushered into a dressing room where I was instructed to disrobe in a modest way. Two female attendants with warm smiles held up a thick blue cloth while I undressed; then without looking, they wrapped my naked body like a burrito. Properly covered, I was handed to an older woman standing inside a large bath of ice-cold water. She pulled me in and held the back of my head to her breast while she instructed me to gaze at the portrait of the Virgin Mary.

"Ask the Mother to come into your heart and purify you. Hold her in your consciousness while you hold your breath." She immersed me completely into the freezing water, like a baptism. When I came up for air, she met my gaze and smiled a beatific smile, like Mother Mary herself. I figured she had the coolest job in the world, being here to facilitate this tender ritual for so many.

After our baths, Diane and I filled gallon jugs from the holy water spigots so we could drink from the sacred springs. I also planned to bring some back for a friend wrestling with chronic, disabling Lyme disease. My sick friend did eventually recover, but whether it was the Lourdes water, the countless other remedies, or the blessing of time that worked, we'll never know.

As Diane and I drove over the bridge and out of town, I was stunned. It would be weeks before I could touch my Lourdes experience intellectually.

Perhaps, like candlelit caresses with a lover, some numinous experiences should be left untouched by the harsh light of analysis.

I came to realize that places like Lourdes are the ultimate example of how some suffering might be too great to be cured, yet it can be carried. Somehow, being lifted on the wings of love by a community united with the intention to heal felt like enough. Maybe only seventy people have ever been cured at Lourdes, but I suspect tens of millions have been made whole.

WHAT MAKES A PLACE HOLY?

As much as I wanted to leave my Lourdes experience unsullied by my analytical mind, after my skeptical scientist part came back online, I had so many questions. Why are some people cured but not others? Do people get better because of the properties of the water itself? Is it imbued with light, information, or consciousness? Is it belief in the water that leads to miraculous cures—a placebo effect? Is it the ritual? Is it the community gathered at places like this? Was there a mineral in the water itself that activated something mysterious? Was the water a conduit for a certain energy amplified at sacred sites, as some Indigenous healers have suggested? Does something in our DNA respond to the prayers for healing that often occur at such springs? Is water the only substance that can help people in this way? What about the sacred dirt reputed to facilitate cures at the Santuario de Chimayo? Although my visit to Lourdes was a holy experience, it didn't answer these questions.

The English word *holy* originates from a proto-Germanic root that means "whole, uninjured." Some healers assert that physical and mental illnesses result from disconnection from Source or whatever we choose to call our Inner Pilot Light. When this happens, they say, disease can be reversed by anything that reconnects the individual to Source, resulting in wholeness and, with it, healing. A holy site could be anything that facilitates reconnection. Some places might be holy because they invoke the mystical with their awesome beauty and grandeur. Some people believe holy sites lie on ley lines that link sacred locations around the world, like acupuncture points forming a matrix of earth energies or "telluric currents" that move underground or through the seas.

Many holy places such as mountainous Machu Picchu, a grand cathedral such as Notre Dame, the pyramids in Egypt, Stonehenge, or the sacred redwood trees in Muir Woods, near my home, are considered a bridge between earth and sky. Some say these sacred points attract lightning strikes, and this supercharges the ground upon which they stand. Perhaps these locations act as metaphysical gateways into altered states of consciousness or dimensions where healing is more accessible.

Before my trip to Lourdes, I attended a workshop about pilgrimages at Grace Cathedral in San Francisco with Cambridge University–trained scientist Rupert Sheldrake and the Episcopalian bishop of California, Reverend Marc Handley Andrus. To prepare us for the experience of walking the cathedral's famous labyrinth, Sheldrake lectured on his theory of *morphic resonance*, a phrase he coined from studying animals who move as a unit, such as schools of fish or murmurations of starlings. He explained why sacred sites might be powerful. He postulated that spaces, like species, might have a collective memory. If hundreds of thousands of people have visited a sacred site, and if a percentage of them have had a mystical experience, then perhaps others who visit the same space are more likely to experience the same. By this explanation, a building newly constructed on land with no historical significance might affect the humans who occupy it differently than a location approached by millions of people with reverence throughout centuries. Perhaps the reverence becomes somehow inextricable from the space itself.

Sheldrake asserts that if many people have been cured in a holy place, cures might become possible for others as a habit of nature. In his book *Science and Spiritual Practices*, Sheldrake writes,

> People in a particular state of sensory stimulation
> resonate with those who have been in a similar state
> before. When we enter a holy place, we are exposed to the
> same stimuli as those who have been there before, and
> therefore come into resonance with them. If pilgrims
> to a holy place have been inspired, uplifted, and healed
> there, we are more likely to have similar experiences
> of spiritual connection. Holy places can grow in
> holiness through people's experiences with them.[3]

After discussing why pilgrimage sites might affect people's consciousness, we circled the beautiful and imposing Grace Cathedral three times on foot. As we approached the labyrinth, a sound healer played singing bowls while the crowd waited to enter. When it was my turn, the man monitoring the queue said, "Have a good journey."

As I navigated the labyrinth, I expanded my awareness until I felt attuned to the struggles and triumphs—but also the resilience and healing—of every human who has ever walked not only this particular labyrinth but the spiritual path. I felt strengthened by this. When I reached the center, I fell to my knees, putting my head on the holy ground like all the other pilgrims who have ever trod a sacred path.

DO YOU NEED TO BE SOMEWHERE SPECIAL TO FIND HEALING?

Maybe it's the morphic resonance of the ancient holy sites that facilitates healing . . . or maybe it's something else. I have had similarly profound experiences in the most unsacred of spaces—a hotel conference room. I was at a New Age spirituality conference in a windowless room full of plastic chairs when the group leader said, "Everyone break into small groups and sit in a circle." Several hundred people swam among the tables like schools of fish until we settled into groups of six to ten people. We were told to choose one person among us as the "healee." The others would be healers. One woman in our group had chronic knee pain and had undergone several surgeries without resolution of her pain. Lydia volunteered to be the healee.

"Once you have your healee," the group leader continued, "let that person share what needs healing. Hold hands in a circle, the healee in the middle. Place one hand on the healee's shoulder and hold the hand of the person next to you with the other, forming an energetic circuit."

We did as the leader instructed, connecting ourselves, Lydia, and the group. The leader guided us in meditation, and then as music played, we closed our eyes and focused our healing intention on Lydia's knee. What followed took me by surprise.

I felt like my head was jerked back, like on one of those roller coasters that accelerate to full speed in two seconds, as if I'd been hit in the front by a wave of something invisible. Along with this physical sensation, I teared up and felt as if a waterfall of love poured out of my chest onto Lydia, reminding me of the heart opening I had felt while watching the processional at Lourdes and walking the labyrinth at Grace Cathedral. I wasn't participating in an ancient ritual or walking around a grand cathedral, yet this group healing practice touched me deeply. I hadn't anticipated a profound experience during a ten-minute exercise in a dingy, crowded, windowless conference room with several hundred strangers. After the music stopped, Lydia thanked us. When other participants pulled out tissues, I realized I wasn't the only one who felt moved. Lydia said her knee didn't hurt for the first time in months. I don't know whether the relief lasted, but for that moment, she was free from pain and felt nurtured and loved. Even those assigned to the "healer" roles described relief from physical symptoms. Maybe you don't need to go someplace special; maybe love heals. Or as Peter, Paul, and Mary sing in "Wedding Song": "For whenever two or more of you are gathered in His name, there is Love."

RITUALS OF HEALING

This New Ager leading groups in a conference room is far from the first to gather people in circles with the intention of healing those who suffer. Prayer circles and faith healings span religions and traditions. Faith healing has allegedly cured people unable to see, hear, or walk as well as those with cancer, HIV, developmental disorders, anemia, arthritis, corns, multiple sclerosis, rashes, paralysis, and various injuries.[4]

Although the Christian Gospels describe many miraculous healings at the hands of Jesus—bringing movement to a paralyzed person by the pool in Bethsaida, giving sight to a man born blind, and resurrecting Lazarus of Bethany—Jesus demonstrated that anyone with faith can do this and encouraged his followers to heal others. Because Jesus was a hands-on healer, many Christian pastors and congregations practice hands-on faith healing. Healing revivals grew in popularity during the early twentieth century and are still popular in some parts of the world. Televangelism often includes group healings, and many attendees have reported experiencing and witnessing miraculous healings at such events. Muslims also practice various forms of faith healing, such as reciting the Quran over water or olive oil and drinking, bathing, or anointing themselves with it. They also place their right hand where there is pain or on their foreheads while reciting "Surah Al-Fatiha." Pentecostal, Evangelical, and New Thought churches also practice group healings, and Christian Scientists and members of the Church of Jesus Christ of the Latter-Day Saints (Mormons) include faith healing in their belief system, sometimes putting parishioners at odds with the recommendations of conventional medicine.

Most ministries endorse following doctors' orders as an adjunct to faith healing, believing God provides conventional medicine and doctors as part of Divine bounty, whereas some, such as Christian Science, advise against conventional medicine even for critically ill children, which has led to tremendous controversy, lawsuits, and even preventable death. A study published in the *Journal of the American Medical Association (JAMA)* found that college students who were Christian Scientists had statistically higher death rates and shorter longevity than their classmates.[5] One review in *Pediatrics*, examining religion-motivated medical neglect looked at 172 cases of deaths among children treated by faith healing instead of conventional methods.[6] Researchers estimated that if conventional medicine had been used, the survival rate for most of these children would have exceeded 90 percent, with the remainder of the children also having a good chance of survival.

Once again, we need not be binary in this regard. If optimal health outcomes are our goal, I'd advocate for faith healing *and* medical treatment for those inclined toward such approaches—neither one camp nor the other but a bridge that has room for both.

Rituals of healing are often married with intention or prayer. Immersion in water, spell casting, sacred attire, music, movement, touch, metaphors, and symbols can create altered states of consciousness that might be associated with transformation and emotional healing. Although religious leaders and the recipients of such healings tend to credit Divine intervention, scientists posit that such rituals might result in the placebo effect. In his article "Placebo Studies and Ritual Theory," director of Harvard Medical School's Program in Placebo Studies and the Therapeutic Encounter (PiPS) Ted Kaptchuk writes,

> Healing rituals create a receptive person susceptible to
> the influences of authoritative culturally sanctioned
> "powers." The healer provides the sufferer with
> imaginative, emotional, sensory, moral, and aesthetic
> input derived from the palpable symbols and procedures
> of the ritual process—in the process fusing the sufferer's
> idiosyncratic narrative unto a universal cultural
> mythos. Healing rituals involve a drama of evocation,

enactment, embodiment, and evaluation in a charged
atmosphere of hope and uncertainty. Experimental
research into placebo effects demonstrates that
routine biomedical pharmacological and procedural
interventions contain significant ritual dimensions.[7]

Surely, my Lourdes experience might be explained by this kind of grand ritual. But what about the group healing in the stuffy hotel conference room? Nobody was undergoing a complex ritual. We were sipping cheap coffee, and the plastic chairs, canned music over loudspeakers, community of caring individuals, and intention of healing made up the entire pageantry. So why did Lydia feel better? If it couldn't be explained by some elaborate ritual or a charismatic shaman, was there an ecstatic contagion or a group energy field? Was this simple practice reproducing a Lourdes-like effect without all the travel, expense, and ritual? Did bringing people together with a shared intention result in an ecstatic transcendence such as what I experienced in that conference room? Could it be as simple as love? Was it possible to produce long-term health benefits by leveraging this kind of healing tool? If so, was the effect permanent, or did it wear off and require repeated doses? What was the optimal dosing regimen to sustain a long-term outcome? Would Lydia need daily or monthly sessions? Or was her knee cured?

Perhaps group healing works because it is essentially a meditation. The science is indisputable that individual meditation improves almost every health condition for the one meditating. But what about group meditation and prayer? Group prayer and healing circles would balance many of the stones in the Whole Health Cairn—Inner Pilot Light, Relationship, Spirituality, and Work/Life Purpose for those who felt called to volunteer their healing intentions. The same applies to all aspects of the Healing Bubble: Love, Gratitude, Service, and Pleasure. Through the subjective lens, it would make sense that healing circles, group meditation, and intention might affect health outcomes. But can we prove it scientifically? To explore this question, we must examine something studied in depth—the power of prayer.

THE SCIENCE OF PRAYER

When it comes to miracles at places such as Lourdes, the Catholic Church would consider it heresy to credit anything but God and prayer. But if the miracles are the answer to prayer through an act of Divine intervention, why have only seventy pilgrims been granted miracles in a century and a half? Given they started rigorously recording Lourdes miracles in 1858, and given that six million people visit every year, those are crummy odds. If God chooses the seventy people who get their miracle out of hundreds of millions, what makes one person worthy while another continues suffering or dies?

Years ago, I had read Larry Dossey's books, including *Healing Words: The Power of Prayer and the Practice of Medicine.* But I had never reviewed the scientific research myself. How effectively had scientists studied prayer as medicine? Were the data reliable? If so, what had science concluded?

I was overwhelmed by the volume of data on prayer and health outcomes. A brief PubMed search of "prayer" delivered 66,599 results. When I entered "intercessory prayer," I still got 106 entries. Given the schism between science and spirituality, I was shocked to see how many scientists had indeed tried to study prayer as a medical intervention!

I returned to Dossey's books. He makes the case, based on his synthesis of the immense amount of hard-to-quantify data, that although the data are not conclusive, there is considerable evidence suggesting prayer as medicine works. Dossey doesn't take a stand on whether prayer works because God listens and answers prayers or because the conditions that come with prayerful behavior are likely to promote healing.

According to Dossey, healthy behaviors that might accompany prayer include austerities that might promote health, such as abstaining from alcohol, cigarettes, illegal drugs, or a diet heavy in meat; social support through community and the alleviation of loneliness; the psychological impact of rites, rituals, and beliefs, which can release suppressed emotions, boost the immune system, and reduce anxiety; placebo effects; the loving presence of those praying, which might foster a sense of belonging and feeling nurtured; the endocrine and immune system boost of being the object of prayer; and the healing physical preparations for prayer, such as meditation, fasts, diets, and abstentions. Citing many scientific studies, Dossey concludes that prayer has been scientifically proven effective, and he makes a case for integrating group prayer into conventional medical treatment by, for example, activating a prayer chain of volunteers anytime a sick person comes to the emergency room.

Intrigued, I paid a visit to Dossey at his home in Santa Fe, New Mexico. Larry is a tall, earnest, and jovial fellow with a Texas accent, a warm heart, a quick wit, a healing presence, and self-deprecating humor who must have made patients feel comforted. With decades of experience exploring energy healing, faith healing, and the power of prayer, he is a wealth of knowledge, able to quote studies at the tip of his loquacious and often hilarious tongue.

When I asked how the medical community reacted to his books, he said he received backlash from both sides—not just the scientists who thought science and spirituality should never be mixed but also religious folks. After reviewing the data, he concluded not only that prayers might have some health benefits but also that it didn't matter what deity you prayed to. Christians, Hindus, Buddhists, and even pagans seemed capable of getting a Higher Power's attention. This makes him unpopular among fundamentalists convinced theirs is the only path to the Promised Land.

Before I left, Dossey shared his favorite prayer, taught to him by a surgeon who routinely recited it before operating: "Dear God, these are your hands. Now don't go and embarrass yourself."

Still seeking answers about the impact of prayer on health outcomes, I discovered that the scientific studies on prayer and healing have been fraught with challenges. If you ask the skeptics, they'll say that one Harvard study hammered the nail in the coffin, disproving prayer's clinical efficacy. The Harvard Medical School "Study of the Therapeutic Effects of Intercessory Prayer (STEP) in Cardiac Bypass Patients" was published in 2006 by Herbert Benson, author of *The Relaxation Response* and a pioneer of mind-body medicine.[8] The purpose of STEP was to assess if intercessory prayer affected the outcomes of patients undergoing coronary bypass surgery. Benson found that patients who knew others were praying for them not only didn't do better, but their outcomes were also worse than those who were receiving prayers but didn't know it or those for whom nobody was praying. This study resulted in a media bomb in *Newsweek*: "Spirituality: Don't Pray for Me! Please!"[9] In a 2008 article in *Explore,* Dossey analyzed this study, discussing why it might have been flawed and why the interpretation of it might have been misguided, but for most scientists, the question was answered: Prayer doesn't work.[10]

I have a different interpretation that accounts for the variability of a practice as subjective as prayer. *All* medicines can have variability. One surgeon can perform the same surgery as another and routinely get better outcomes. One doctor can give a pill with a hug, words of encouragement, and healing touch, and another can give the same pill with a scowl, a pessimistic attitude, and a hand that never leaves the door. As suggested in the venerated *British Medical Journal,* which I discuss at length in *Mind Over Medicine,* their patients might get different health outcomes not because the pill was different but because the doctor and their attitudes and expectations of a positive outcome were.[11]

Applying the principles of science to prayer is likely to have even more unpredictable and unmeasurable variability, making it hard to compare apples to apples. One analysis in the *Indian Journal of Psychiatry* examined the data of studies that meet the gold standard for the investigation of the efficacy of medical interventions—the double-blind, randomized, controlled trials.[12] They discovered that the data are all over the map. Sometimes prayer helped. Sometimes nothing happened. Sometimes it seemed to make things worse. As good scientists are inclined to do, the researchers wrestled with how to make sense of such conflicting data, posing a series of hilarious, forehead-smacking inquiries worth reading in the original study.[13]

As the researchers pointed out, the limitations of current scientific methods are obvious when it comes to measuring subjective qualities—such as whether one person praying is more sincere, moral, focused, or favored by God. How would a scientist control for such potentially important variables? Wouldn't it make sense that these variables might affect outcomes?

Whenever someone says, "Please pray for me," I always call my friend Mary. When Mary says she'll pray for you, she means it. If you had a choice between Mary or me when it comes to prayer, you'd want to pick Mary. Mary does not take praying for someone lightly. She prays *hard,* literally begging God on your behalf. If anyone has earned the ear of God with her devotion, dedication, and discipline, it's Mary. If you put the two of us in a study, science would have no way to discern the difference between me, admittedly lazy at praying, and Mary, a prayer Olympian.

This isn't to suggest we should abandon science but to recognize and admit that science has its limits, and some aspects of medicine are more easily measured than others. When it comes to aspects of Sacred Medicine, you might have to rely on all your Whole Health Intelligences, not science alone, or simply sense into what feels good and what seems to ease your symptoms, even just temporarily. Science is based on statistics—and you are not a statistic. As statisticians would say, you are an "n of 1." In other words, although science can help us make blanket recommendations, you can't predict what will work for any individual based on group probabilities and statistics. If prayer helps you, use it! If it doesn't, avoid it.

By the time I went to Lourdes, I was five years into my exploration of Sacred Medicine, and it was clear that demystifying the mysteries of healing might be an unachievable, perhaps laughable, goal. The more I applied science to the sacred, the more the mystery smirked at me, but that didn't quiet my inquisitive mind or keep me from trying to make sense of these healing methods.

Could unexpectedly good health result from making a healing pilgrimage, asking loved ones for prayers, or sitting in a circle and intending healing for someone? *Maybe.* Should people pray instead of getting proven medical treatments? No! That would be reckless. These medicines work best in tandem rather than in a binary, either/or way. We'd be wise to apply them together based on the wisdom of our Whole Health Intelligences. Can I explain how visiting sacred sites, group healings, healing intention, and prayer work? I can speculate but can't prove or disprove how they might work scientifically. Is there any harm in going on a pilgrimage, sitting in a group sharing healing intention, or asking for healing prayer? Not if you're not refusing proven conventional medical treatments because of it.

If you've felt drawn to a pilgrimage site, you might consider putting your whole heart into preparing emotionally, spiritually, physically, and financially for such a trip. Assuming doing so involves no financial hardship or undue physical risk, it can't hurt and might help. You never know—you might be Lourdes's seventy-first documented miracle!

Pilgrimage

Pilgrims often feel drawn to a specific location, but any place can be a pilgrimage site. Trust that if a pilgrimage is part of your Prescription, you'll know by tuning into your Whole Health Intelligences. If you're unsure, research options—or try muscle testing it (see chapter 8). If traveling far from home isn't financially or physically feasible, consider applying the principles of a pilgrimage somewhere nearby. Anything can be treated as a Sacred Medicine pilgrimage if you approach it with the consciousness of healing.

Walk to the pilgrimage site if possible, or at least walk the last mile if you're able-bodied enough to do so. When you arrive, circumambulate it clockwise three times to anchor the experience. Hold the paradox of healing in your heart: be clear in your intention to heal *and* surrender attachment to outcomes, trusting that whatever is aligned for your highest good will happen. Remember, healing might go where it's most needed rather than where you most want it.

Bring an offering to the sacred site: something meaningful to you that feels like a sacrifice, whether it took a long time to prepare it, requires monetary deprivation, or holds precious memories or sentiments. If it feels right, offer a song as you walk and lift up prayers of gratitude in advance for any blessings that arise from your pilgrimage.

Group Healing Rituals

If your religion offers faith healing, prayer circles, or hands-on healing from pastors or volunteers, tune in to whether you wish to add such a healing treatment to your Whole Health Prescription. If you're spiritual but not religious, you might feel more comfortable gathering with friends and family for group healing or shared intention. Try this practice, which I lead regularly in my workshops.

1. **Create sacred space.** You can sacralize the space with your prayers, intention, and music. Or create a simple altar using candles, flowers, or objects from nature.

2. **Choose a healee.** Invite the healee to share what needs healing, and ask if they would prefer safe touch or not.

3. **Gather in a circle.** Sitting on the floor or in chairs, encircle the healee. The number of people is not important, although I find that anywhere from six to twenty can be powerful.

4. **Together, close your eyes, drop into your hearts, and make a connection to Source, to the healee, and to each other.** Use whatever meditation practice you prefer to "drop in" and connect to whatever you might call Divine energy. If you don't have a meditation practice, try grounding yourself into the earth as if plugging in an electrical cord and allowing earth energy to come into your heart from your seat. Then imagine opening yourself to heavenly energy through the top of your head. Let earth and heavenly energy meet in your heart and pour out of your chest like a waterfall. Send a loving thought to yourself first, such as "May I be well and free from suffering." Then focus on your heart and send this blessing out to the healee or whoever needs healing.

5. **Lay-on hands (optional).** If the healee wants touch, allow this healing energy from your heart to move into your hands, laying them on the one in need of healing. If the healee would prefer not to be touched, or if you're practicing this remotely, see them in your mind's eye and offer the practice from a distance.

6. **After you feel the connection, play at least one uplifting instrumental song.** My favorite for group healings is Thomas Bergersen's "Colors of Love." You can also let the healee choose the music, creating their unique field of resonance.

7. **Offer your prayer.** You might pray for what the healee requests. Or you can try the one my teacher taught me—"Let us pray for that which is most right," acknowledging that "most right" is a mystery to our limited human minds.

8. **Move aside.** After the energy is "running," get out of the way. If you're sensitive, this might feel like vibrations, tingling, or a rush of emotion.

Chapter 2

THE ENERGY CURE

was new to my inquiry into Sacred Medicine when someone who knew about my research handed me William "Bill" Bengston's book *The Energy Cure*, which tells the story of how Bill's curiosity about energy healing led him to the laboratory to study the effects of hands-on healing on mice he had injected with breast cancer. Having witnessed one unexplainable cure after another at the hands of mysterious healer Ben Mayrick, Bill wrote, "At the risk of sounding biblical, I witnessed scenes in which the blind regained some vision, the deaf could once again hear, the lame could walk, along with a string of cancer cures that the medical profession summarily dismissed as spontaneous remissions." However, Ben couldn't cure warts or colds.[1] His best results were with young people with aggressive cancers not yet treated with chemotherapy or radiation. Some people responded to Ben's "treatment" quickly. Others slowly. Some not at all.

Bill asked Ben, "Are you some sort of freak, or is this something that can be learned by others?"

Ben had no idea, but he allowed Bill to interrogate him with hundreds of questions. Ben's responses were visceral, immediate, and intuitive. Bill says he was "tuning in to something."

Thinking like a scientist, Bill understood he couldn't prove Ben's treatment caused these cures, given how many factors were not controlled for scientifically. Bill noticed that when many people are sick, they make all sorts of changes—taking supplements, changing their diet, and seeking out interventions they believe will help cure them, including conventional medicine. How could he determine scientifically whether Ben's treatment or all these other influences made their illnesses go away? How could he be sure it wasn't some placebo effect?

Bill figured if he got Ben into a lab, working with easier-to-control rodents, he could prove Ben's "hocus pocus"—not diet, environment, yoga, or other medical interventions—was responsible for the cures. Bill shared his intentions with David Krinsley, head of the geology department at City University of New York at the time. Despite his skepticism, David offered to help Bill set up his first laboratory experiment.

Initially, Bill arranged the study design, and Ben agreed to cooperate as the healer. Twelve mice would be injected with a dose of mammary cancer, scientifically proven to kill 100 percent of mice within fourteen to twenty-seven days. The plan was for Ben to do his hands-on healing treatment on the twelve mice, holding their cages for an hour with each treatment. As a control group, another cohort of mice would receive a sham treatment. Even one mouse that outlived the maximal life span of twenty-seven days would break scientific records.

After considerable effort, expense, and string pulling, Ben bailed, explaining that his "guidance" had withdrawn its consent. Bill had his doubts about this, sensing that Ben was afraid to risk failing and have his alleged superpowers scientifically disproven. However, Ben offered to help Bill learn how to reproduce what he did so Bill could study himself. What followed was a six-month process of Bill grilling Ben about each step, something Bill glossed over in the book but that I tried to pin him down about when I flew to the East Coast and took a ferry to Bill's home on Long Island, where I tried to get to the bottom of what happened. When I asked Bill how he figured out how to reproduce whatever Ben was doing, Bill said, "That's like asking people how they walk. You don't know how you walk. You walk! How can I walk like *you* walk? I kept asking questions."

Ben told Bill, "I feel something going through me."

Bill asked him, "Where does it come from? How can you reproduce it? Are you special, or can anyone do it?"

Ben said, "Anyone can do it."

"Does it require belief?"

"No."

"Is it your left hand or your right hand?"

"I'm right-handed, but my left hand does the healing."

"Are you *trying* to heal?"

"No. I'm observing it. Healing just happens."

"Does visualizing a positive outcome matter?"

"Yes . . . but no. Visualization isn't enough. Positive thinking won't cut it. Positive thinking is about belief. This is not about belief. If you make it about belief, you blame the sick person and assume they can't visualize well enough. Belief isn't relevant. Skeptics can heal. Nonbelievers can be cured. Manifestation doesn't help."

"But does visualizing a different future help?"

"Yes," Ben said. "But you can't dwell on anything. Visualizing things you want in the future can help you heal, but not if you dwell on the outcome. You have to visualize multiple unrelated things. Sure, you might have an image about having good health or helping someone heal, but you need to get off that image and go to the next one. What else do you want besides fixing your sore knee or helping someone fix theirs? Sure, go ahead and see yourself or the other person playing tennis, but then see something else you want. You, the healer, not the person you're trying to heal. Be selfish. Think about yourself. You can want to heal someone because it's fun, but focus on something else you want. Don't get stuck on the image of healing, or it won't work."

"Is it two images back and forth, or are there lots?"

"At least twenty," Ben said. "Less than twenty, and you dwell on the images. If you dwell on something, then you're bringing in the conscious mind. You're trying to *get past* the conscious mind. That's when the cool stuff happens."

Bill explained to me:

> We started playing with that—making up pictures in our minds of twenty things we wanted—or more— and then speeding up our images. We'd mess with each other. Ben would speed it up, and then I would speed it up, and we'd fool around and wonder what we could do as we flashed through the images faster and faster. We called it *cycling*. It was very playful.
>
> I started treating people with Ben. We'd play with cycling and then put our hands on people while we did it. It was like a game. He'd let me practice on minor aches

and pains. We were observers, with no attachment to the outcome, just goofballs fooling around. Ben didn't think it was him that was healing someone. He was around while healing happened but didn't think it was coming from him. He wanted to be worshipped in every other part of his life but not while his hands were on people during a healing. It's like his ego disappeared. He was like a virtuoso musician. If you play the piano, you might have to practice, but at some point, you must let go. Ben let go. I started letting go too. *That's* when it works.

I had so many questions, and Bill, bless his heart, tried to answer them, although he cautioned that he didn't know all the answers. He was clear about one thing, though: "It's important to distinguish between *intention* and *attention*. If you're even considering putting your hands on someone sick, you have the intention. Attention is where you get messed up. All healing ought to be mindless. Healing is somehow considered more sacred than walking. Walking is a miracle."

CAN HEALING CURE CANCER IN MICE?

I wanted to know more about the experiments, and Bill was happy to share. He explained that he entered his laboratory at Queens College and St. Joseph's College with a batch of mice he had injected with cancer. He treated a whole cage at once, but it was time-consuming to cycle from cage to cage as Ben had taught him. Bill figured if Ben could teach *him*, why not enlist some skeptical graduate students who knew nothing about healing so Bill wouldn't have to hold a bunch of mouse cages for hours upon end? Bill didn't believe the mice would be cured, and the students thought they were being duped into a gullibility study, but lo and behold! The mice treated with hands-on healing in the first study had full remissions (100 percent). Problematically, four of the six control mice treated with sham healing also remitted (66.7 percent).[2]

Because we know from decades of data that 18–80 percent of study participants get better when given placebos in the form of a sugar pill, saline injection, fake surgery, or sham treatment, evidence-based science requires that new treatments undergoing efficacy studies prove the treatment works significantly better than a placebo. If the placebo effect is high, it's hard to prove a treatment is efficacious. But the results of Bill's study were perplexing. Why were the mice in the placebo group getting better? Never in the known history of science had even one mouse injected with this particular dose of lethal cancer survived, making it the ideal model for studying potential cancer treatments. So how could the group getting the sham healings be cured too? If the healing wasn't curing the cancerous control mice, then what was?

Although Bill never fully solved the placebo problem, he did discover that taking the mice offsite, away from the researchers, seemed to allow them to die on schedule, although the control mice that remained in the lab still got better. By Bill's fourth experiment, eleven mice were in the experimental group. Ten out of eleven remitted (90.9 percent.) Seven of the eight onsite control mice had remitted (87.5 percent). Zero of the four control mice offsite remitted (0 percent).

Bill hoped this would win him the Nobel Prize, but instead, nobody seemed to care that he had proven that hands-on healing, even with skeptical graduate students, could cure well-proven "incurable" cancer in mice. He barely managed to get the study published. In 2000, Bill's study "The Effect of 'Laying on of Hands' on Transplanted Breast Cancer in Mice"[3] did get published in what is considered by some a fringe publication: the *Journal of Scientific Exploration*. Buried as it was in a periodical few people read, it didn't garner much attention. But that didn't prevent Bill from performing more mouse studies, giving cancer to a total of ninety-seven mice. Forty-four of forty-eight mice treated with hands-on healing remitted (91.7 percent). Thirty-three of forty-one control mice onsite in the same laboratory remitted (80.5 percent). Zero of eight offsite mice remitted (0 percent).

Years later, Bill presented his research to a roomful of oncologists and researchers. His talk led to an invitation to take a sabbatical from his position at St. Joseph's College in Brooklyn and continue his mouse research at the University of Connecticut's Center for Immunotherapy. Bill designed nineteen research studies, but things went painfully awry. Although seeming to welcome Bill, the university did not follow through in providing a supportive environment. After everything that could go wrong did, he concluded he was unwelcome among other cancer researchers, who not only did not believe in what he was studying but also didn't seem curious. Bill thinks his research threatened the worldview they held dogmatically dear.

Bill isn't the only scientist studying energy healing and its effects on cancerous mice. He is also not the only one bumping up against institutional resistance because of the nature of what he is studying. As examined in biofield researcher Shamini Jain's book *Healing Ourselves*, Gloria Gronowicz, a professor of surgery and orthopedic surgery at the University of Connecticut, performed several groundbreaking placebo-controlled studies on Therapeutic Touch—a hands-on energy healing technique believed to ease pain and facilitate relaxation, wound repair, and recovery from illness—and its relationship to cancer growth, both in vitro and in vivo in mice. Her study of the impact of Therapeutic Touch on bone, tendon, connective tissue cells, and bone cancer cells found that not only did the Therapeutic Touch affect cell growth far more than sham treatments did but it also was intelligent. Healthy cells proliferated, while cancer cells shrank.[4] She then studied the effect of Therapeutic Touch on mice injected with breast cancer cells, also using a sham treatment as a placebo control. The mice treated with Therapeutic Touch but not the ones treated with the placebo showed reduction in tumor metastases, although the tumors did not disappear as they had in Bill's mice.[5]

CAN HEALING CURE HUMANS?

Although mouse studies are promising, the question remains: Can we prove that this way of treating cancer in mice works for humans? So far, all we have are intriguing, unscientific anecdotes. Bill reported to me that treating humans by cycling has resulted in many cures, notably of hard-to-treat cancers such as pancreatic and retinoblastoma. "The more aggressive the cancer, the more this method seems to work. Don't know why. It doesn't do anything for benign tumors though. I can't explain that either. You can throw a sugar pill at a wart, and it'll go away, but cycling doesn't touch warts. Pancreatic cancer, however? I 'fixed' one last month."

Bill reports successful treatment of ovarian torsion, improvement in arthritis symptoms, and the instantaneous healing of his daughter's crushed finger after it was caught in a car doorjamb. He taught his daughter how to cycle, and she successfully treated his injured knee and gallstones that had caused an acute attack—two conditions his doctor said would require surgery. Bill has been symptom-free ever since.

Bill has also experimented with storing "healing" in water and cotton, then using the water and cotton to treat by proxy. One woman who had some of Bill's cotton created an unanticipated control study. When attacked by a cat, she applied the charged cotton to her neck and chest. She didn't have enough cotton for the gash on her hand. The footlong gashes on her neck and chest turned white within a couple of hours, whereas the hand gash developed a red scab. Several days later, the throat and chest wounds were healed with no marks, but her hand took several weeks to heal and left a pink scar still visible a month after the wound closed.

Bill says he can't treat himself with cycling, but he claims to have treated himself for corneal abrasions and corneal detachment, using cotton he had previously charged. Since then, many of Bill's students and practitioners have also experimented with treating not only other people but also themselves using previously treated cotton someone else cycled on.

Although Ben and Bill experimented with many medical conditions, cancer is what the Bengston Energy Healing Method seems to treat best. Previous surgery for cancer does not seem to interfere with the success of his treatment, but he'd had less success with those who had already undergone radiation and chemotherapy. I admit that red flags went up for me when Bill said these conventional cancer treatments might be incompatible with cycling as complementary therapy, and he understands the concern. When time is of the essence, energy healing seems harmless as an adjunct to cancer treatment, but if it causes people to delay efficient and well-proven methods, it could be life threatening. When I asked him if he could explain why cycling might fail after chemotherapy or radiation, he said he thinks cycling is about healing, and chemotherapy and radiation are about killing. If healing and killing are applied together, maybe they cancel each other out, he postulated.

"But hell if I know," he concluded. He encourages his students to prove him wrong and claims some have seen success with cycling as an adjunct to oncology treatments that also include low doses of chemo or radiation.

Aside from cancer, according to Bill, other conditions have a good prognosis using the Bengston Method. It seems to work better with young, otherwise healthy people than with older people with many comorbid conditions. Injuries are most treatable when fresh, "before the mind cements itself around the notion of being injured or disabled." The longer it takes to develop a condition, the longer it takes to treat and the less successful the treatment. For example, conditions such as arthritis, which develops over many years of degeneration, do not respond as well as rapidly growing or quick-onset conditions, such as bacterial or viral infections, aggressive cancers, or a fresh injury.

The Bengston Method seems helpful with Alzheimer's disease but less so with Parkinson's, suggesting that it works better when taking away what should not be there (cancer, beta-amyloid plaques) than replacing something that's absent (dopamine-producing nerve cells). Practitioners have had success with asthma, allergies, autoimmune disorders, chronic pain, and even veterinary illnesses.

WHAT IF SOMEONE DOESN'T *WANT* TO BE CURED?

One phenomenon that has bewildered Bill and other Bengston Method practitioners is the rage reaction some people have when they are cured of a potentially life-threatening condition. Bill says he's witnessed this many times. A desperate friend convinced a begrudging cancer patient to try the Bengston Method after everything else failed and the doctors had given up. Giving it everything they had, Bill and other practitioners have sometimes even moved people into their own homes so they can treat them once or twice per day, effectively "blasting" them with healing.

Bill says it's the darnedest thing. The cancer will go away. The doctor will confirm it's gone. The Bengston Method practitioners are ready to celebrate the great results of their hard work. And the patient is *pissed*.

One practitioner wrote a letter to Bill about a patient named Sarah. In their first session, she sensed Sarah was depressed but also that she had accepted her cancer and had faith she was safe in God's hands. Sarah came in for frequent sessions. She started feeling worse. Concerned the cancer had spread to her brain, she went in for more testing. Not only was it not spreading; it was disappearing. When Sarah learned her cancer was diminishing rather than spreading, she canceled her Bengston Method treatments. Sadly, a few months later, she killed herself. In an email forwarded to me, her practitioner wrote, "I thought it was interesting that she was getting better despite not really wanting to and although she didn't think she could. She was pretending to want to get better for everyone else's sake. Which I guess isn't much different from the person who gets mad when they get cured."

I suspect some people consciously want to be cured or to stick around for their families, but maybe life is hard, traumas are heavy, and some desire buried in the unconscious wants a socially acceptable exit plan. This made me think about one of the core principles of medical ethics: informed consent. Unless the patient is a minor, it's considered medical malpractice and a boundary violation, not to mention morally wrong, to intervene with a treatment for patients' bodies without their explicit consent. In other words, the patient always has the right to stay sick or die, and nobody, even people with good intentions, has the right to interfere.

Bengston Method training includes a rigorous ethics lesson around practicing "cycling" only on those who consent to treatment. But what if patients are only consenting because they feel pressured to please family members? If we had a way to seek consent—or not—from those deeply buried parts of the unconscious that might view a life-threatening illness as a valid exit plan, would patients who are cured still get mad?

Perhaps part of healing requires treating a wounded will to live. In physician Arnold Hutschnecker's remarkable book *The Will to Live*, he recounts stories of how the will to live bolsters health in patients and how, when it wanes, our health might suffer or we might even die. Whatever Hutschnecker knew must have worked for him—he died in 2000 at 102, having survived a sex scandal with a patient and the infamy of being Richard Nixon's psychiatrist.

I wondered how much this "will" factor influenced those who said they wanted Bengston Method treatment but seemed upset when they got better. Perhaps if we can't help people get excited to stick around for a longer, more vibrant life they're likely to love, we should keep our healing to ourselves and let them die with dignity.

WHAT IS HEALING?

When I asked Bill to explain what he thinks happens when he cycles, he said what he often says—"Hell if I know!" But he took a stab at it, telling me,

> Everybody calls it "energy healing." But it can't be energy.
> Healing works across distance. You can use your hands,
> but it's not required. Distance doesn't affect it at all. It's a
> nonlocal phenomenon. What does that tell us? If there's

no respect for distance, then there should be no respect for time. . . . If I'm shining a light, the light gets dimmer the farther away from it you get. All energy diminishes with distance. Healing doesn't—so it can't be energy.

"What is it?"
Bill shrugged and said,

> I think it's *information*. I've got data that indicate the insertion of information into a physical system. If I run random number generators in a room, they no longer put out random numbers when healing is happening. I tested this informally when we were doing magnetometer studies.[6] I treated the random number generator directly, as if it were a "client." Nothing. We ran the random number generator in a room with five cages of cancerous mice. That's when the random number generator "responded" by (apparently) the insertion of information/reduction in entropy/ sensitivity to the treatment. We did this from time to time, and it remained consistent *until* the mice were cured. Then, no response from the random number generator. My tentative conclusion is that this pattern is consistent with the thought that healing is a response to need. It may be a reduction of entropy in a system that makes it no longer random because I'm inserting information when I'm healing. Are information and energy interchangeable? Is energy also information? If it's information, how is it inserted? I have a hypothesis but can't prove it. I'm looking for a physicist who can help me, but I haven't gotten there yet.

Bill continued:

> Healing is driven by the healee. It's a response to a biological need. When the mice with cancer have a need, they go to the healer's left hand. If you spin the cage, they still move to the left hand, but only when they're sick.

The minute they're better, they lose all interest in the
left hand. Kids and pets do the same thing. A boy with
retinoblastoma came right over and stuck his forehead
on my left hand—and his tumor went away. Adults stop
doing this. They think it's crazy. Kids and animals are way
easier. Mice are even easier. Cell cultures are the easiest.
If we put cotton that we've charged with cycling next to
ordinary cells, nothing happens. But if we put the cotton
near wounded cells, they respond genomically. If they
have motility, they swim toward the cotton. The problem
is, we can't find a gizmo that can detect what "it" is.

Bill is irritated that I have titled my book *Sacred Medicine*. "It's not
sacred, Lissa. It's natural. Healing happens all the time. You don't have to
get into a spiritual mindset and pray to a deity. I swear by my logo." He
handed me his business card, which says, "Be playful" on one side and
"Avoid ritual" on the other.

Ritual will kill anything you're trying to do. If you're
engaging in some ritualized form of healing, you're
thinking, "First I bow on my knees, then I lift my eyes
to the sky, then I spin my crystal three times, and last
time I did this, the cancer got cured." Now you have
a ritual. A ritual is any activity meant to bring about
some consequence. You're doing it for safety, to lock
something in. You're giving up power through the ritual,
rather than harnessing it the way you think you are. If
you do this, you'll focus more on the performance of
the ritual than on the playfulness that made it work the
first time. It's like beginner's luck. How do you stay a
beginner? You avoid ritual. Don't make it sacred. You'll
have forgotten what you did it for. Don't even heal
to be a good person. Heal because it's fun. . . . Quit
trying so hard. Be mindful, and then be mindless.

As much as Bill claims this medicine isn't sacred and considers it more
a function of nature than God, he tips his hat to spirituality. "Perhaps by
touching the Source, I can give my patients what they need to heal, because

the Source offers an infinite number of simultaneous existences transcending time and space. Perhaps there's a place where you crushed your finger and a place where you did not; there's a place where the finger heals and a place where it does not. These places are probably close to each other, so if we act quickly before your thoughts have had a chance to harden around a negative reality, maybe we can somehow back up to before the crushed finger time."

FUTURE RESEARCH DIRECTIONS

As for what's next, Bill is interested in the potential to scale healing and perform clinical trials in humans, more difficult to control for than mice. Although he treated his mice in batches, most of the practitioners using his method are working one-on-one with clients, which is inefficient, expensive, and hard to scale. He's excited about the possibility that healing could be stored and transferred in cotton or water as well as converted into a sound frequency that might cure cancer without the presence of a healer. Bill is having a tough time finding a laboratory that will let him test this, but he is dogged in his determination to discover the answer. If he can do it, he wants to release this healing MP3 for free on the internet and see if it helps cure people with cancer. His fantasy is to give the middle finger to the cancer pharmaceutical industry and make healing accessible and free to anyone in the world who wants it.

I was a pain in the ass for six years of interviews with Bill over the course of researching his work. He tolerated my challenges with self-deprecating humor and eventually (albeit reluctantly) agreed that humans are not mice, and there might be a psychospiritual underpinning to why humans get sick, as opposed to the healthy mice, whose only trauma was getting injected with cancer by Bill. Introducing Bill to *Radical Remission* author Kelly Turner's research on the emotional, psychological, and spiritual underpinnings of people who have better-than-expected recoveries from "incurable" cancers, I hypothesized that treating people with "cycling" without also treating traumas and lifestyle stressors that might predispose people to illnesses such as cancer might bolster their life force but only cure them temporarily. My hypothesis was that, like any blood transfusion received by a bleeding patient, evidence of disease might disappear. But if they're still leaking life force, the disease would reappear as a different diagnosis. Bill admitted this might be possible, and with me cheering "Go Bill!" he's added to his research plan markers to assess emotional, psychological, and spiritual well-being in the humans he's starting to study.

As our umpteenth interview wrapped up, I asked Bill if he could summarize his understanding of the efficacy of the Bengston Method for treating humans. Bill said,

> The clinical problems with treating conditions as a "complementary" therapy rather than as an "alternative" therapy is what drove me away from treating humans with Ben into the lab with my rodents thirty years ago. As you know, most clinical cases in "uprights" are so complicated. There's virtually no way to parse out the effects of hands-on healing over vitamin C. For example, my partner, Margaret, and I recently treated the wife of a doctor friend of ours who was diagnosed with stage-four pancreatic cancer. Knowing the prognosis, they didn't want to go the traditional route. So they came to visit us and got "zapped." We treated her ourselves but also applied charged cotton and treated water . . . yadda, yadda, yadda. But in the real world the "yadda" also included upping this vitamin, changing that diet, etc. So did we fix her? I can't claim anything other than her cancer is gone and conventional medicine didn't do it. Good for her, but not sufficient for science.

As frustrated as I felt, I admired his unwillingness to hang his hat on any certainty or exaggerate claims he couldn't prove. In the realm of Sacred Medicine, I discovered that "I don't know" is a trustworthy and valid answer. It's also a reliable sign of an ethical healer and a good scientist, someone humble in the face of mystery rather than full of braggadocio and false certainty.

BILL AND BEN: AN UNCONVENTIONAL LOVE STORY

One summer night as the sun was setting, over wine and dinner on Bill's wraparound porch in Long Island, I asked him what ever happened with Ben. Bill explained that he and Ben had a falling out after Bill started curing cancer himself. Ben blamed Bill for cutting him out of the mouse research, but Bill insists Ben backed out. Many decades had passed since Bill had heard from Ben, until after a long plane ride across the Atlantic returning from London, Bill crashed exhausted into bed.

> I intended to just take a nap, so I set the alarm for seven o'clock. But in my jetlagged oblivion, I accidentally set it for a.m., not p.m. I slept right through. At eleven p.m., I sat bolt upright, startled to see a glow in the middle of the room. The dark shades were down, so it was dark, and a glow like a floating ball of light was so bright that it lit up the whole room. I knew it was Ben. I don't know how I knew, but I knew with every ounce of certainty in every cell in my body. I reached out and said, "Ben."
> It was pure love. Ben's asshole tendencies somehow melted away, and all that was left of Ben was love. I found out later that this was exactly when he died.

Bill got quiet, and I thought he might cry, when he sat up straight, cleared his throat, chuckled as he glanced at the setting sun, and said, "So that's all I've got. That and a lot more unanswered questions."

"But wait! One more thing."

Bill looked at me suspiciously and gestured as if to say, "Whaddaya got?"

"What about love? Isn't healing about love?"

Bill shook his head and said, "Now you're way above my pay grade . . . and dammit, I don't have a clue."

I haven't got a clue either, but maybe cycling shifts us into a pleasurable state of wish fulfillment, lifting us out of the energetic sludge of fear, scarcity, doubt, unmet longing, and the mind's efforts to solve problems it needn't solve. Maybe imagining wish fulfillment provides that pleasure boost from the Healing Bubble of the Whole Health Cairn while simultaneously lifting some emotional weight. Maybe if the person cycling cares about helping someone who is suffering, the service aspect of the Healing Bubble lights up. Maybe those grad students loved those mice, something a curmudgeon like Bill would have been reluctant to admit.

Who knows? It's clearly above my pay grade too. But I learned how to cycle at one of Bill's workshops in case it might prove useful. A few months later, a neighborhood gardener I'll call Hugo fell off a tall ladder onto a sharp rock. He was screaming in pain while I examined him with my hands and stethoscope. I was sure he had broken a rib and suspected he might have punctured his lung, which can cause a tension pneumothorax that can rapidly lead to death. I called 911. The emergency medical response team sent a helicopter, because we were far from a trauma center, upon hearing that he had no breath sounds on one side.

When a lung gets punctured and starts leaking air into the pleural space, it can compress the heart, making it incapable of pumping blood. Death can come swiftly. Although I had been trained decades earlier to use a kitchen knife to stick between someone's ribs and let the air out in case of emergency, I was too scared to try it at home because I'd inserted chest tubes but never tried the kitchen knife trick. What if my diagnosis was wrong and I killed him?

I was afraid Hugo was going to die in my arms before the helicopter arrived. With no chest tube in site and no drugs, with my nervous system in fight-or-flight stress response, all I could remember from what I had learned about Sacred Medicine was how to cycle. Closing my eyes, putting my hands over Hugo's chest, and bringing to mind my list of twenty-something wishes, I started cycling, but not before crying inside, "God, help me do this!"

Hugo screamed, but as I cycled, his howls faded. Wrapping my arms around him and cooing, I flashed through my most selfish wishes, trying not to dwell on my wish to see Hugo bounding back across the street in a few weeks, completely healthy, with no disability. When the paramedic took him out of my arms and listened to his chest, he said, "Good call, doc. Sounds like at least a partial pneumo," and rushed him into the helicopter.

When I called to check up on Hugo, the doctor said, "I can't explain it. Our guys were all prepared with a tray, the operating room prepped for a thoracotomy if necessary. But by the time he got here, he had breath sounds and was laughing. We did a chest X-ray, and he has a broken rib but no pneumothorax. Guess the paramedics were off on their diagnosis. Or maybe the guy has a guardian angel."

A few weeks later, the image I had cycled of Hugo bounding across the street flashed through my mind as I saw him, fully recovered, climbing a tree. I told Bill what had happened, and Bill said, "I hope you remembered the golden rule: Be playful. Avoid ritual."

The mechanisms of how this cycling practice might lead to physical healing are not yet understood, but if you're struggling with a disease doctors are unable to cure, perhaps this technique belongs in your Sacred Medicine toolbox. When people are sick, they are often cycling toxic, fearful, and doom-and-gloom imagery, which floods the system with stress hormones such as cortisol and epinephrine, shutting off the body's natural self-healing mechanisms. However, imagery of wish fulfillment likely produces a biochemical soup of dopamine, endorphins, oxytocin, and other healing hormones. Why not try? It's free. It's harmless. At worst, this technique might help you feel happier. At best, you might experience unexpected healing. And if some of those wishes just happen to come true, that's just icing on the cake, right?

The Bengston Method™

The method Ben and Bill developed together, which was used to cure cancer in mice and has anecdotally cured many conditions in humans, is based on mental image cycling. When Bill and the Bengston Method practitioners he has trained practice cycling as a form of healing for humans, they recommend that the healee also practice cycling to have "skin in the game." Try it yourself if you feel inspired!

1. **Make a list of at least twenty of your ego's greatest desires.** Be selfish! The items must be measurable, something you will know to check off your list if you fulfill the desires.

2. **Take each item on your list and translate it into one image.** If I want a red bicycle, I might see an image of myself riding one, coasting down a hill.

3. **Boil down each image into one word or phrase.** My one word might be *bicycle*.

4. **Make a list of your one-word images.**

5. **Spend time "savoring" each image.** Take at least ten to fifteen minutes per image to allow yourself to imagine feeling all the emotions and sensations you might feel if you were fulfilling this desire, acting "as if" in your mind's eye.

6. **Cycle the images.** This is the challenging part. Flash each image through your mind's eye like a slideshow. Start with one image per second. It's hard to explain how to cycle the images without listening to Bill explain it in depth. It's not a memory exercise— randomize the images in your consciousness, as if you're shuffling the deck.

7. **Speed up the pace of the cycling.** When he teaches this technique, Bill starts by playing a drum slowly. *Boom . . . boom . . .* he speeds up, and finally, he plays a metronome that beats up to 100,000 times per second. You can't "see" the images anymore at this speed of cycling.

8. **Heal while you cycle.** While the mind is busy cycling imagery, the hands can be used to heal. Apparently, this can also be used remotely—hands free.

To learn Bill's cycling method in more detail, listen to his Sounds True audio program *Hands-On Healing* or attend one of his workshops.

Chapter 3

THE ENERGIES OF LIFE

As "out there" as the Bengston Method might be, studying with Bill Bengston satisfied the skeptical scientist in me. His rigor, unwillingness to jump to conclusions, and understanding of what is scientific and what is not comforted the parts of me that value certainty. But there aren't many Bill Bengstons in the world of Sacred Medicine. Many energy healers don't think like scientists, aren't open to being studied scientifically, and routinely answered with glib remarks such as "I just care about curing people" when I pushed for more scientific rigor.

I understand this sentiment while I simultaneously desire to merge such responses with science. Nevertheless, I have come to respect and value the subjective aspects of healing the scientific method hasn't evolved to include (*yet*). I resonate with energy healer Ellen Meredith in *The Language Your Body Speaks*:

> The scientific mindset calls for objectivity and discourages
> subjectivity. This means that all the information that
> arises within you—your inner knowing, your experiential
> insights, your personal experience, the personal story
> line in which the health challenge developed—is
> considered mostly irrelevant. . . . By asking doctors to
> turn off their intuition and rely on evidence, I believe
> the medical profession is hampering the way the mind

is designed to work: Right-brain intuition guides our
journey, and left-brain logic works out the details of
the itinerary. What would happen to medical care if
doctors were encouraged to use both evidence *and*
intuition to guide their choices, and they could use
both medical and alternative remedies as needed?[1]

Ellen's book is entirely nonscientific, and she owns it, yet I considered
her suggestions potentially helpful for those who might be struggling
with illnesses not responding to treatment. She justifies her approach:

This is a nonscientific form of discourse. You might
ask yourself whether it bothers you to not have science
repeatedly cited as an authority. Can what I am saying
be true if I don't cite some study that proves it? I am not
saying science is always wrong, nor am I rejecting science.
Instead, I think focusing solely on science deflects us from
understanding the communications of our bodies and minds.
It undermines our confidence in our ability to participate
in our own healing, and it curtails ways of knowing.[2]

I agree with Ellen in that science appeals only to our mental intelligence, yet if we rely solely on science, we run the risk of being stripped
not just of our intuitive intelligence, as she suggests, but our valuable
emotional and somatic intelligences as well. I reached a point in my journey when it was time to explore the more subjective aspects of healing,
which science doesn't fully know how to study yet.

Stories and firsthand accounts often fall into this category of subjectivity. They are not scientific, and even thousands of comparable ones do
not add up to evidence. Yet science often lags behind stories, which are
sometimes at the forefront of what's possible. Stories can guide science.
If enough of them catch the attention of open-minded and curious scientists such as Bill, you might be lucky enough to wind up with data. To
dismiss stories categorically as unscientific would be foolhardy if we're
going to unravel the mysteries of healing.

With that disclaimer, I'll share a remarkable story. Melanie was believed
to have advanced ovarian cancer when she visited an energy healer for
a session intended to help   prepare energetically for the surgery she

had scheduled for five days later. She was told to "get her affairs in order" because her doctors were concerned she might not survive, given how weak her immune system appeared. The hands-on healer assessed Melanie energetically and had a strong intuitive sense that the cancer had not metastasized. Although Melanie's energy was dim and her aura collapsed close to her body, the only place that looked like cancer to the healer was localized to Melanie's left ovary. The texture, vibration, and appearance of the energy coming through her ovary seemed responsive when the healer applied her methods. She could see and feel them shift as she worked on Melanie, and by the end of the session, the pain that had plagued Melanie for weeks disappeared.

The healer told Melanie what she had experienced and questioned whether it was necessary to rush into surgery because she agreed with the doctors that Melanie's immune system might indeed be too weak to survive. Plus, the healer felt confident, given how responsive Melanie's body was to the minimal intervention she had tried, that the tumor's growth might be reversed without surgery.

Given her decades-long experience and understanding of how risky it is to ever suggest that someone with a potential cancer diagnosis might benefit from delaying surgery, this healer knew she was in uncertain territory. She was careful to use strong disclaimers when suggesting Melanie might delay the surgery, knowing she could be putting Melanie's health at risk or arrested for practicing medicine without a license. Melanie responded to the possibility of canceling the surgery with horror, but the healer felt hopeful given the way Melanie's body had responded to minimal intervention. Could Melanie delay surgery by just two weeks, the healer wondered? Melanie scheduled another session for the next day and said she'd talk it over with her husband.

That evening, the healer received an earful from Melanie's outraged husband, who called the healer a quack and threatened her, saying she would never have another chance to give his wife false hope. Before the healer could explain, he'd hung up.

The healer called again, and Melanie answered. She said, "Melanie, don't postpone the surgery, but please keep your appointment tomorrow. You don't have to pay. You have nothing to lose. I believe in what I am saying. I *want* you to bring your husband with you. Find a way!" She didn't expect to see Melanie again, but the next day, Melanie arrived with her scowling husband. Learning that the healer had offered to do the session at no cost quelled suspicions that she was a con artist out to take advantage of his wife.

The healer asked Melanie to lie down on the massage table and then scanned her energy field. This time, the healer saw a dark, dense energy over Melanie's left ovary, and when she put her hands over it, the healer felt like her hands were moving through mud. Hoping to ease Melanie's husband's skepticism, she asked him to place his hands a few inches above Melanie's body where her ovary was. She instructed him to move his hands in a circle. She demonstrated a motion that tends to draw energy out of the body. To his great shock, he felt something he couldn't see. Within two minutes, his hand pulsed with pain. As the pain increased, his wife reported hers was abating.

By the end of the session, Melanie was pain free and feeling significantly stronger. The healer taught Melanie's husband a healing practice he could perform on her at home. Melanie and her husband were so surprised they temporarily postponed the surgery. They insisted that Melanie's doctors repeat her imaging tests before they went through with it. After ten days of daily treatments from Melanie's husband and three more sessions with the healer, the doctors repeated the tests. The tumor was *gone*.

ENERGY HEALING IN THE HOSPITAL

I met Melanie's healer—Donna Eden—at the University of California–San Francisco (UCSF) hospital long before I heard Melanie's story. When I told my physician friend I was going to the hospital to watch Donna treat a sick friend, this doctor knew who she was, although I had never heard of her. It turns out Donna is one of the most famous healers in the United States, runs one of the oldest and most respected energy medicine training programs in the modern world, and has written the flagship do-it-yourself self-healing book about the subject, *Energy Medicine*. Given how I was focusing on the subjective aspects of healing, I considered her synchronistic appearance in my life Divine timing. Donna came to the hospital at UCSF to treat a mutual friend during a life-threatening medical emergency. With a curly mop of strawberry blond hair and a huge smile, Donna looked like a cherub grown into an adult woman. I could almost see her halo in the sunlight streaming through the window. She appeared so luminous and youthful that I was shocked when she revealed her age. She personified what New Agers must mean when they say, "She has such good energy!"

Donna approached my friend, whom I'll call Eric, in a matter-of-fact manner and put him on a massage table she had brought to the hospital. I watched her manipulate his body in ways I didn't understand. She used strange jargon we don't learn in medical school when referring to the human body, phrases borrowed from Traditional Chinese Medicine (TCM), such as triple warmer, strange flows, meridians, and governing vessel as well as lingo I had heard elsewhere, such as chakras. I had no framework for what she was doing with Eric, but I watched with intent curiosity.

I don't know what Eric's frail body looked like to Donna when she scanned him energetically, but Donna got to work manipulating one knee over one leg and moving his arms in opposite directions, as if she was performing a strange massage. She thumped on his chest and pressed on "sore spots," spending time doing something I couldn't track and didn't understand.

Eric's doctors had warned us that he might die quickly from the acutely life-threatening complication of his cancer and prepared us to possibly lose him within the next forty-eight hours. I can't prove Donna's treatment helped Eric, but he did survive the immediate medical emergency, along with conventional medical interventions. Perhaps she saved his life in the short term, but neither energy medicine nor conventional medicine was enough to cure his end-stage cancer. Despite all attempts to prolong his life, Eric died within a year, leaving us grieving.

ENERGY HEALING AS A FIRST RESPONSE

One of Donna's stories of healing really struck me. While visiting Mexico, Donna encountered a gruesome scene: A young woman had been hit by a bus. Its back tires had stopped right over her pelvis, hip, and upper legs. Donna was the first to arrive at the accident and rushed to the girl's side with her hands as the toolbox containing her energy medicine tools, while others called the paramedics.

Donna found an unconscious girl whose life force was leaving her. Her aura had completely collapsed, and Donna could see the energies draining out her feet. Because the situation was so dire, she focused on what could be done to keep the girl alive until the paramedics arrived. Sitting at her right side, Donna began holding triple-warmer points, meant to stabilize the girl's energies and alleviate immediate shock. Signaling to a local boy who arrived at the scene, she showed him how to hold the same points on the left side of the girl's body. The two of them quite literally held her fragile life force in their hands until the acute shock started to reverse.

Finally, Donna felt a power surging under her hands, as if the young woman's life force was coming back online. Donna was moved to hold her neurovascular points, and she showed the boy how to hold the end points of the heart meridian to support the girl's cardiovascular system as best he could. By the time the paramedics arrived, and the bus driver had come to his senses enough to see that he needed to either move the bus forward or back up to take the weight off the girl's body, Donna had completed several other emergency interventions.

Donna intuited that the bus needed to back up rather than move forward but that the driver should wait until she did one more intervention so the girl could survive having the thirty-two-passenger bus roll over her again. When Donna tuned in to the girl, the girl opened her eyes briefly, then closed them again. Donna took this as a sign that she could handle it now. Donna told the bus driver to back up slowly, which he did, while Donna held points on the girl's forehead. Then the paramedics rushed in with a stretcher and raced the girl to the hospital. After the bus driver hugged Donna, she got back into her car and wept, holding her own neurovascular points and breathing deeply until she felt she could drive.

The next morning, Donna went to the hospital to check on the girl. The doctor, who had heard about the strange blond *gringa* at the scene of the accident, said in English, "You are the one who helped Maria at the accident. Something wonderful happened there. Somehow her blood coagulated and stopped her internal bleeding. Did it have something to do with what you did? It probably saved her life. What did you do?"

Donna replied, "This is what I did," and put her fingers on the doctor's forehead. She said she'd never seen appreciation turn more rapidly into bewilderment.

Because she has trained thousands of practitioners, Donna has also heard countless stories from those who have studied her method, such as the experience of Tim Garton, a forty-nine-year-old world-champion swimmer who first had non-Hodgkin's lymphoma and then prostate cancer. Both cancers had been treated with conventional medicine, but his widespread lymphoma recurred. Doctors tried a bone-marrow and stem-cell transplant, which was not successful. The only treatment option left was an experimental injection, Retuxan, which Tim received but which doctors didn't put much hope in.

Then Tim sought out energy medicine from one of Donna's students, Kim Wedman. Tim's sessions included a basic energy-balancing routine; meridian tracing; a chakra clearing; work with the electrical, neurolymphatic, and neurovascular points; a correction for energies meant to cross over from one side of the body to the other that are not crossing; a daily assessment of other basic energy systems; and finally, corrections for anything deemed out of balance. Kim also empowered Tim to treat himself with a twenty-minute, twice-daily energy medicine protocol.

Returning to his oncologist, Tim was told that conventional medicine had nothing left to offer him, but to determine how fast the cancer was spreading, further testing was done. To everyone's surprise, Tim was cancer-free! Was his remission the result of Kim's energy treatments, the single Retuxan shot, the green juices and herbal teas he started drinking at Kim's prodding, or all three? Nobody could say, so doctors continued treating Tim with Retuxan injections every two months, Kim gave him energy tune-ups as needed, and he kept drinking his juice. He finally passed away sixteen years later at seventy years old, twenty-five years after his initial cancer diagnosis.

WHEN HEALERS "SEE" ENERGY

It wasn't until years later that I began studying Donna's work more intently for my book. When I was remembering that time together in the hospital, I wondered what patients looked like through her unusual way of seeing. She wrote,

> For as long as I can remember, I had a capacity for
> sensing the body's energies more vividly and distinctly
> than most people, including an ability to see its energies
> as colorful fields, flows, and swirls. Much later, I learned
> that what I see corresponds with maps and descriptions
> found in ancient healing traditions. So I am not alone
> in this ability. I feel certain that the individuals who
> mapped these energies had a similar type of perception.
> In fact, the ability to respond to the direction and

polarity of magnetic fields of extremely low intensity, well established in homing pigeons and a variety of other animals, has now been detected in humans in laboratories at Cal Tech and the University of Tokyo.[3]

What I'd give to spend one day seeing the world the way healers like Donna do! One healer I encountered explained that these heightened sensitivities might develop as a way of surviving childhood, often as the result of trauma. The child learns to develop extreme empathy and extra-sensory capacities—seeing, hearing, and even smelling things others can't or "reading" energy to avoid an abuser (for example). This heightened perception becomes a survival tool. After the trauma ends, the gifts linger. Hearing this saddened and moved me. It also led me to ask many of the healers I interviewed if they'd be willing to share their trauma histories. Sure enough, most of them revealed horrifying traumatic histories that broke my heart and evoked an upwelling of compassion. They said they were grateful for the gifts, although the torture was hell.

I asked Donna if this theory was consistent with her understanding of how and why some people "see" energy. She agreed this might be a piece of it, but perhaps it is a natural gift we lose if it's not acknowledged and developed in childhood. She wrote in an email to me:

> I believe that infants see or vividly sense auras and other subtle energies from the start. If this ability isn't reinforced by the culture or by the parents, it fades into the background "noise" of growing up, acquiring a language, learning how the culture requires its members to think and act, establishing an identity, etc. In less complicated cultures, which are closer to nature, this commerce with the energies in the environment becomes part of how the world is understood, part of intuition, not a separate skill or ability. . . . I know that some healers who see energy believe that it is because they were traumatized early in life that they developed this ability as a survival mechanism. This suggests the way dissociation develops. Some children who are abused escape the trauma by creating a separate world, sometimes separate personalities. But my seeing energy didn't develop along a trauma path. While many healers have had more

than their share of trauma—many share the journey of the wounded healer—I didn't suffer major traumas during my childhood. I grew up with a wondrous mom. Mama could always see energy. She assumed that everyone sees energy. She thought it was normal. She would discuss the energies she saw as casually as describing the leaves of a tree. As a result, my sister, brother, and I all grew up seeing energy. It was reinforced in us and seemed perfectly natural.

HEALER, HEAL THYSELF

In the process of writing this book, I interviewed, studied with, and observed nearly a hundred healers from all over the world—in the cities and suburbs of the United States; in the towns and metropolises of Europe; in Indigenous villages in North America, Peru, Africa, Bali, Australia, Colombia, and Thailand—and I visited many of them on their home turf. Whereas Indigenous healers often undergo rigorous selection processes by their tribes, are put through often dangerous and traumatic initiations, and experience extended training as apprentices, a large number of healers I met in the West developed their techniques out of sheer necessity to treat *themselves* for conditions conventional medicine couldn't adequately address. Donna was no exception. In 1959, at age sixteen, she was diagnosed with multiple sclerosis (MS). Periodically unable to walk, she experienced chronic pain and terrifying intermittent "spells" during which she became paralyzed for up to twelve hours. At the age of twenty-seven, she had a heart attack, and her doctors told her the damage to her body from her MS was irreversible. They said her organs were breaking down, and she probably had only a few years left.

Although Donna could see energy for as long as she could remember, it never occurred to her to use this ability for healing. However, faced with a grim diagnosis—and two young daughters she intended to stay alive to raise—Donna focused her intuitive understanding of the body's energies on her illness. She noticed she could shift the energy flow in her disabled legs by using her hands to reduce her chronic pain. Desperate, she began experimenting. She made passes over her skin that moved the energies, circled her hands over particular spots, touched specific points, and moved her body into certain postures. Doing so changed how she saw her energies, providing something like biofeedback, which matched her symptom relief.

Although some relief was immediate, it took six months of intensive work until she found reproducible ways to systematically move her energies and get them flowing and balanced. Finally, she could consistently walk, although it would be several years before the intermittent spells stopped. By her mid-thirties, she was symptom free and has remained so for forty years. Obviously, she proved her doctors wrong by not dying from complications of MS.

Having become her own guinea pig, Donna realized she might help others suffering from serious illnesses that did not respond to conventional treatments. She found that when she helped people the way she had helped herself, some experienced remarkable results. She treated thousands of clients and taught others to do so. They, too, reported promising results, suggesting that it was the method and not solely Donna that helped people heal. As a result, Donna launched Eden Energy Medicine (EEM) in 2005, which has trained more than 1,600 certified practitioners who work with clients across the world.

WHAT IS ENERGY MEDICINE?

When I pose this question to energy medicine practitioners, they almost universally answer: "It's *all* energy." When asked to explain what they mean, their language differs, but generally, Sacred Medicine practitioners make a distinction between "subtle" and other types of energy—such as electrical, magnetic, light, or mechanical—readily measured and accepted by mainstream science. In "Exploring Multiple Meanings of Subtle Energy," former president of Holos University Bernard O. Williams defines it as "different forms of energy more subtle than conventional physical instruments can detect. In this sense, the concept comes from traditions that accept the human ability to see or feel forces that are not physically measurable."[4]

Although most mainstream science denies the existence of subtle energies, at least in relationship to healing or medicine, the fundamental understanding among energy medicine practitioners is that energy ranges from invisible particles and waves to densified energy as matter—including the human body—as well as the energy of thoughts, beliefs, damage from traumas, and even emotions. These healers operate with the premise that waiting to work with the diseased body at its densified physical level, as a surgeon would, misses the chance of preventative treatment before disruptions in the body's "energy field" condense into physically manifested disease. Although most ethical energy healers agree that conventional medicine is necessary to address immediately life-threatening physical manifestations, they usually argue that by the time disease appears, disruptions in the energy body have preceded it—and that disease might have been avoided had those energies been manipulated earlier. Energy medicine practitioners, including TCM doctors, view physical disease as the result of a long-standing energy condition that might have begun as early as childhood or even, perhaps, in a past life, or a generational condition passed down via energy fields.

These healers posit that disease begins as blocks in the natural flow in the "energy body," the invisible layers and pathways that surround and interpenetrate the physical body. They believe that, if these blockages are identified and treated at the energetic level, disease might be prevented before it's physically apparent. They also believe that treating the energy body when physical disease is present can facilitate and hasten a cure by restoring the natural flow of life-force energy, as Donna did with Melanie's tumor.

Systems of energy anatomy differ from one healing practice to another, but most agree discrete energy centers and pathways of energy moving in and around the body hold certain qualities, such as stuck energy caused by trauma that can predispose the body to disease. When flow is restored, diseases related to these blockages might remit.

Energy medicine in the United States runs the gamut. Nurses apply Therapeutic Touch to postoperative patients in the recovery room. Hands-on healers often work undercover as massage therapists. There are Reiki practitioners in integrative medicine clinics, along with every possible kind of sound healer, color therapist, crystal healer, chakra healer, aura healer, magnetic healer, intuitive healer, faith healer, psychic healer, remote healer, sacred geometry healer, spiritual healer, and neoshaman. And that doesn't even include the acupuncturists, Ayurvedic healers, Tibetan medicine doctors, yogis, craniosacral therapists, chiropractors, and others who claim to work with qi, prana, energy, or some other form of flowing life force believed to be manipulated by healers to "move" energy.

Whether you can teach someone to be an energy healer or whether it's a natural gift is disputed.[5] But that doesn't prevent healers from trying to reverse-engineer healing methods into something teachable. Many of the expert energy healers practicing in the United States today were trained by rigorous pioneering programs such as EEM, Barbara Brennan's Hands of Light school, Janet Mentgen's Healing Touch, Dolores Krieger and Dora Kunz's Therapeutic Touch program, and Mikao Usui's modern-day Reiki. Yet many of these contemporary schools of energy medicine are syncretic, cherry-picking (and some might say culturally appropriating) elements of long-established ancient healing traditions, such as Ayurveda, TCM, and Tibetan medicine.

Some healers train over many years before becoming skilled at their art, such as those who study and become certified in acupuncture and TCM. Others, like Donna, learned how to heal their own illness, developed a method, and hung up a shingle. Some learned to heal at their grandmother's knee or apprenticed with an expert outside of any official training program. Some have attended a weekend workshop or taken a daylong online course. To label such varied degrees of experience with one term—energy medicine—is the equivalent of suggesting that board-certified medical doctors and kids who play doctor are both practicing medicine.

This is part of the challenge when it comes to objectively measuring the efficacy of energy healing modalities. Are Donna's students going to get the same results as Donna herself, just because they're all using "her" technique? What if Donna is to energy medicine as Mary is to praying? If I learn EEM, will I have any chance of being as masterful as Donna, or will my energy medicine skills be as lazy and potentially ineffective as my prayer?

Skill and proficiency aside, what about the subjective aspects of the healer's presence, consciousness, empathy, communication, connection to Source, and open heart? Science has no way to measure and control for such things, yet those aspects of healing might be why alternative medicine is a multibillion-dollar industry. People are willing to pay for what they might not be getting from their conventional, burned-out, rushed, traumatized doctors: time, presence, healing touch, even love. Yet this lack of ability to measure a healer's proficiency subjectively can make energy medicine a dangerous free-for-all.

What's more, there are both differences and similarities in how healing systems describe and teach human energy anatomy. The terminology you're likely to hear if you seek the help of an energy medicine practitioner is not what I learned in medical school, and you're not likely to hear it at your doctor's office. We didn't study these aspects of energy anatomy during gross anatomy in medical school because there's nothing to dissect and no way to prove they exist. Yet energy medicine practitioners rely on these systems, and as is the case for healers with unusual vision like Donna's, some say they see this energy anatomy as clearly as a surgeon sees a blood vessel.

Donna places particular emphasis on nine types of energy that are part of the human energy anatomy, corresponding with healing traditions from Indigenous practices of China, India, Ireland, Scandinavia, Tibet, Fiji, and Native America. For the purposes of establishing terminology and reviewing energy anatomy, I've summarized them here.

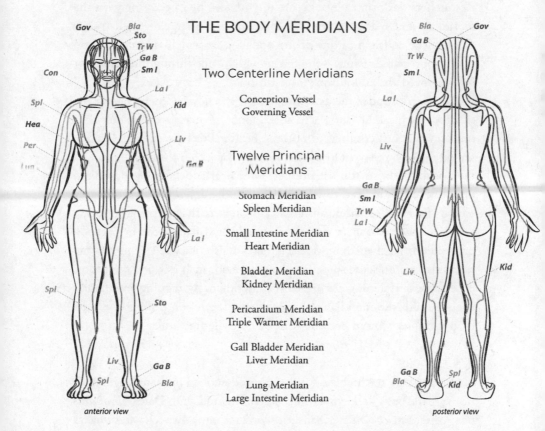

THE BODY MERIDIANS

Two Centerline Meridians

Conception Vessel
Governing Vessel

Twelve Principal Meridians

Stomach Meridian
Spleen Meridian

Small Intestine Meridian
Heart Meridian

Bladder Meridian
Kidney Meridian

Pericardium Meridian
Triple Warmer Meridian

Gall Bladder Meridian
Liver Meridian

Lung Meridian
Large Intestine Meridian

anterior view

posterior view

1. Meridians

These fourteen pathways, as mapped in TCM, are believed to move life-force energy throughout the body, connecting invisible reservoirs of heat, electromagnetic, and other subtle and hard-to-measure energies. Meridians lie along the skin's surface and move deeper into the body and around the organs, like an energetic circulatory system. Conventional medicine does not acknowledge the existence of meridians, but those who have written about the science of TCM assert that although meridians cannot be dissected like arteries or nerves, they are explainable biological phenomena and can be located in the body's largest unacknowledged organ—the connective tissue, called the *interstitium*, or the bodywide matrix of collagen, fluid-filled spaces, and fascia just below the skin, which surrounds all our organs and could serve as a way an electrical charge can propagate through the collagen network.[6] Researchers posit that acupuncture might work by interacting with the meridians and manipulating the "piezoelectric charge," which travels through the collagen in one of the body's most widely distributed and rarely appreciated tissues—the fascia, which runs throughout this newly recognized and ubiquitous interstitium.

TCM works under the assumption that the flow of energy along meridians, which can be stimulated at acupuncture or acupressure points, is not only real but essential to optimal health. Practices such as Qigong are meant to be preventative, keeping the *chi*, or *qi*, flowing. Although most acupuncturists still use needles, some healers believe needles might not be necessary to keep your meridians healthy. Energy healers often say, "Energy flows where attention goes" and suggest that learning to locate meridians and trace their course—manually or visually—can be part of a daily preventive medicine practice. You can also practice tracing the meridians when you sense something might be off, such as when symptoms arise in organ systems governed by that meridian. By aligning your hand's energies with the meridian's energies, "like the moon pulling the tide," Donna claims you can become your own needle-free healer.

2. Chakras

If meridians are the highways, the chakras described in many yogic traditions are the body's energy stations. According to Cyndi Dale's *The Subtle Body*, the term *chakra* is a Sanskrit word meaning "wheel," and chakra teachings were mentioned in the ancient Vedic texts of India. The chakras are commonly described as at least seven whirling vortices of energy situated along the center line of the body, starting at the perineum and moving to the crown of the head. An unusually sensitive healer might feel or see heat, pain, or something like stickiness over one of these chakras, suggesting emotional pain from a past trauma or physical pain as the result of a diseased organ related to that chakra. Each chakra is believed to govern the organs in its vicinity, and balancing and clearing them is said to have physical and psychological impact.

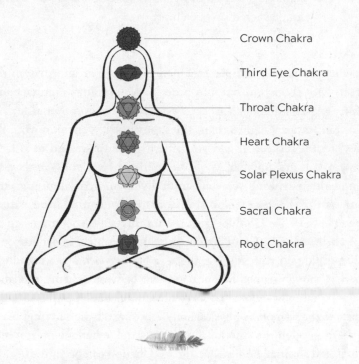

Crown Chakra

Third Eye Chakra

Throat Chakra

Heart Chakra

Solar Plexus Chakra

Sacral Chakra

Root Chakra

Cherishing and Connecting the Chakras

Adapted from Donna Eden's *Energy Medicine*[7]

Although full chakra balancing might require the help of a healer or at least the more detailed instructions offered in Donna's book, these two do-it-yourself exercises can help you nurture your chakra health at home.

Try cradling a chakra, sending it loving gratitude, and holding it with your hands, like soothing a baby.

If you place your right hand on one chakra and your left on another, you can enter a prayerful state. Spend at least three minutes letting these energies merge, as if your hands are jumper cables. For example, power disconnected from compassion and love is part of what's destroying the world. Connecting the heart chakra and the power chakra could help you amplify your power with the kindness and compassion of an open heart.

3. Auras

Imagine you are surrounded by an energetic egg of information that interacts with the world but also protects you, serving simultaneously as a filter and an antenna. This egg typically extends around as far as your arms can reach in all directions. If it's too close to your skin, your boundaries are not protected, and you'll be hypersensitive and at risk (think "empath"). If it's inflated, you'll be at risk of violating other people's boundaries, engulfing everyone around you, and consuming more than your share of the space (think of what a "force of nature" some narcissistic types can be). Like Goldilocks, you want this egg—your aura—to be *just right*, believed to be about eighteen to thirty-six inches beyond your skin.

Depending on who you ask, the aura has between seven and dozens of layers. Although names are not consistent between systems, the labels for the seven rainbow-colored layers of the aura include the etheric body (the closest to the skin of the physical body), moving outward in rings like those of a tree through the emotional, mental, astral, etheric template, celestial/causal, and spiritual bodies. Because dysfunction can occur in the layers of the aura before disease manifests in the physical body, many believe working with these energetic layers has significant potential for diagnostic and preventive clinical applications as well as treatment for disease.

Aura-reader-turned-empathy-researcher Karla McLaren describes auras in scientific terms for those more comfortable with such language. In an email, Karla explained auras:

> It's about the proprioceptive system, which maps our bodies in space and creates our external "peripersonal" space. Your proprioceptive system is connected to your interoceptive system; proprioception helps you map and become aware of your peripersonal space, while interoception helps you map and become aware of your interior space.

What if your aura is in bad shape? Putting your attention on it is a good start. By imagining it is your birthright to have this clear egg of space surrounding your physical body, you might feel more expansive and protected. You might be more able to guard your sacred energetic space from intrusion, while simultaneously protecting yourself and others from inadvertently penetrating someone else's sacred space. Your aura is your business. Other people's auras are their business. Unless you ask for an aura reading, no one has the right to penetrate yours without consent—you have the right to protect it.

Shoring up your aura might require psychotherapy if your boundaries were violated during childhood. But you can begin by visualizing your aura as a bubble and filling it with whatever color you feel drawn to. You can also fill your aura with song, a calming image, or a lovely fragrance or taste.

4. Electrics

The electrics, which involve the movement of electrons and protons, are the densest of the subtle energies (such as the aura, chakras, and meridians) and the subtlest of the dense energies (such as magnetic fields) that we can measure. The electrics bridge the various energy systems of the body.

I hadn't heard of the electrics in other systems I researched, so I asked Donna about them. She said, "I've never met anyone who couldn't feel the electrics. They are the least subtle of the energies we work with. I've not heard of others who talk about it, but because it is a more tangible energy, I can't imagine that others haven't discovered it. It may be that people use terms like 'electrical energy' when they are attuned to it."

5. Celtic Weave

Many traditions include the notion of two energy channels crossing a central channel seven times at the chakras. In the West, we represent it as the *caduceus*, the mythological winged staff of Hermes with entwined serpents wrapped around it, crossing seven times. These woven energies are like infinity symbols, spiraling in figure-eight patterns in fractal patterns in nature and in our bodies. This pattern appears on the microscopic level as DNA and on the macroscopic level as the brain hemispheres crossing over and controlling the opposite sides of the body. This pattern is, according to Donna, "the weaver of your force fields."

Some healers say they hear this weave as a musical sound or resonance. As a simple practice, you can hold your arms out in front of you, drawing figure eights while bending your knees, in a rudimentary Celtic Weave dance.

6. Basic Grid

If the root chakra is at the bottom of the vertical axis of the body while standing, the basic grid is near your back if you are lying down horizontally. Whereas the chakras might spin from inside your body out into the aura and the environment beyond your body, your basic grid is contained inside your skin. When intense trauma shakes the body, psyche, or soul, the basic grid acts like a shock absorber to keep trauma from frying your motherboard and destroying the entire energy system. Many healers describe this grid-like structure differently, so although there is relative consensus about meridians and chakras, there is considerable variability in the understanding of this bit of energy anatomy. Donna suggests this system is so foundational, it is best facilitated with expert help, whereas others don't even acknowledge its existence.

7. Five Elements

Many healing systems, such as TCM, contain some version of the five elements—usually water, wood, fire, earth, and metal—sometimes associated with the five seasons. The water element is associated with winter, wood with spring, fire with summer, and metal with autumn. The earth element is considered a fifth season, but it is actually an umbrella term for the times of transition—solstices and equinoxes. We know illness arises from many factors, and each human is unique. If we're strong in one element/rhythm and weak in others, we might be prone to illnesses, just as certain psychological patterns are associated with specific illnesses. Your dominant element/rhythm also influences your personality, your relationships, and nearly every other aspect of your life.

8. Radiant Circuits

The radiant circuits (also known in TCM as the "extraordinary vessels" or the "strange flows") are the energies of bliss. They can be strongly influenced by thought and intention, tending to go to the part of the body you are thinking about. Although they might function like meridians, they are not limited to specific pathways but can jump around.

Self-hypnosis, guided imagery, affirmations, gratitude practices, nature immersion, good news, and laughter can all activate radiant circuits.

Because laughter activates radiant circuits and signals to "triple warmers" that all is well, radiant circuits might explain why laughter helped Norman Cousins, who used laughter as medicine for a debilitating disease, as described in his book *Anatomy of an Illness*. Radiant circuits can turn your energy around on a dime, which we've all experienced from something as simple as a shift in perception or a gorgeous sunset. One of Donna's asana-like exercises, called Connecting Heaven and Earth, similar to exercises taught in Egypt, China, and India, is said to quickly activate the radiant circuits.

9. Triple Warmers

A term borrowed from TCM, *triple warmers* have qualities of both a meridian and a radiant circuit. Rather than staying in their lane, like a typical meridian does, triple warmers jump across meridians like a radiant circuit, hooking up with other meridians and organs in conjunction with the hypothalamus (the thermostat of the nervous system), which regulates whether the system is in relaxation response or fight or flight. When all is well, triple warmers strategically distribute heat and energy in the body. When fight or flight gets activated, triple warmers prepare the body for threat, which affects the immune system. This can be both protective and destructive. Most confusingly, the mechanisms of triple warmers can attack through an autoimmune disease or show up as an allergy. Triple warmers often decimate whatever is in their midst and have a challenging time distinguishing friend from foe. Although triple warmers tend to cause physical illness when they are overactive, less commonly, they need a boost, as in anaphylactic shock.

Donna says, "[A] triple warmer has no interest in your happiness or your spiritual development—only in keeping you alive. Unfortunately, its information bank about what is required for survival has not received a major deposit in several million years."[8]

Donna's book includes methods for keeping triple warmers healthy. Try this one: Wrap your right hand around your left side above your hip. Wrap your left hand above your right elbow, which is near where the triple warmer meridian passes. Hold this position for at least three deep breaths; repeat on the opposite side.

HABIT FIELD

Donna describes the habit field as a force of nature, as real as gravity, that carries information and organization like a blueprint of the organism's biological as well as spiritual development. This field moves little, shows little color, and has a remarkably steady rhythm. Donna wasn't sure how to interpret this field until she heard Rupert Sheldrake describe morphic resonance and fields. In an interview in *Scientific American*, Sheldrake defines morphic resonance and fields in this way:

> Morphic resonance is the influence of previous structures of activity on subsequent similar structures of activity organized by morphic fields. It enables memories to pass across both space and time from the past. The greater the similarity, the greater the influence of morphic resonance. What this means is that all self-organizing systems, such as molecules, crystals, cells, plants, animals, and animal societies have a collective memory on which each individual draws and to which it contributes.[9]

The habit field carries the blueprint of an oak tree in an acorn. It helps salamanders regenerate lost legs. The habit field is a blueprint for the whole organism. The habit field is meant to resist change and preserve patterns, conserving what evolution created. But because our world is changing so quickly, Donna suggests we might need to override the habit-maintained programs of our bodies if we want to keep up with all the insults our bodies, psyches, and souls are exposed to in modern society. Your habit field is what can keep you stuck—not only as it relates to illness or injury but also at the level of life purpose, relationship to abundance, intimate relationships, and collective dysfunction, such as the impacts of systemic racism and colonization.

Effectively, this is the field that effects transformation—a paradigm shift changing everything. You're at the mercy of your blueprint and have, to some degree, a fixed destiny unless your habit field shifts—then anything can happen.

CLINICAL APPLICATIONS FOR EDEN ENERGY MEDICINE

I asked Donna and her husband and coauthor, energy psychologist David Feinstein, to help me understand the best clinical applications of EEM. They explained that the approach focuses not on illness or its symptoms but on blocked, scrambled, or disharmonious energies. The symptoms guide the practitioner to assess the state of the body's energies (with pain or a failing organ being particularly informative). But medical diagnosis is secondary to how the treatment is oriented. The target is systemic change brought about by balancing and harmonizing energies. This approach can ease or completely eradicate an illness, but the interventions are not focused on symptoms and disease. It's hard to compare the holistic energy-based paradigm to reductionist, symptom-based conventional medicine, which focuses on which symptom-relief treatments work for which conditions.

I also asked how one might best include EEM in a personal Prescription and which kinds of illnesses it might work best for. In an email to me, David wrote,

> While virtually any medical condition is going to benefit from harmonizing the body's energies, EEM has been successful with certain conditions for which conventional medicine doesn't have effective interventions, such as autoimmune illnesses, certain immune deficiencies, and other systemic conditions. EEM might be a first line of treatment for conditions such as fibromyalgia, chronic Lyme, MS, chronic pain disorders, irritable bowel syndrome, migraines, food allergies and chemical sensitivities, mixed connective tissue disease, electromagnetic hypersensitivity, and chronic depression. More invasive treatments might then be applied with whatever symptoms remain. EEM can be a secondary intervention when conventional medical treatments may be remarkably successful, such as many medications and surgeries, but which produce unwanted side effects. If you break your leg, you want it set in the emergency room. But if you want to manage the pain more naturally or

help the bones mend more quickly, energy medicine can make a significant difference. We often recommend it as a complementary treatment for conditions requiring radical medical interventions, such as organ transplants, artificial joints, pacemakers, chemotherapy, radiation, and of course surgery and medication. It is also a powerful tool in an integrative medicine approach in treating any challenging physical condition, such as cancer or Parkinson's.

Donna's email reply to me was more emphatic. Although she didn't disagree with the specific points in David's response, her answer to "What is Eden Energy Medicine best for?" included every diagnostic category in the International Classification of Diseases. In the more than ten thousand clients who had ninety-minute-plus sessions with her in the twenty-four years she had an active practice, she saw EEM help, though not necessarily cure, nearly every physical and mental health issue imaginable, at least as an adjunct if not always as primary treatment. (If you want to learn more about Donna and watch free videos of her energy-maintenance techniques, visit edenenergymedicine.com.)

THE SCIENCE OF SACRED MEDICINE

I began this chapter with the disclaimer that science has had little success proving beyond a doubt the existence of subtle energies, much less whether manipulating them with healing hands can reliably cure disease. But has there been any science insight at all?

I titled this book *Sacred Medicine* and use that term to refer to energy healing because most healers employ spiritual language—not scientific lingo—when discussing their healing. The majority of healers explain their work as a kind of meditative practice or prayer, referencing some version of connecting to Source and letting healing run through them as a conduit. Many explain that they have to "get out of the way," putting their egos aside so they can be a clear channel for Divine love or the Buddha field or something sacred that uses them to facilitate healing in others. The scientific community, however, doesn't use the words *sacred medicine*; they call it *biofield science*, using the term proposed in 1992 by an ad hoc committee of complementary and alternative medicine (CAM) practitioners and researchers convened by the Office of Alternative Medicine (OAM) at the National Institutes of Health (NIH).[10] The committee defined *biofield* as "a massless field, not necessarily electromagnetic, that surrounds and permeates living bodies and affects the body."[11]

I've already talked about Bill Bengston's science, but let's go back in history a bit. Before scientific materialism rigidified to the point of a stultifying lack of curiosity about the science of healing, some legitimate data came out of the laboratory of Bill's hero Bernard Grad, a research oncologist on the faculty of McGill University in Montreal whom Bill nicknamed "The Great Grad." During the 1960s and 1970s, Grad extensively studied Oskar Estebany, a hands-on healer from Hungary skeptical of his own healing powers and humble enough to volunteer to be studied scientifically. Grad performed experiments on mice induced to have goiters (enlarged thyroid glands). The mice treated by Estebany still got goiters, but Estebany's treatment significantly slowed their growth. Grad had Estebany "treat" scraps of cotton and wool, then used them to treat the mice without Estebany's direct contact. These mice also showed significantly slower rates of goiter growth.

Other scientists also got involved in studying Estebany, including Justa Smith at Rosary Hill College in Buffalo, New York. Smith gave Estebany test tubes containing the enzyme trypsin to treat. The longer Estebany treated the test tubes, the faster the enzyme trypsin catalyzed the activity of proteins. Perplexingly, Estebany's effect on other enzymes caused the enzyme activity to slow down. Smith then made a unifying and surprising conclusion: *Estebany's effect on the enzyme activity always either accelerated or slowed in the direction that would induce greater health in the organism.*

At New York University, Dolores Krieger had Estebany treat the blood of sick people, who then demonstrated an increase in hemoglobin compared with the blood of the control group, suggesting an immune response.[12]

Since then, researchers have attempted to use evidence-based science to establish the legitimacy of energy healing. Shamini Jain, founder and director of the Consciousness and Healing Initiative (CHI) and assistant professor in the Department of Psychiatry at the University of California–San Diego, studied the impact of noted energy healer Rosalyn Bruyere's biofield healing methods on the debilitating fatigue breast cancer survivors suffered that did not resolve after treatment. The effects of Bruyere's healing were compared with the effects of unskilled sham therapists who laid their hands on patients in similar ways but without healing intention or manipulating the biofield. Within only eight one-hour healing sessions, the levels of fatigue of the survivors in Bruyere's treatment group dropped to normal, whereas those in the placebo group were not significantly more energized.[13]

Susan Lutgendorf, a professor at the University of Iowa, monitored natural killer cell activity, comparing Janet Mentgen's Healing Touch method applied to cervical cancer patients going through chemotherapy and radiation with relaxation alone. Only those treated with Healing Touch maintained their natural killer cell function, a critical part of the immune system necessary to fight off cancer during chemotherapy and radiation.[14]

In a systematic review, "Biofield Therapies: Helpful or Full of Hype?," Shamini compiled and analyzed sixty-six clinical studies of biofield therapies (Healing Touch, Johrei, laying on of hands, Reiki, spiritual healing, Therapeutic Touch, and others) that met her rigorous criteria.[15] She concluded that biofield therapies:

- show strong evidence beyond placebo of reducing pain (thirteen clinical trials evaluating patients with arthritis, carpal tunnel syndrome, chronic pain, fibromyalgia, neuropathic pain, and osteoarthritis all had consistent, significant benefit);

- show moderate evidence of treating acute pain in cancer and hospitalized patients, with more studies needed;

- show promise for improving mental health, but the data are insufficient;

- affect our biology, including blood pressure, brain activation, cortisol rhythm, heart rate, heart-rate variability, and salivary IgA levels.

Although none of these conclusions will blow anyone's socks off or win a Nobel Prize, it's worth noting that three different universities and a prestigious medical center in the United States (Harvard University, Indiana University, the University of Connecticut, and the MD Anderson Cancer Center) are all studying biofield therapies and comparing them with sham control treatments—with promising results. Discoveries are being made that show how energy healing can affect tumor growth, death, and migration as well as related cellular immune function in different types of cancer in both animal and cell culture studies.[16] Not only do biofield therapies show impact at the cellular level, but also several studies suggest that there is an intelligence to this kind of healing, influencing cancer cells and regular cells differently.[17] This science alone upsets the applecart of our mainstream worldview about modern medicine. So far, the only way we've known how to have this kind of impact on cells, especially cancer cells, is through drugs and other technological interventions. All these healers are doing is intending to heal and then transmitting healing directly to cells. *Take a moment to let that sink in.*

CAN WE EXPLAIN A MECHANISM FOR HEALING?

Can scientists propose a mechanism for how biofield healing might work? Countless theories have been proposed, but all of them are still in the realm of the speculative. Some researchers believe it's all mere placebo effect. Others propose a mechanism by which low-level electromagnetic fields (EMFs) affect biological receptor systems that might be located in the interstitium. The idea of healing being propagated through a living matrix has been around for decades, so this recent discovery of the interstitium as a bodywide organ could help explain the physiology of acupuncture and movement practices such as yoga, Qigong, and tai chi that move the fascia and affect the interstitium.

Others, including Bill, theorize that biofield effects might be non-local, nonlinear, and more "information" than "energy." By definition, *energy* is "the capacity to do work" and should drop in intensity with distance. However, those who claim to practice distance healing say that distance has nothing to do with it. This is where scientists who study such things venture into the dicey territory of the "quantum," a term often misused by healers in ways that leave legitimate scientists rolling their eyes. That said, quantum entanglement, or the capacity for separated objects to share a condition or state, famously called "spooky action at a distance" by Albert Einstein, might eventually help explain how distance healing could work. Although the answer is still a long way off, I recommend reading Shamini's rigorous review of the science we do have in her book *Healing Ourselves: Biofield Science and the*

Future of Health.[18] I also recommend checking out the CHI website if you like to nerd out on data like I do. Read the free "Subtle Energy and Biofield Healing: Evidence, Practice, and Future Directions" report cocreated by countless CHI scientists and healers as a sort of state of the union of our understanding of what we can prove and what has yet to be unraveled.[19]

Shamini suggests we consider the science of biofield healing from more of a systems-thinking approach, opening ourselves to a both/and explanation rather than an either/or that requires us to validate one theory at the expense of another. Reminding me that the paradoxes of healing can hold multiple truths as simultaneously relevant, she writes,

> We know placebo effects are real, we know EMFs
> seem to play a role in physical healing, we know
> distant healing and intention have real effects on
> biology, and we know quantum mechanics experiments
> support the idea of nonlocal information transfer.
> What if all these things are simultaneously true?[20]

WHY SCIENCE MIGHT STRUGGLE TO VALIDATE SACRED MEDICINE

Although we might lack clear scientific evidence to support the claims of healers and patients that Sacred Medicine can cure humans of everything from cancer to paralysis to Alzheimer's, there might be a valid reason for this paucity of reliable information. Many healers cite a conspiracy by the medical-pharmaceutical complex to suppress evidence that Sacred Medicine works for financial motives and the corruption of greedy capitalists who don't care about patient well-being. Skeptics argue that the lack of overwhelmingly clear clinical data is because energy healing is hogwash. Rather than polarizing into one camp or the other, I'll make a speculative case for why the deck might be stacked against proving the legitimacy of Sacred Medicine as effective, evidence-based medical intervention, not through any malicious conspiracy but simply through the limitations of the current scientific paradigm.

1. No pharmaceutical companies stand to profit from proof that energy healing might work, so there's little motive beyond pure scientific curiosity to study it.

2. Researchers, scared of mockery by institutions where they might not have tenure, are understandably hesitant to risk their reputations, livelihood, and long-term security by studying topics viewed with contempt by mainstream academia.

3. Some science has become dogma, the antithesis of science. Dogma puts science into the realm of a fundamentalist religion, and science should not be a religion. Peer pressure to study only the sciences we accept as "real" (aka purely materialist) casts those who genuinely wish to learn more as heretics. Medical science is still based on materialism and makes little room for the metaphysical, spiritual, or energetic aspects of healing. To understand more, read "Manifesto for a Post-Materialist Science."[21]

4. Researchers courageous even to take on studying Sacred Medicine lack funding.

5. As keepers of the dogma, reputable journals are often reluctant to publish even impeccable science in areas they deem "paranormal," thereby silencing or exiling to fringe journals the good science that does get funded.

6. Energy healers tend to be skittish around scientists and have often been traumatized by skeptics who dismiss their gifts and mock their life's work. Many report feeling "off their game" in the clinical sterility of a laboratory, under the harsh observation of skeptics.

7. It is possible that a laboratory is a nonconducive environment for reproducible results.

These factors do not even take into consideration the upset applecart of quantum physics and how this discovery might affect the evidence-based medicine model of science.

1. What if the assumption that we can objectively separate the treatment given from the people giving it is categorically false?

2. What if it is not possible to separate the treatment group from the placebo control group if the participants in the trial are in some way bonded to each other with what Bill calls "resonant bonding?"[22] What if anyone bonded to anyone else in the group might affect each other's outcomes? What if the placebo effect, still not explained scientifically, is a result of this resonant bond? If we can't fully separate the treatment group from the placebo group, and they might entangle with each other in ways that corrupt the data, how can we possibly differentiate the snake oil from the medicine in a reliable way?

3. Science has not yet figured out how to objectify, quantify, and measure the subjective. Yet subjective experience is a real human phenomenon. We try to measure the efficacy of subjective interventions such as psychotherapy and prayer. But how can we objectively measure things that rely on the consciousness, presence, and skill level of the practitioner? Are we really expecting such factors not to influence the outcomes?

Overlay these obstacles with the legitimate pushback from publicly traded companies and institutions that give lip service to patient well-being but are required by law to unapologetically prioritize the financial bottom line and fatten the pockets of shareholders over helping you—the patient—become miracle prone, and "Houston, we have a problem." Suffice it to say that we don't really know how well Sacred Medicine works because, at this point, the headwinds are making rapid scientific progress in these fields inch forward. What we can say is that the field is deserving of more study, and desperate patients conventional medicine has failed to help are using it with or without evidence that it works.

Will you be one of those people who claims to benefit from some sort of energy transfusion? Is it possible that some of these approaches could relieve at least some of your suffering? You won't know until you try.

Chapter 4

PLEASURE PRACTICES AS MEDICINE FOR THE BODY

A consideration of energy-transfusion-enhancing Sacred Medicines would not be complete without touching upon what I call "pleasure practices." If your life force is depleted, pleasure can transfuse you energetically as powerfully as any biofield healer, so it's in the Healing Bubble of the Whole Health Cairn. The best part is that many kinds of energy transfusions—such as dancing, singing, making art, performing a ritual, doing yoga or meditation, and engaging in humor and sex—are free, accessible, readily available, do-it-yourself Sacred Medicine practices used for purposes of self-healing and community healing by Indigenous cultures for millennia. If you're on a healing journey, I cannot recommend enough adding such practices to your Prescription for Healing for the purpose of transfusing yourself with life force. I do consider pleasure practices a kind of energy medicine because they bolster life force and affect the will to live, perhaps by activating the radiant circuits some healers reference.

There are countless books and scientific studies about the health benefits of yoga, meditation, sound healing, laughter, and even sex as medicine for the body, so I won't review that data, although during my Sacred Medicine research I did study a variety of pleasure practices as tools for the medicine bag. I even got certified as a "laughter yoga" instructor and giggled with cancer patients at the University of California–San Francisco's

(UCSF) Osher Center for Integrative Medicine. Just as Norman Cousins laughed his way from an "incurable" illness to good health in *Anatomy of an Illness*, some of those cancer patients swore group laughter was making them well again.

As part of my own healing journey, back when I had fully weaned myself from seven drugs and then again when I was healing from the dog-bite injury, pleasure practices became a huge part of my Prescription. I returned to singing, which I had always done as a young person but had largely abandoned during my years as a doctor. I began playing singing bowls and chanting along with them and joined drum circles and vocal groups who sang old folk songs together. I even recorded a CD. (You can download one of the ceremonial songs I use for earth rituals from thesacredmedicinebook.com.)

I also dove back into every dance form I could find—Nia, Journey Dance, Soul Motion, Ecstatic Dance, S Factor—anything that didn't require going to a smelly club or getting bumped by drunk people. Someone recommended I check out a dance community in Sausalito based on Gabrielle Roth's Five Rhythms and later renamed Open Floor by Kathy Altman and Lori Saltzman. This dance community was a valuable part of the healing journeys of everyone in it.

I knew getting back in touch with somatic intelligence and movement practices was essential to good health and full of energy transfusion possibilities, but I was never so aware of the potential of dance as energy medicine as when my friend Jarman Massie, one of my favorite Open Floor partners, got tonsil cancer. As part of his regular practice, Jarman had spent years dancing regularly alongside me and hundreds of others in a sweaty gym. Jarman was usually out there in the center of the dance floor, showing off his Solid Gold moves and lighting up the room with his grin and unapologetically unrestrained enthusiasm. But on this particular night, Jarman was frail, pale, and barely able to smile because his lips were cracked and scabbed. Still, he held his arms out in hug gestures to us all.

After being in peak physical form as a professional dancer, Jarman had wasted away to 130 pounds as the result of his cancerous tonsils, which left him unable to eat during grueling radiation and chemotherapy treatments. When Jarman received his diagnosis, he told his best friend he wished he could attend his own funeral, and his friend nodded. "That can be arranged."

He gathered us in a church to celebrate and energize Jarman's healing, to perform our music for him, to memorialize him, to raise money for treatments he couldn't afford, and of course to dance. Hundreds of us got weepy during shared testimonials and live performances of world-class music. We didn't want Jarman to die, and he didn't want to leave, but it was a powerful testament to a well-loved man to hear all the things we often only say about someone in eulogies after they leave their body. Jarman was visibly moved, as were we.

This set the tone for what came next, a surprise to Jarman. He was invited into the nave of the church. Chairs and pews had been removed, and the church had been transformed into a dance floor. The men stood along the perimeter of the room, while the women, bedecked in colorful silk scarves, surrounded Jarman. He looked shy until he realized the women were flirting with him in a sexy scarf striptease, and then his grin returned. We encircled him with our scarves, gyrated our hips, batted our eyelashes, and poured life force into him with our hearts and bodies, all the while feeling supported by the men, who held space around us in an outer circle. The slow, sensual music sped up, and we filled with a wild energy, legs kicking, arms whirling, butts circling in a frenzied momentum that culminated in a kind of group energy-gasm. At one point, Jarman was arched across the chair that supported him, one toe pointed on the ground, the other extended high in the air in a full split, arms thrown back in ecstatic surrender, his chest open to receive.

The music faded to a whisper, and the women brushed Jarman with kisses of our scarves before withdrawing to the outer circle and letting the men penetrate the center. Drums beat, and men pounded their feet and chests in unison as they approached him, like warriors. They collectively lifted him out of his chair and held him over their heads, where he lay as if in a coffin, his arms crossed. The music grew somber, and I got teary as I prayed we wouldn't have to do this for real.

Then the music livened, the energy shifted, and Jarman kicked a leg in the air, saying, "If I have to do this, I'm dancing my way home!"

The men put him in the center and stepped back. Jarman danced like his life depended on it. This man, who could barely walk into the church, now undulated, kicked, and twitched his hips like Elvis. He continued for almost three hours, and we took turns fueling his revelry and being fed by it in return. At the end of the night, sweaty and pink in the face, Jarman said, "*Heaven.* This is heaven here now. Thank you all for this love-dance-healing."

The idea that some suffering might not be curable, but it can be carried, comes to mind when I remember this emotionally evocative, heart-opening moment of deep connection in community. Paradoxically, when we carry our suffering together in community, some people do wind up mysteriously cured—even those who don't feel more whole. We didn't know how this story would end for Jarman, but being present in that moment is one of the most gorgeous memories of my life. We were all part of something larger than ourselves. Jarman gave all of us permission to tap into our own suffering—and together we received the chance to heal the loneliness of bearing our suffering in isolation.

As I went home that night, sweaty and ecstatically connected with my senses, I thought, "*This* is Sacred Medicine." If only every cancer patient could receive *this*. I knew the way you just *know* things that Jarman would survive. Five years later, he's still dancing and cancer-free.

A few years later, I brought the doctors in training in the Whole Health Medicine Institute to Open Floor to dance with me. We were so happy, intimate, and cuddled together after a year of working together, grooving and jiving in our little love bubble, when the founders, Kathy and Lori, approached us with admiring faces, asking, "Who *are* you people?"

One of our new graduates said, "We're doctors!"

I explained they were learning about Sacred Medicine options for helping people conventional medicine doesn't know how to cure. The founders' faces lit up. They know Open Floor is medicine, but few doctors recognize it as such. These doctors were glowing—the medicine was healing them too.

DANCING AS PRAYERFUL MEDICINE

Before my dance community was called Open Floor, we called it Sweat Your Prayers. My dogmatically Christian mother did not understand how having this much soulful, tearful, rageful, and sometimes even erotic dancing could possibly be prayer. I explained to her what my teachers told me—that the dance is how we talk to God, and the stillness after the movement stops is how we listen. As has been practiced by Indigenous communities since the dawn of time, dancing and praying can be one and the same because our bodies lift up our blessings and pleas for help, and our stillness opens up our receptivity and gratitude. Both the movement and the stillness are sacred prayers, like the out breath and the in breath. Praising with our bodies, moving sometimes painful emotions through them, and being vulnerable before the Divine within ourselves and with each other are all forms of prayer. In the stillness that opens up our meditations at the end of the dance, we listen, receiving guidance, opening to embodied ways of knowing and hearing God talk back.

We also commune with each other in this prayerful way. Healing cannot happen in isolation; healing is, almost by definition, a relational activity. Yet many of us are challenged to heal in relationship because so many of our wounds happen there, causing attachment injuries and boundary confusion. How to work in connection with another person without losing our sense of self must be part of any embodied spiritual practice. If I have to leave myself to be with you, I can't heal. If I must leave you to be with myself, this won't work either. How do we find the balance between intimacy in solitude, with others, *and* with the Divine? Dancing together can help us learn this not only cognitively but also through the body. This is part of being an embodied human.

Dance as medicine is not a New Age phenomenon. Our ancestors around the world have always used dance in ceremony for healing, to cast out evil spirits, to invoke blessings, to celebrate the changing seasons, and to call in the rain. Kathy and Lori explain that dance turns healing on its head because the dance is the teacher, medicine, and healer. The healing lies in our willingness and capability to be with all parts of ourselves *and* everyone on the dance floor—together, whether we can accept whatever arises or not.

The scaffolding of the Open Floor practice is fourfold: physical embodiment, emotional tolerance, mental constructs, and soul retrieval. The physical dimension focuses on range of motion and sensate awareness. Where are you in your body, and how might you expand that range? You also work with arising emotions evoked by music, other people, and situations in your life. You allow *all* emotions—there are no bad or wrong ones. The point is to allow feelings to move in and through you, to build your tolerance for the feelings you don't like. They might shift from fixed and frozen to fluid . . . or not. The mental constructs help us use the mind not to escape thoughts but to allow imagination and creativity to flourish on the dance floor. Why would we want to exclude our brilliance from our dance? The shadow of the mind is revealed when we become calcified in our belief systems, but dancing can help shift beliefs about ourselves and each other. In Open Floor practice we ask, "Where is our choice point?" Many of us feel that how you move on the dance floor is how you move in the world, so we practice having more fluidity and choice in both places. Soul is our unique purpose and contribution this time through.

I'm not the only one who has had embodiment and somatic intelligence traumatized out of me. We live in a disembodied culture because trauma causes us to *leave* our bodies. It's a defense mechanism and, in extreme cases, a survival skill that can save you. Yet you can't heal the body without being in it. In spiritual circles and certain meditation practices, we often attempt to transcend our bodies, believing only the spiritual aspects of consciousness have merit. Open Floor helps you become physically, emotionally, mentally, and soulfully embodied, allowing you to examine the relationships outside yourself. We need to relate and belong.

Open Floor is not the only practice to use dance for medicine. San Francisco Bay Area dancer Anna Halprin, who is 100 years old as I write this and is still dancing, used dance as healing during the AIDS epidemic from the 1980s to 1990s and continues to teach dance as a form of medicine. Debbie Rosas considers her Nia dance a form of healing as well. S Factor founder Sheila Kelley teaches pole dancing as a healing practice and a way to reclaim exiled aspects of our often-traumatized sexuality. I invite you to tune into your Whole Health Intelligences and try this medicine.

Dance Your Medicine

If this embodied medicine appeals to you, see if your community has an existing dance practice group like Open Floor, Five Rhythms, Nia, S Factor, or other conscious dance communities.[1] Some offer online classes, so get creative! If you don't have access to a dance community, start one! Invite friends to dance with you. Be your own DJ or ask someone to do so. Making a healing playlist and allowing your body to respond to the music can be fun, nourishing, and full of sound-healing medicine. Which songs bolster your life force, help you feel emotions you need to move, uplift you, soothe you, and facilitate your reconnection to Source? Whatever the music, allow your body to move naturally and unselfconsciously with it.[2]

HEALING WITH INTENTIONAL CREATIVITY

Although song and dance got left by the wayside during my medical training, art and creativity were always part of my medicine—and I still use them for medicinal purposes. When I was pre med in college, I also majored in creative writing. When I started medical school, I bought a set of watercolors at the drugstore and taught myself to paint. When I was a full-time OB/GYN, I practiced medicine all day and painted with beeswax (encaustic) all night. I always said medicine was my hemorrhage and art my transfusion. It was an obsession until I quit working in the hospital and my manic need for an art transfusion settled down. I still live a creative life, but after I stopped hemorrhaging, my urge to paint, which I still enjoy as a playful hobby but no longer do professionally, shifted to other creative outlets such as writing and cooking.

One of the most nourishing phases of my healing journey began before I quit my hospital job and ended with an art show called *The Woman Inside* at Commonweal, a retreat center with a gallery space where Rachel Naomi Remen taught the Cancer Help Program. I spent years making plaster sculptures of women before and after their breast cancer treatments. The women would come to my house, disrobe while I cast their torsos, laying my hands on them and sculpting their bodies with medical-grade plaster gauze scented with lavender oil while singing to them or listening to them discuss how they felt about their bodies. When we were finished, I'd invite them to bathe in my tub and get dressed. I'd interview them about "the woman inside," listen, and write narratives of the beauty I saw within each woman on scrolls of rice paper that I dipped in beeswax. Their stories hung alongside the sculptures.[3]

One of my closest friends and art playmates, Shiloh Sophia McCloud, understands art as a pleasure practice and healing medicine as well as anyone I know. For more than twenty years, she has been facilitating healing through the arts with women, many of them survivors of trauma, at MUSEA: Center for Intentional Creativity. She traded San Francisco's corporate world and art school for a "chop wood, carry water" mentorship with the artist Sue Hoya Sellars, a back-to-the-lander since the 1970s. Still in her early twenties, Shiloh went from high heels and high tech to hiking boots; living in a trailer in Mendocino County; running naked in the woods; and digging red earth from the hills to make clay, paint, and write stories.

Sue, also a mothering figure to Shiloh, wanted her to learn the goodness of diligence. One day, Shiloh playfully complained she didn't understand why she needed to dig the earth out of the hillside to make clay. Why couldn't they go to the art store like normal people?

As Shiloh wedged the clay, Sue asked,

> What do you care about seeing changed in the world?
> Solving the problem of global hunger? Poverty? Ending
> violence against women and children? Sex trafficking
> and gender inequality? Get clear on what your heart
> cares about, and put that love into the clay as you wedge
> it. Imagine your love going to those who need it most,
> *right now*. Your love is going into the clay as you wedge.
> The particles of matter are being impacted by your
> intention. As you intend it, it begins to happen—right
> then. Believe this. This is how the universe works.

In that moment of infusing healing energy into the clay, Shiloh *got it*. She infused the clay with passion, sending love and a desire to end violence against women and children. The clay itself, and Shiloh's heart, were awakened in that moment. Shiloh *knew in her body* that the molecules of the clay were responding to her energy and that anything she made from that clay would carry that intention. Whether she infused it with neutrality, hostility, or healing love, it would be transformed, so why not infuse it intentionally with healing?

Shiloh edited a much longer story here as a way to honor Sue and share Sue's Intentional Creativity teaching with you, dear reader.

The Feast Table of Love

Shiloh Sophia McCloud

A young woman artist is going for a visit to see her teacher, the Master Artist, who lives in the deep woods at the top of a mountain. The teacher greets her warmly and reveals her latest creation—a luminous table shining in the sunlight in the middle of the studio. The teacher caresses the smooth wood with her weathered hands, saying, "This table is really special to me. To us."

The student asks, "Will you tell me what is special about this table?"

"Every work of art has its own story. But first, some tea." The ritual of making the tea is done in silence except for the crackling wood, the whistling kettle, the spoon stirring the wildflower honey and fresh goat milk into the clay cups. The student and teacher are sitting at the new table together, sipping tea as if in ceremony.

The teacher begins:

> There is always a catalyst when you are
> making art. Sometimes inspiration comes
> from nature. Or it may come from a desire
> to transform suffering. A spark for creating
> is ignited and chosen. Then my imagination
> reveals choices. What is my intention for this
> work of art? What am I carrying in my heart?
> What ideas am I reconciling within myself?
> Where can I ease pain? And then there are
> the more logistical inquiries: What medium
> and tools am I called to? What is the shape
> of this creation?
>
> The intention for this table arose when
> I looked in my heart to see what suffering
> needed tending within myself and in the
> community and the collective. I opened
> to insight, and quite clearly the vision of
> my heart went to those who do not have
> enough to eat. I trust the impulse of the
> vision, perhaps because right now I have
> enough. There have been times when I
> didn't have enough food myself, so this
> ache is very real for me. As I made this, I
> included nourishment, for them and for me.
> Making art can be a kind of praying.

Tears rise in her eyes about the past and the struggle of making a living as an artist and how grateful she is for what she has today and how art has been her medicine.

Suddenly, the honey-colored table seems so full of life. The student feels it humming in her body. The teacher says, "The artist heals herself by making art intentionally that helps others heal. Being with compassion in a big way changes her. I imagine that there is an energy traveling from these creations to tend the suffering of others. All thought is energy. All energy has power. Where will we place that power?"

The teachers asks, "What kind of healing will you infuse into your work?"

Feeling it in her whole body, the student says, "I long to ease pain and violence for women and children."

The teacher nods yes. This has been important to her too. "Once a decision is made about the intention, it shapes the form. Making art in this way with Intentional Creativity serves my own desire to create as well as centering around an idea that matters to me. I flesh out my intention and the design in my notebook, woven with my desire to ease suffering. I begin to feel the flow of inspiration increase. I experience an amplification of energy in my body. The works of art become resonators and carry a charge."

The student feels expanded. Her skin is star sprinkled with little bumps. She begins to wonder how she can pass these ideas on to others and instantly feels a quickening.

The teacher goes on. "As I work, I revisit the purpose of this table. Suddenly, I see a vision, not just of the people I imagined coming to eat at this table but of other people as well—ones I don't yet know. I include their energy. My choice activates the flow of energy that contributes to the healing of the whole. We are all related, but this is not just an abstract concept; each one of us who does our work contributes to the consciousness of the whole. I am making this table for love, from love. Love is in the table—literally and energetically. Artists have always stretched their visions this way, making the impossible possible through imaging the possibility we could not see before. I will always be a part of this table. Whether or not others who sit at this table know it, love resonates *from* this table."

The teacher runs her hands over the table again. "Intentional Creativity calls us to sacred responsibility, to mend what is broken. Something powerful happens to us, through us. We are changed, and we learn to care about more than just our immediate needs. To make something with intention is ancient, a tradition that belongs to all beings. This table is not just about who can eat here or make art here. You have an incredible opportunity to live life being nourishment for others. Not as a kind of obligation and not because people need your help—although they will—but because nourishing others will nourish you too. In the case of the artist, this often happens through an offering of creativity, beauty, resources, ideas, and of course stories like this.

"There will always be great needs in the world that will call you to tend them. Just as you have needed me, I needed my teacher. My teacher took me in and fed me when I had very little food to eat. She taught me when I had no money to pay for lessons. She gave me a sense of worth when I had very little. She treated me as an artist when I had only just begun to create, and I was so young. I have passed this on to you."

The teacher smiles upon her student and says, "Now, you can tell the story of this table."

The young woman brings her hand to her chest in surprise. "I can?" she asks. "How can I tell this story? This is an honor . . ."

"I am giving you this story and this table. You are an artist. You will feed many more than I, with more than literal food." The teacher nods her head with assurance of her choice.

"I will tell the story of the Feast Table," the young woman promises.

NOT JUST CLAY AND ART

Over time, it dawned on Shiloh that if we applied Intentional Creativity to everything in our lives—not just the clay or our art but also how we deliver medicine, educate children, love, and govern—life could fundamentally transform.

This practice of putting healing intention into food, art, and rituals designed to help the earth is consistent with Indigenous spiritualities.

A friend of mine lived at the Taos Pueblo with her Native American husband, and she explained that everything that happens in a traditional home in the pueblo is rooted in prayer. The corn is planted and harvested, the deer hunted and gutted with prayer. The corn is baked into bread, and the venison is made tender in a stew infused with prayer. You don't merely recite a blessing before the meal, as is often done in Jewish, Muslim, or Christian homes. By the time you eat, the food and the prayer have united, and you are believed to be physically ingesting prayers.

Just as in Laura Esquivel's *Like Water for Chocolate*, in which the protagonist, Tita, yearns for the lover she can't have, putting all that painful longing into the food she cooks and making the people who eat it cry, the ancients weren't being metaphorical when they said they were putting love into their food, weaving, or beadmaking. The idea that you can "feel the love" someone puts into her cooking is not just sweet talk. I've experienced it directly when Shiloh's chef husband, Jonathan, imbues his cooking with love and serves it at the original Feast Table of Love.

This is the opposite of how most Westerners typically grow food, make art, or treat the earth—through mass production, poisoning the water supply and the land, and unapologetic exploitation. Perhaps Shiloh's Intentional Creativity offers us a way back to what our Indigenous family has been practicing since the earliest art was made. For our ancestors, it was likely natural to imbue everything with an intent to teach, share, or tell a story, as in the case of prehistoric cave paintings and carvings. Whether we're creating art, food, herbal remedies, poetry, or dance, the intention we imbue in them can affect what we make in ways that amplify their Sacred Medicine properties.

We should never underestimate the power of encouraging dancers or artists to gather with the intention of healing as a pleasure practice and energy transfusion that bolsters life force. During the series of personal, national, and worldwide traumas of 2020, I started a Zoom community called Healing with the Muse to help people cope by singing, dancing, drawing, meditating, writing, reading poetry, listening to music, and practicing Internal Family Systems, which I discuss in chapter 11. Mostly we feel, love, ease trauma, and engage in sacred healing practices together, something we decided to continue after that painful year ended. Perhaps you'll discover some playful ruckus and muse time is just what the doctor ordered![4]

Heal with Creativity

Consider what needs healing. Maybe it's your body, mind, or emotions. Maybe it's someone you love who is suffering. Maybe it's a social justice cause near and dear to your heart. Maybe it's the earth. Using whatever creative outlet you love most, put all your healing intention into the creation of this art form. Whether your medicine is painting, drawing, pottery, music, dancing, cooking, or any other form of creativity, pour your love, care, and healing intentions into whatever you make. Don't feel shy about incorporating your trauma into the creation, just as in *Like Water for Chocolate*—and then remaking it, painting over it, sculpting it, and alchemizing your pain into something beautiful as a physical gesture of what has been transformed. Trust that whoever interacts with what you've made will, in some mystical way, experience healing just by being with whatever you've made. Not only will the creative process heal and affect the creator but also it might touch the heart of those who interact with it.

Chapter 5

RESACRALIZING NATURE

During my Sacred Medicine journey, I'd become quite the guinea pig. I'd been strapped under giant magnets. I'd attended faith healing revivals where ministers touched the foreheads of sick people who then fell back as if shocked unconscious into the arms of attendants who dutifully caught them and laid them on the ground. I'd had coca-leaf readings and shamanic healings from Peruvian *paqos* in a Q'eros village where I lived in a hut with the villagers at 15,000 feet in the Andes. I'd visited Qigong experts from China, including one who appeared to manifest herbs out of the palms of her bare hands and another who claimed that must be a fraud because an ethical Qigong master would never show off that way. I'd received "casting of the bones" readings and shamanic healing sessions from several Indigenous healers in Africa. I met with and learned from Aboriginal healers in Australia. I visited Hawaiian kahunas and studied with the late Robert Elphin Smith, a medical school professor who trained with a Hawaiian kahuna for four years before returning to the mainland and teaching medical students what he learned.[1]

I had sessions with energy healers; received a hug from the "Hugging Saint," Amma; and went on a drug-free psychedelic journey induced by sound alone with Corine Sombrun, a Parisian musician and sound healer who, as the first Western woman to be initiated as a Mongolian shaman, was rigorously studied by neuroscientists. I'd had countless divinations with rattles shaken over me, my stars read, and my palm analyzed. I'd been served a variety of herbal brews (although for a variety of reasons, not for lack of opportunity, I said no to all the mind-altering ones). I'd attended meditation retreats reputed to cure illnesses. I'd bathed in sacred springs and drank allegedly miraculous waters. I'd been saged, slept in a teepee, made tobacco offerings in the Bighorn Medicine Wheel with members of the Crow nation, offered prayers in their sweat lodge, and participated in their pipe ceremonies. I'd had my aura cleared and my chakras balanced and experienced psychic readings and dozens of hands-on healings. I'd read hundreds of books and articles—most of them riveting—few scientific.

Despite being a privileged kid in the candy store of mystical experiences, New Age faith, and Indigenous wisdom, one impulse coming from my Whole Health Intelligences that I hadn't yet indulged was a trip to Bali, to which I felt strongly drawn. When I was offered the opportunity to teach a writing workshop there and stay afterward to study Balinese healing, I jumped on it.

One of the students in my workshop—Casi, a Sri Lankan who had settled there—invited me to move into her spare room and make it my headquarters while I explored Balinese healing. Our first order of business was a trip to a famous healer and Tantric guru reputed to cure incurable diseases. Casi and I had risen early so we could go to the market, where we purchased *canang sari*, banana-leaf baskets of flowers that are ubiquitous offerings in Bali. These baskets are not just offered to temples, healers, and sacred sites in nature but placed on every doorstep, in every taxi, on electricity generators, in rice fields, and in front of businesses. Every morning, as an act of sacrifice and meditative labor of love, women spend considerable time and effort weaving them.

The canang is more than an offering. The practice comes with a complicated ritual of blessings, incense, and a special prayer for each flower. If you're at a temple, it also includes blessings of rice and holy water that the priest sticks to your forehead in a gooey mix. Although the canang is part of everyday life in Bali, Casi and I had taken a spiritual shortcut. Because we hoped to get to the healer early enough to avoid the wait, we bought our canang readymade from a Balinese woman at the market and stuffed each basket with the appropriate amount of cash.

When Casi and I arrived at dawn via motorbike, we were met by two barking dogs. Twenty people were already in line ahead of us. We were ushered into the *shala*, the outdoor gazebo-like structure where the healings would take place. While waiting for the arrival of the healer, still meditating to prepare for a day of healing, we were encouraged to meditate, too, to help his healing become more powerful.

When the healer arrived, a man moved toward him, but the healer said, "Ladies first" and chose one of the women. "Man makes baby for three seconds. Woman makes baby for nine months. Woman has all the power. She goes first." We laughed.

The thin, white-haired healer sat on a chair, and the woman sat on the floor with her back to him. Apparently, there are no HIPAA privacy rules in Bali. All healings were witnessed by everyone else, even when seekers were wrestling with vulnerable issues such as sexually transmitted diseases, mental health disorders, and unwanted pregnancies.

The healer palpated the woman's head and face with his fingertips—her temples, cheekbones, the bridge of her nose, her ears, the sides of her head, and her scalp. A Dutch physician apprenticing with the healer explained in English that this practice was intended to find pain points. When he palpated certain spots, her face twisted in pain. He said, "Anxiety. You have anxiety."

He asked her to lie down on a straw mat. Approaching her left foot with a black piece of wood that looked like something you'd stick in a hair bun, he began poking between her toes while he announced, "This spot bladder. This spot heart. Here neck and back, here liver, here spleen." He got to one spot. "This one hormones."

She screamed and writhed when he pushed her toe with the stick.

He pressed his finger into her shins. "Anxiety," he said, and whispered something into her ear that made her cry. Then he began his treatment. Standing at her feet, he called out numbers to his apprentice. He silently waved his arms over her. He bent to his knees and, taking out the same stick he'd used to poke her foot, traced shapes on her body, running the stick down her midline, encircling her breasts, bifurcating one leg and then the other. When he was done, he returned to the sore spots he used to diagnose her and made a dramatic and exaggerated movement with the stick, showing that he could push as hard as he wanted, and it no longer hurt. We were to take this as proof she was cured.

When it was my turn, the healer palpated my head, sticking his fingers into my ears and pressing into the recesses between my facial bones. He found no area of concern. Before he asked me to lie down on the mat, he looked me in the eye and said, "You have trauma."

Well, yeah. Who doesn't? I'd been through a hell of a year of unexpected, tragic, and violent deaths, losing six people I loved.

I nodded.

He said, "Forget the past. It's over. Trauma over. Live here. Peace in your heart." He drew a circle around my heart with his stick.

If only it could be that easy.

He palpated my feet and found no sore spots. He announced with a grin, "You all good! All perfect! Only world worries. You carry world worries on your head. You get headaches?"

I laughed. He was right about that. An empath with childhood boundary wounding, like some of the boundary-wounded sensitive healers I've interviewed, I sometimes feel the suffering of the oppressed in my body and psyche. I feel the torture of animals going extinct. I feel the shrinking biodiversity and extermination of so much of nature. I feel the injustices visited upon the Black and Indigenous people and how wrongly they've been treated in my country. I feel the sexual exploitation of women and children all over the world. No, I don't get headaches. But the healer was right. I had world worries on my head.

He was surprised that I had no headaches. "All those world worries should give you headaches."

Nope.

He put his hands on my head. "All these world worries, let them go. Don't doubt. Trust. Don't doubt. Trust."

Could I? Could I keep caring but stop carrying the burden of thinking I should be doing something to alleviate suffering? Could I let go and trust that it's all handled and let the activist in me relax? I wasn't sure I was ready for that, but it felt calming to imagine doing so.

He said, "Spirits say, 'You're fired.'"

"Fired?"

"You're fired. You're fired from saving the world. The Universe doesn't need you to be in charge."

I took that in, allowing it to land in my heart, all the while noticing my resistance to his instructions. What about my righteous anger at how innocent people were dehumanized? What about all the ecocide? What about the white supremacy and racism in my country? What about the economic disparities growing between the haves and have-nots of the world? Was I supposed to zone out and pretend there were no crises?

If I didn't leverage my power, privilege, and platform to use my out-
rage to fuel social change, what was I supposed to do? Sit back and
watch humanity destroy the biosphere and succumb to my child inher-
iting a planet potentially inhospitable to human life? Was my impulse
to serve a trauma response, my savior complex acting up, as it had often
done in the hospital? Maybe I *was* fired! What a relief that would be!
Was I getting a hall pass? Or was this guru encouraging me to act like
an ostrich and bury my feelings in the sand?

The healer must have sensed my doubt. He said, "You've done enough.
Spirits are pleased. You're fired. You get to enjoy life. No more world saving. No more worries on your head. Relax, play, trust all is well."

Wow. All I had to do was relax and play? *Seriously?* Was this what the
spirits had said, or had he just figured out how to say things foreigners
liked so we referred our friends, wrote about him on social media, and
filled his canang baskets?

The healer asked his apprentice to give me a blessing, calling out four more
numbers. Were these hand movements choreographed by number? What
did they mean? The Dutch physician waved his arms about and performed
the blessing with tenderness in his moist eyes. When he had finished, the
healer instructed me to rise, beckoning me with his finger. I crawled over to
him on the floor. He whispered, "Someone is coming to love you and bring
you joy." It sounded like a fortune cookie, but I wanted to believe it.

After three years of being mostly single, interspersed with some brief
experiences of heartbreak, I'd gobble up that fortune cookie even if it was
just a line.

He reiterated, "Your service on this earth is enough. You are free to play.
Go have fun."

The healer looked at his apprentice and said, "She all good."

Casi was next. She had been suffering urinary tract infection (UTI)
symptoms for more than a month. Ardent about natural healing, Casi
was averse to antibiotics, but her holistic remedies weren't working. She
sensed that her bladder symptoms had metaphysical underpinnings and
suspected she knew why they were showing up but wasn't sure how to
get rid of them. As is so often the case, awareness and insight into what
might be predisposing the body to illness, although valuable, does not
necessarily translate into healing.

This is where I tend to part ways with the antimedicine camp. I'm all for
natural healing when it works, but have you ever had a UTI? It *sucks*. If I

had a UTI that wasn't responding to hydration, cranberry juice or tablets, and high doses of vitamin C, I'd be the first to check in with my Whole Health Intelligences and, assuming I got the green light, take a dose of antibiotics to knock out UTI symptoms within forty-eight hours, then follow up with some probiotics. I told Casi that UTIs are super-easy to treat with conventional medicine, and she was willing to go see a doctor if this guy's treatment didn't help. She figured she'd give the healer a shot before putting her microbiome at risk from the havoc antibiotics can wreak.

Casi didn't utter a word to the healer about why she was there, but when he poked around her scalp, he found a sore spot. He also hit a spot on her foot. When he pressed, she screamed and recoiled in pain, contorting her leg and twisting her spine.

"Bladder," he said.

After her treatment, he whispered something into Casi's ear, and she smiled. Using his stick, he demonstrated—with a mischievous grin and theatrical flair—that the pain at the bladder spot was gone.

Casi's symptoms resolved immediately and didn't recur while I was with her. As for me and my world worries, well . . . I relaxed for a few days until I learned whom my country elected president in November 2016, something nobody I knew thought could possibly happen. My world worries spiked; I considered not returning to the United States, which no longer felt like home.

INTRODUCING MYSELF TO THE NATURE GODDESSES

Reluctant to return to a country soon to be "led" by Donald Trump, I entertained the idea of expatriating during his administration, but that was a decision my daughter, her father, and I weren't prepared to make. In the interim, I flew to Malaysia for a quick in-and-out at the airport so I could get another thirty-day visa and extend my stay in Bali. I needed to leave the spiritual Disneyland of Ubud and see what I could learn from North Bali, away from the tourists. My British friend Emma traveled with me to a beautiful eco resort in Tejakula, where few white people venture because it is far from the luxury hotels and famous temples. Here Indigenous Balinese who have mixed their traditions with Hinduism practice a more earth-based spirituality.

In North Bali I mentioned my interest in learning from Balinese healers, and a Buddhist monastic from Malaysia whom I'll call Aida offered to take me to see her godfather, a Hindu high priest as well as Indigenous Balinese shaman and traditional healer, a rare combination. When I arrived at his temple, I was offered a cup of black coffee and asked to wait with the others until the medicine man completed his morning prayers. When I was ushered in, Aida, Emma, another friend, and I formed a circle around the healer. When it was my turn, he sat me square in front of him, looked at me for a long time, then laughed his ass off!

I felt self-conscious and bewildered, but his laugh was so contagious that we joined him. His laughter triggered a coughing attack, and when I saw blood in the sputum he spit into a tissue, I said, "Shouldn't you get a healing for yourself?" He ignored me and laughed and coughed some more.

He said that the goddess Durga, a warrior goddess who cuts away everything that is not love, had my back, but I needed to make sure she didn't "sit on me" all the time. Other goddesses wanted to sit on me, apparently, and they wanted to take turns. When I asked which goddesses, he looked at Aida and rattled off a list, which she translated by explaining that he wanted her to take me on a pilgrimage to three different temples to meet the goddesses who inhabited those places. Those goddesses wanted to know me better, to check me out. If they liked me, and I was lucky, they might choose to take turns "sitting on me." He said the nature goddesses of my country might also want to sit on me and that I should take what I learned from Aida at the temples and do the same thing when I returned home, making offerings and prayers at the temples in nature in my country, introducing myself to the goddesses when I got a chance.

Bali is full of simple and ornate temples in nature. Every big tree has a temple where people make offerings. Every waterfall or lake or volcano or hot spring has at least one, and usually a whole series of temples, to which you make offerings before visiting the object of beauty in nature, praying to the gods and goddesses who look out for these natural wonders and asking their permission to enter the space. To skip doing this in Bali is considered raping the goddess. As with sex, it is only ethical to penetrate with consent, or karma will get you.

I explained we didn't have temples in nature in the United States like they do in Bali.

He replied, "Make some."

Aida taught me to craft a simple canang out of banana leaves and flowers, then we went to the grocery store to buy fruit. The first temple we visited was high on a hill in a grove of twisted trees, coiled with snakelike vines that kept startling me because I had already seen a cobra slither through one temple in Bali. Aida ushered me through many parts of the temple, where she instructed me about which prayers to say. A Hindu high priest wearing all white met me at every stop, anointing me with holy water and putting wet rice on my forehead.

The next temple required more preparation. I spent an entire day with a local Balinese family, sitting in their *shala* while the matriarch taught me how to make the grandest of offerings, an intricate craft that included killing and roasting a duck, weaving flowers into mats and boxes, and preparing countless exotic fruits in specific ways. What they created quickly and masterfully took me ten times longer, and my attempts at weaving made the children laugh as they hastened to correct my mistakes. In Bali, the firstborn child is named Wayan, and three Wayans from the village all gathered around as I floundered through my attempt to make a temple-worthy offering.

Over the next week, I brought canang and other offerings to introduce myself and honor the goddesses the traditional healer had suggested I visit. I started with one of Bali's most important lake temples, at the base of a sacred volcano. Would this lake goddess find me worthy of sitting on? If so, how would my life be different? What would I have been like if I had grown up with this worldview?

Next, I made offerings at the forest mountain temple, where banyan trees wove around the stone statues. I've always loved trees. Would the forest goddess want to sit on me?

The third temple was one of the most significant and unknown sea temples of Bali—another way to get spiritually wet! I had to time my visit for low tide so the priest could perform a water purification ceremony while a natural spring was accessible from the base of the temple. After placing my offerings at the temple and praying, I was asked to slip out of my temple clothes and change into water clothes, which in my case were a T-shirt and shorts because swimsuits are considered immodest. While I knelt in front of the spring, the priest used a ladle to pour water over my head until I could hardly breathe. I felt a lightness of being as the priest lifted me off my knees and gazed at me with kind eyes, motioning for me to enter the ocean and swim to the horizon. The priest instructed me to let the ocean free me from my hubris, something Aida and her godfather had also suggested. Was I so full of hubris that people who knew nothing about me could detect this defect?

Years later, in the hardest part of trauma therapy, I would become aware of my proud, striving, caregiving, over-responsible, and overconfident parts, full of hubris. I learned that I came by this tendency naturally as the child of a narcissistic mother. I also came to understand the psychology of the "gifted" child and how hubris wasn't my fault—it was a trauma response. But at the time it was easier to believe it might be possible to invite the hubris to wash away, to be cleansed from my shadow by the ocean without digging into my traumas, to become (perhaps magically) someone the sea goddess of that temple might choose to sit on.

The priest invited me to open myself and merge with that sea goddess, if she felt like she wanted to. Perhaps I imagined it, but I experienced the softness of her presence, the gentleness of her potential feminine impact on me. It was a stark contrast to the fierce love of the warrior Durga, whom the traditional healer said had my back. I wondered whether these three visits to the goddesses of the lake, the forest, and the sea might soften my edges and round out my relationship to the feminine after modern medicine hardened me into someone powerful and competent but prideful, more masculine than many men. Time would tell . . .

EARTH RITUALS FROM THE PERUVIAN Q'EROS

The Balinese offerings to sites in nature were similar to the earth offerings I learned to practice from the Q'eros people in the Andes of Peru. I was drawn to the Q'eros by what I read about the ancient mysticism of these descendants of the Incas, believed to hold a transformative and potentially globally healing worldview. The mystical tradition of the Andes is rooted in the complexity of how human beings and nature are interrelated, which many modern humans seem to have forgotten. Like most nature-based Indigenous spiritual traditions, the Q'eros are animists who believe everything has consciousness and divinity, not only humans and animals but also plants, mountains, lakes, and stones. Just as humans might be insulted if they gave you gifts and you failed to express your gratitude, Q'eros believe the spirits of nature give us gifts, such as water, abundant crops, shelter, good weather, and health. We shouldn't feel entitled or take such blessings for granted. Instead, we should express our appreciation for even the smallest of nature's gifts. When we don't, things get off kilter and problems arise, including illness.

The primary spiritual principle of the Q'eros is *ayni*, or sacred reciprocity. They believe we must give and receive from nature in equal measure. If we are greedy, and we take more than we return, we will suffer. Disease is seen as the result of an interruption in this harmonious relationship, a violation of ayni. Therefore, the first step in treating illness or adversity is to restore this balance. We are designed to cooperate with nature. Just as we inhale oxygen produced by plants and exhale carbon dioxide the plant kingdom needs, we are intended to live as if we love nature and nature loves us back. Although we might think of giving and receiving as two ends of a spectrum or a transactional concept, ayni is considered a circular flow, like inhaling . . . exhaling.

If you're only exhaling, endlessly giving, as many codependent types, empaths, and helping professionals do—if you resist inhaling and have trouble receiving what you need—you're likely to become sick, anxious, resentful, and depressed and possibly die young. Likewise, if you're only inhaling, or taking, as self-absorbed or narcissistic types do—exploiting other humans; maximizing profits at the expense of kindness, fairness, or justice; or raping nature and taking from *Pachamama* (Mother Earth)—the flow of life force will be interrupted. Too much exhaling or inhaling will make you and the planet sick.

Ayni includes daily gratitude practice, even if scarcity strikes. This is not artificial gratitude or justification for "toxic positivity," in which we pretend to be thankful and deny our misery, pasting on a smile when we're angry or disappointed. We must always be honest with ourselves when something we have the power to change *needs* change, and we must feel what we feel without faking it. Ayni is a genuine acknowledgment that, even in the worst of times, we still have breath and water, earth still gives us gravity so we don't float away, the moon waxes and wanes, and tides rise and fall. Birds sing. We have one another. There is always something to evoke awe and open our hearts as long as we resist the tendency to take these blessings for granted.

When we forget to honor the gifts we receive, or when we worry about what we lack or don't like, our nervous systems get stuck in chronic repetitive stress response, switching off the body's natural self-healing mechanisms and predisposing us to disease or premature death. Yet in the modern world, we live in a culture of "not enough." In the Q'eros world, if someone is sick, one of the first interventions recommended by the paqos is an offering. Rather than inhaling and asking for what we want from the spirit realm (such as cure from disease), an offering comes first as a gesture to restore balance. Offer thanks and heartfelt gratitude for nature's blessings; breathe out prayers and spend time communing with the spirit world. If we are aligned, and the spirits grant us grace, we might be blessed with a cure. We do not give to the nature spirits because we want something from them. It is not a sneaky manifestation trick. We give because it is spiritual law. We give because we have received so much. Cures come as gifts, not transactions. Just as oxygen comes from the plants, an unearned grace, we give our gifts to Pachamama or the *apus* (mountain spirits) without expectation of reciprocation.

When I started studying the Q'eros cosmology, it made sense that mental and physical illness would be one of the side effects of this disruption of the balance between humans and nature. We know from copious scientific studies the power of gratitude practices to affect mental well-being and physical health, so it makes sense that a practice of earth offerings mixed with eco-friendly life choices, environmentally conscious voting choices, and rituals that prioritize harmony with nature might be ingredients in a recipe for healing.

THE KOGI'S WARNING TO "YOUNGER BROTHER"

The Q'eros belief system is similar to that of holy men—called *mamas* or sometimes *mamos* (translated as "sun")—of the Indigenous Kogi people and their three sister tribes, descendants of the advanced civilization of the Tairona culture who now live in the Sierra Nevada de Santa Marta, in Colombia. The Kogi base their life and culture on the belief that Aluna, their version of Pachamama, is the creator of all nature. Like the Q'eros, they also worship the sacred mountain Gonawindua, which they believe is the heart of the world. They view themselves as the Elder Brother, the caretakers of this beating heart, and they consider modern civilization the Younger Brother, who lost touch with the heart of the world many years ago.

The mamas are strictly raised from childhood to hold these highly respected roles, serving as spiritual leaders, healers, and intuitive guides. Children chosen to be mamas spend the first nine years of their lives in a cave, attended only by their mothers and elder mamas so they can attune to Aluna before being exposed to the outside world.

Known to many as Guardians of the Earth, the four tribes of the Sierra Nevada de Santa Marta, including the Kogi, believe that the land they care for is like a compass representing the rest of the planet. If rivers run dry, plant life is destroyed, and animal species go extinct in the heart of the world, the same will happen elsewhere, they believe. When they discovered that the encroachment of modern civilization was affecting their sacred land in ways that could have global implications, they paid attention. In order to protect their culture, they allowed outsiders into their villages until the Kogi, horrified by what was happening to the planet, allowed Alan Ereira and a small BBC crew to film the 1992 documentary *From the Heart of the World* as a desperate plea to Younger Brother. Their prophetic message to the world was clear: Wake up! It's time to give up your self-destructive ways. Honor the planet before it is too late. Then the Kogi retreated back into isolation and refused to let outsiders in for many more years until rapidly increasing environmental devastation led them to realize that Younger Brother had not heeded the warning and was still behaving in ways sure to lead to ecological catastrophe.

They contacted Ereira, who no longer worked for the BBC. He was given a firm assignment from the Kogi—to make a second documentary as a last-ditch warning, and in the beautiful film *Aluna*, the Kogi opted to share their secrets in hopes that Younger Brother would listen. Their primary message was to stop imposing human will on nature, to stop trying to dominate it. Stop the ecocide. Instead, the Kogi invite us to ask, "What does nature want?" and to honor it as having its own intelligence and capacity to repair itself, just as the human body does.

Aluna contains several scenes of Kogi men crushing shells inside gourds and Kogi women weaving bags intended to create a new future. But how could crushing shells and weaving bags prevent future environmental devastation? I studied their cosmology and won't butcher it by trying to oversimplify it here, but what I took away was similar to the fundamental teaching of the Q'eros: When we are out of balance with nature, there might be consequences that include mental or physical illness.[2] This understanding further affirmed that as part of any healing journey, restoring this balance with nature through our love, caretaking, "green" practices, prayers, ceremonies, humility, and time in wild places *and* community, we can right our systems when they get out of balance.

EARTH AS HEALER

After learning that the energetic frequencies some scientists claim to have measured from the hands of healers are similar to those emitted by the earth as Schumann resonances—electromagnetic peaks in the extremely low frequency (ELF) portion of earth's spectrum that can be generated by phenomena such as lightning—I was curious to make scientific sense of some of the Q'eros's healing systems. Could I tie my rudimentary understanding of how healers might tap into Earth's seven to ten Hz pulse to jump-start healing in other humans? In *Energy Medicine*, James Oschman theorized that meditation can train the pineal gland to take over as a sort of pacemaker for the brain, putting it in an alpha-wave state and allowing Schumann resonances to come through.

Healers often describe experiencing altered states of consciousness. Many are longtime meditators and spiritual practitioners. Might it be possible that the hands of the person who enters this meditative state can quiet the typically high beta brainwaves of the actively thinking mind enough to channel Schumann resonances in a way that entrains the patient into those same resonances? Perhaps, in some way we don't fully understand, whatever might be emitted from that person's hands could somehow stimulate cellular injury repair, perhaps by acting as an antenna for Schumann resonances in a way that amplifies the signal through a biological organism. Wouldn't it be cool if when healers enter meditative states, it allows the micropulses of the earth's geomagnetic field to come through them, amplify the resonances, and entrain the patient into the earth's field? Might this explain advocates of *earthing*, laying the body directly against the earth or walking without shoes, to treat disease?

Some time ago, I met Clint Ober, the father of the earthing movement, at a conference. Surrounded by people dressed in suits, he wore jeans and a T-shirt and walked around barefoot. After giving me his spiel about why we need more direct earth contact as a healing practice, he gave me a copy of the documentary *The Grounded*, directed and filmed by Steve Kroschel, a naturalist and *National Geographic* filmmaker who claims to have personally benefited from earthing practice. Earthing is described as a means to receive healing from free electrons by lying on bare earth or walking barefoot. The movie focuses on a village in the Alaskan wilderness where sick people started putting their bare skin directly on the soil and claiming to experience remarkable healing. They explain that this might work because we are all bioelectrical beings living on an electrical planet, but we have lost our natural electrical grounding, thus predisposing us to illness. Although the documentary is full of wild claims I *want* to believe but have trouble buying, what if there's some truth to it? If healers can quiet the high beta brainwaves enough to sync with Schumann resonances, can they effectively do the same thing for healees without requiring them to walk barefoot across a pebbly earth?

Might this explain part of why the Q'eros *despacho* ceremonies, in which paqos make offerings while the whole village sits in a circle on the ground, can bring not only spiritual connection but also physical healing? Although it's part of the principle of sacred reciprocity, what if the ceremonies are also intentionally (or unintentionally) keeping the tribe healthy by entraining everyone into Schumann resonances? Might entering the liminal space of ritual and sitting on the ground and absorbing the sun's vitamin D create a field effect of the earth healing people directly as an intrinsic preventative medicine or treatment? Would it make sense that ancient people, who had no access to modern medicine, might have known something about getting and staying healthy that we modern folks might have forgotten?

Can we prove such a wild hypothesis? After returning from Peru and scouring my notes, I found that in 1969, physicist Robert C. Beck embarked upon a decade of research studying the brainwaves of healers including shamans, psychics, dowsers, Christian faith healers, and Hawaiian kahunas. Regardless of their backgrounds or how they described their healing techniques, they shared one thing: They uniformly registered brainwave activity around eight Hz when in the altered state they entered for healing. Beck also found that while they were healing, their brainwaves became phase- and frequency-synchronized with the Schumann resonances.[3] Wouldn't it be poetic if what the Q'eros do out of love and gratitude for nature jives with what might heal the body through the earth?

During the peak of the 2020 Covid pandemic, when countless New Agers and Covid deniers insisted they'd be immune to the coronavirus if only they kept their vibration high and were posting memes like "Vibe up!," a smarty-pants part of me wanted to run around screaming, "Keep your vibe down!" But I saved my snark for emails with Bill Bengston and found I wasn't the first to reach this conclusion. Bill sent me a copy of an article he cowrote with Luke Hendricks and Jay Gunkleman, "The Healing Connection: EEG Harmonics, Entrainment, and Schumann's

Resonances."[4] In his email he said, "An interesting theme in your speculation is the idea that quieting your mind might put you in the territory
of a *lower* frequency . . . all those who speak of 'raising your vibration'
virtually never consider that the opposite might be the case!"

Whether the earth cures illness or not, the ritual of despachos and other
earth offerings must be married with environmentally wise living if we
wish to be true stewards of our planet. A despacho can't undo the damage
our environmentally destructive habits wreak or clear the *hucha* (heavy
energy) we might incur individually and collectively. Performing despacho when someone is sick wouldn't reverse harm, but it might make us
care more, which might cause us to change our behaviors. Maybe sitting
on the earth and offering gratitude can thaw our frozen hearts, opening
them to sacred reciprocity, which so many of us seem to have forgotten.

WALKING IN THE SACRED MANNER

As part of my Sacred Medicine discovery process, I read Mark St. Pierre's
book *Walking in the Sacred Manner: Healers, Dreamers, and Pipe Carriers
Medicine Women of the Plains* at the recommendation of our Crow guide,
who had offered to teach my daughter and me about his people's spirituality and medicine. Del led us through a ceremonial smoking of the
sacred pipe, a rare honor not typically offered to women, a custom he as a
pipe carrier believes must change. According to tribal elder Grant Bulltail,
quoted in a local newspaper, for the Crow the pipe is a gift from the sun,
or maker: "Smoking the pipe expels bad energy, empowers the smoker,
and restores harmony with nature."[5]

Del also broke custom by inviting my daughter and me to a co-ed
ceremonial sweat lodge. We stayed in a traditional teepee and learned
to make the customary tobacco offerings to honor sacred sites. We were
taught how to prepare colorful bundles of tobacco, tie them together
with string, and infuse them with our prayers. This was a preparation
for our pilgrimage to one of the Crows' most revered "sacred hoops," or
medicine wheels, the Big Horn Medicine Wheel in Northern Wyoming.

The Big Horn Medicine Wheel is a deeply mysterious place believed
to align with the stars, sun, moon, and various other celestial bodies and
events. It is also the origin of the story of why the Crow people have
inhabited this region for thousands of years, of how a vision of a tobacco

seed in the Big Horn Mountains guided a Crow leader to travel with many of his people from the Midwest to begin a new life in the place we now call Wyoming.

The Big Horn Medicine Wheel is now managed by the National Park Service. Visitors can walk the fenced perimeter of the medicine wheel, but only Native Americans can enter. We were granted access at Del's request. There, he led us through a series of rituals—sage, prayer, and walking the perimeter of the medicine wheel clockwise three times before approaching the stone altars. After preparation, Del invited each of us to allow intuition to draw us to a cairn where we would offer our tobacco ties and receive the wisdom, insight, and blessings of each altar, all imbued with significance. Del, my daughter, and I cycled through the altars, praying, offering, and opening to receive guidance.

As I prepared to leave the medicine wheel, I was flooded with painful emotions about being a white person of power and privilege, of how my people had disrespected and tortured Del's people. I flashed back to photos and stories I had seen and read of peaceful Northern California Native Americans shot and killed in sport by white "gentlemen," as if fox hunting. I was overwhelmed by grief, shame, and rage. What must happen to suppress human empathy to such a degree that we are capable of mass cruelty and dehumanization? The medicine wheel brought all those images flooding back until the trauma wave moved through me and my peace returned, but not without residual unease. By the end of our journey around the medicine wheel, I felt like I'd been on a long pilgrimage.

We took home some of the tobacco ties because they were believed to be imbued with the energy of the medicine wheel. I brought mine back to California and set them on my home altar beside my *mesa* (medicine bundle) from the Q'eros. Then, changing my mind, I felt moved to take them all into my backyard, to consecrate the land on which I lived, land stolen from the Miwok nation. I offered thanks—and apologies—to the land and its original caregivers.

BRINGING INDIGENOUS CONSCIOUSNESS HOME

After making offerings to nature in Indigenous villages all over the world, I returned home with so much devotion in my heart and a commitment to honoring the ocean, mountains, rivers, and Pachamama and, as I was instructed, to pass on what I'd been blessed to learn. I climbed to the top of Mount Tamalpais and entered a quiet forest I'd frequented but never thought of as a place of worship. I announced aloud, "I am here to do despacho for you and honor sacred reciprocity. I will be your caretaker and perform a ceremony to show you how much I love you."

As I spoke, the forest came alive! Wind stirred the trees, showering me with dew. Quail fluttered as a hawk flew overhead. Coyotes howled in hallelujah. A rush of love poured through me as if the forest and mountain were excited. I fell to my knees, full of apologies, but what rose to meet me was vast grace, unconditional love, forgiveness, and acceptance. I felt like the prodigal daughter returning to welcoming arms waiting for just this moment.

Although I have received permission from all my teachers to share their teachings, I don't want to be the next overprivileged white person who exploits Indigenous healing. I could never come close to replicating the rites and rituals of someone who grew up with them. Because these traditions are contextualized within a culture, they don't readily translate to Western minds and methods. To attempt this would require a "dumbing down" that could be insulting to those who shared their practices with me.

With that disclaimer, it would be an oversight not to honor my commitment to these Indigenous healers and offer some of what I received from the world's medicine bag with anyone who might want to apply these practices to healing.

Make Nature a Temple

You don't have to do the traditional Balinese canang or perform an entire despacho ceremony or spend days praying into tobacco ties to treat landmarks in nature as if there is an invisible temple where you can make offerings, asking for consent before penetrating the holy places. You can take this mindset into your consciousness and practice it in any way that feels comfortable. Instead of feeling entitled to swim in a lake or enjoy the shade of a tree, approach it as if there is a god or goddess inside. Honor that deity. Let it know you recognize its presence. Ask permission to enter and engage, to play and savor. Offer a gift of prayer, flowers, food, song, or even a lock of your hair. The greater the effort and sacrifice on your part, the more likely nature will "receive" your offering as an act of sacred reciprocity. Customize the practice in a way that feels authentic. The medicine is in how you resacralize your relationship to nature, restore appreciation for all that is, and honor it. Your inner shift of consciousness is medicine. You never know how those nature goddesses might heal you if they choose to sit on you to reward your devotion!

Part Two

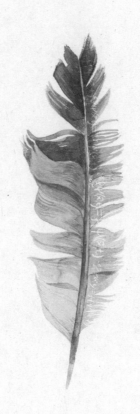

SHINING LIGHT ON
THE SHADOW

'm all for you bolstering yourself with energy transfusions when you're life-force anemic. If a healer, practice, or community can lift your spirits, help you feel better, and relieve your symptoms, even if only temporarily, do whatever helps. Many of the practices in part one work with manipulating subtle energies; the power of personal or group intention; the boost from tuning in to nature; the impact of pilgrimage on the mind-body-spirit connection; and the legitimate health benefits of dance, art, creative expression, and other forms of pleasure practice.

These are wonderful medicines. If you are privileged enough to have access to them, go for it! Just be careful not to confuse temporary relief with a cure—and be sure you don't break the bank grasping at wild expectations that you could be the next miracle. At some point, as much as you might lean toward the light and hope to be spared more pain, the shadow is likely to eclipse you. It's not just the pain or shadow you might be turning from in yourself, which could be the ticket to true healing; it's also the shadow of spiritual healing as a pass from emotional pain. It's the shadow of corrupt healers and communities devoted to healing (which sometimes bear a striking resemblance to cults). It's the shadow of our emotion-phobic, white supremacist culture and how greed and the monetization of spirituality can hijack healing. Although it might feel good to chase the light, at some point in your healing journey, pain is likely to catch up with you. If optimal health is our goal, we'd be wise to quit running and turn toward the pain, welcoming it and getting curious about what it could teach us about what still needs healing.

Whereas part one focused on practices meant to uplift your spirits and strengthen your life force, in part two, I explore the darker aspects of Sacred Medicine. So . . . grab your flashlight, and let's go spelunking in some of its murkier recesses. Learning how to do this will help you detect false light and recognize true healing in others and yourself.

Chapter 6

FEELING IS HEALING

spent my time with the Q'eros in 2014, the Kogi in 2015, the Balinese in 2016, and the Crow in 2018. In between, I explored half a dozen other Indigenous earth-healing offering practices and worldviews, and this way of inhabiting our planet fundamentally changed me. Not only was I becoming increasingly agitated about how we were treating our home and its Native people but also I was beginning to feel my shame, rage, grief, and humility as a white person. The Donald Trump election amplified this rush of emotions not just for me but for many Americans, whose activism bubbled up through the numbness of apathy and passivity.

When I'd arrived in Bali, and Balinese people asked me where I hailed from, they'd respond to my answer of "California" with "Ah . . . naked sexy Hollywood," to which I'd laugh and shake my head. "Not *that* California." After Trump was elected, when people asked me where I was from and I told them, they'd shake their heads with worried expressions and say, "Ah . . . *Donald Trump*," looking at me with pity as if I'd just told them I was afflicted with a disease. I felt humiliated and furious.

For me, 2016 marked the end of a long phase of *spiritual bypassing*, which John Welwood, who coined the phrase, defines as using spiritual beliefs and practices to hide or repress emotions and avoid conflict. As I look back with more than a little nostalgia, I see that using my spirituality to avoid feeling the painful emotions of my past traumas began in 2006, right after my daughter was born. My father died two weeks later, and I quit my job in traditional Western medicine soon afterward. I felt unsupported in my choice by many people in my life who thought I was "merely" having a midlife crisis and should just go buy a fancy car or have an affair like normal people.

Because of my wounding, I did not have the emotional resources to cope with that much intensely painful emotion, so I sought out spirituality and felt so much better after I embarked upon that path in earnest. This anesthesia was an intelligent defense mechanism that helped me cope and kept me functioning, but although my spirituality bolstered my life force and transfused me so I could function, it failed to *heal* those traumas. I had been medicating myself with what I now call "bliss hunting"—pilgrimages, silent meditation retreats, yoga classes, kirtan, ecstatic dance, Tantric lovers, energy healers, art, and rituals in nature and temples—one energy transfusion practice after another. I painstakingly covered my wounds with a bandage of spirituality. But when the bandage was ripped off in 2016, the wounds were still raw. Underneath all that "love and light" was a slurry of pain it would take years to heal. Only then would the energy drains stop leaking my life force.

Leaving Bali to come back to the United States after the 2016 election was culture shock. For the first time in my life, I no longer felt like I belonged in my own country. I clung to instructions I had received from Aida's godfather—to bring Balinese consciousness to my homeland, to make offerings and pray to its goddesses, and to see whether I was lucky enough to have any nature goddesses sit on me.

I was too triggered to return to business as usual, so my daughter met me at the airport, and we made pilgrimages to twelve US national parks, where we performed our version of the *canang* ritual to help me transition. In Bali, you would never just approach a sacred landmark in nature, much less approach a nature goddess through a camera lens while taking a selfie, without at least having made offerings. If what the Balinese believe is true, Americans regularly "rape the goddess," feeling entitled to do as we wish with little reverence or even respect for sacredness. I'd been equally guilty of such entitled behavior—hubris, indeed. I'd always loved nature and considered myself an environmentalist, but I had not thought of nature as being alive and having consciousness until I stayed with the Q'eros. My time in Bali anchored animism as my dominant religion.

Moving so quickly from observing the way the Balinese revere nature to seeing how Americans in their own national parks disrespect or even exploit it, as if it's nothing but an Instagram backdrop, made me angry. That anger fueled a growing sacred activism that would replace my bliss hunting. Meditation retreats turned into giving my meditation feet by participating in Standing Rock Sioux protests. I took my yoga off the mat to #MeToo marches. I danced my way to taking a stand against immigrant abuse. My prayer turned into blogs I wrote about Black Lives Matter.

I don't regret all those spiritual bypassing years. All that spiritual practice allowed me the spaciousness to engage in my growing activism with a calmer nervous system, healthier body, and greater capacity to resist polarization while still taking a firm stand. In order to do this, I needed the painful emotions beginning to seep up from the wounds I had yet to heal, but it wasn't easy to learn to feel them.

I clung to the words of Daniel Schmachtenberger, a founding member of the Consilience Project, who spoke at the Transformational Leadership Council gathering I attended. He said:

> Every negative emotion is a response to care and love. If you feel angry, find what it is that you hold sacred and ask, "How is what I hold sacred getting violated?" See the sacredness in it and ask, "Am I willing to make sacrifices to protect that sacred thing?" That's when it's appropriate to use your will, aligned with what you love. To do this, you'll need your mind, your heart, and your gut. Your mind needs clarity on what it is that you love and hold sacred and are willing to protect. Your heart needs to feel heartbroken because what you care about is being hurt. Your gut will give you the courage to do something about it. Think about and feel into what is most sacred to you. What will still matter after you're dead? What are you devoted to and willing to sacrifice your comfort for—because it matters so much and you love it so much? Ask yourself, "If this is really what I care about, what should I be doing to be congruent with my own self, my own deepest values? What am I doing now that is different than that? How do I close that gap?"

Schmachtenberger asked us to move beyond shock and start to *feel*. Feel our grief, our rage, our heartbreak, our despair, and our helplessness.

Feel our compassion for those suffering and give it feet. Let those feelings move through us until they compel us to go beyond complacency, to stop meditating for social justice and take sacred action, to leverage our privilege to *do something* to make things right. But the truth was that my ability to feel all those emotions had been handicapped, replaced by spiritual beliefs that denied, rejected, and bypassed emotions too painful for my delicate sensitivities to handle. I gave lip service to action, but was I really giving my compassion feet?

As a longtime spiritual seeker, I considered myself an empathetic person, or at least someone who tried to be kind. Much of my spiritual life revolved around working through my triggers, taking responsibility for my reactivity, and opening my heart to extend compassion to those who triggered me, even when they mistreated me. I hadn't realized I was spiritualizing my trauma-induced conflict avoidance, distorting healthy compassion, and practicing what *Spiritual Bypassing* author and reformed-cult-leader-turned-psychologist Robert Augustus Masters defines as "blind compassion." I felt like I was punched in the gut when I read his definition of blind compassion.

> Blind compassion is rooted in the belief that we are all doing the best we can. When we are driven by blind compassion, we cut everyone far too much slack, making excuses for others' behavior and making nice situations that require a forceful "no," an unmistakable voicing of displeasure, or a firm setting and maintaining of boundaries. These things can and often should be done out of love, but blind compassion keeps love too meek, sentenced to wearing a kind face. This is not the kindness of the Dalai Lama, which is rooted in courage, but rather a kindness which is rooted in fear, and not just fear of confrontation, but also fear of not coming across as a good or spiritual person. When we are engaged in blind compassion we rarely show anger, for we not only believe that compassion has to be gentle, we are also frightened of upsetting anyone, especially to the point of their confronting us. This is reinforced by our judgment of anger, especially in its more fiery forms, as something less than spiritual;

something that should not be there if we were being truly loving. Blind compassion reduces us to harmony junkies, entrapping us in unrelentingly positive expression.

With blind compassion we don't know how to—or won't learn how to—say no with any real power, avoiding confrontation at all costs and, as a result, enabling unhealthy patterns to continue. Our "yes" is then anemic and impotent, devoid of the impact it could have if we were also able to access a clear, strong "no" that emanated from our core. When we mute our essential voice, our openness is reduced to a permissive gap, an undiscerning embrace, a poorly boundaried receptivity, all of which indicate a lack of compassion for ourselves (in that we don't adequately protect ourselves). Blind compassion confuses anger with aggression, forcefulness with violence, judgment with condemnation, caring with exaggerated tolerance, and moral maturity with spiritual correctness.[1]

I felt nauseated when I first read this passage, but I feel tender for myself now, hugging myself rather than judging myself for my confusion. My self-image at the time was quite inflated, but underneath was a core sense of "not enough." I didn't realize I was deserving of love just because I have a spark of divinity in me that makes me—and everyone else—inherently worthy of belonging. I thought I had to earn love by tolerating the intolerable and proving my loyalty, by demonstrating how "spiritual" I was, even when people treated me badly and I should have held them accountable for such mistreatment. I didn't know any better back then, but I do now, and I want to make sure you are not needlessly suffering by harming yourself with blind compassion, dear reader. Doing so can put you at risk of getting and staying sick, so that tendency needs to be healed if optimal health is your goal.

To protect ourselves from emotional and/or physical abuse, we need access to our healthy, well-boundaried anger. But in my case, anger had been shut down back when I was barely two years old by a mother who judged my anger as "un-Christian." After I left the church at eighteen, I was influenced by Buddhist teachings that reinforced my anger-phobia. I recall a plaque I read at a Tibetan Buddhist retreat center:

For a Buddhist practitioner, the real enemy is within—our mental and emotional defilements that give rise to pain and suffering. The real task of a practitioner is to defeat this inner enemy. . . . It is important to cultivate mindfulness right from the beginning. Otherwise, if you let negative emotions and thoughts arise without any sense of restraint, without any mindfulness of their negativity, then you are giving them free rein. They can develop to the point where there is simply no way to counter them. However, if you develop mindfulness of their negativity, then when they occur, you will be able to stamp them out as soon as they arise. You will not give them the opportunity or the space to develop into full-blown negative emotional thoughts.

It made sense to me that we must maintain vigilance over our negative thoughts, beliefs, and feelings in order to avoid getting overtaken by stress and violence-inducing reactivity, hostility, judgment, polarization, and condemnation. The Dalai Lama said, "Anger destroys our peace of mind and our physical health. We shouldn't welcome it or think of it as natural or as a friend."[2] If the revered Dalai Lama said we shouldn't tolerate anger, then it must be so.

Even though I wasn't raised Buddhist, I had been conditioned to take as gospel spiritual teachings like this. As a young child, if I expressed emotions such as anger, jealousy, disappointment, or even sadness, my mother did not do what twentieth-century English pediatrician and psychoanalyst D. W. Winnicott described as what the "good enough" parent should—acknowledge my healthy human emotion, validate it as normal, mirror it back to me, help coregulate my nervous system so I didn't feel flooded and overwhelmed, and show me that my little child body could handle feeling those emotions without dying. Instead, she would shut me down lickety-split, shaming me for my intense emotions and ordering me to be a good little Christian girl, which translated into a mild-mannered child who smiled, appeased, complied, and generally behaved in ways meant to make me easy on the experience of others (and reflect positively on my mother for raising such a pleasant, well-behaved child). Because of that, from a young age I stopped feeling about half of the normal human emotions, leaving me vulnerable to abuse by predatory men who took advantage of my compliance. These patterns also put my physical and mental health at risk, leaving me with physical symptoms and suicidal thoughts.

Not having access to the emotional intelligence that might have protected me, I grew into a damaged adult, which left me experimenting on the spiritual path with others and not taught how to cope with strong emotions, such as anger, in a healthy way. If people got angry in my "spiritual but not religious" circles, they were "polarizing" rather than "unifying" or weren't "nondual" enough, which we interpreted as "less spiritually developed." Those of us who had the capacity to see both sides, resist polarization and judgment, and extend compassion, even to those we disagreed with, tended to perceive ourselves as spiritually superior.

When I read Laurence Heller's book about NeuroAffective Relational Model (NARM), *Healing Developmental Trauma*, I was stunned to realize that the suppression of anger and exaggerated tolerance I had developed for abusive people was not a sign of spiritual maturity but a side effect of developmental trauma. Others included being out of touch with my body and my emotions; difficulty attuning to my own needs; trouble reaching out and asking for what I need from others, challenges with knowing I deserve to rely on others and trusting others enough to let myself lean on them; and a damaged capacity to set and enforce appropriate boundaries, say no, and speak my mind without guilt or fear. I was not spiritually advanced; I was hurt.

Don't get me wrong. Spiritual bypassing is only one of many defensive strategies that help us avoid painful emotions we didn't learn how to fully feel as children. You can do it the good, old-fashioned way—addiction to busyness, substances, social media, hoarding, or sex. You can overintellectualize, micromanage, eat, or squelch your feelings. You can sublimate them as you kick the dog or fake a smile. You can be passive-aggressive. Those strategies are widely recognized and examined—and there are treatment programs for most of them.

Spiritual bypassing gets discussed less, yet we must understand its role as we continue to examine the landscape of Sacred Medicine, where it tends to flourish. If our intention is to relieve needless suffering and open ourselves to healing, which require resisting the tendency to exile *any* human emotion from the scope of our wholeness, we need to unpack this.

WHAT IS SPIRITUAL BYPASSING?

Masters defines it as "the use of spiritual practices and beliefs to avoid dealing with our painful feelings, unresolved wounds, and developmental needs."[3] Spiritual bypassing is not only seldom discussed but also downright celebrated. Spiritually bypassing teachers have sold millions of copies of their books, and because the practice encourages us not to feel our painful emotions, these teachings can make us feel better . . . temporarily. They might even save our lives if we're actively addicted, suicidal, wrestling with an eating disorder, or otherwise trying to cope with our pain, using unhealthy strategies that, although intelligent in design, can wear out their usefulness and cause us (and others) harm.

The problem is that emotions do not go away; they get trapped in the body and can lead to mental and physical illness. And spiritual bypassing tendencies are not sustainable. They function as a stopgap measure—a kind of emergency relief that might serve as balm on wounds too bloody to treat. But spiritual bypassing doesn't heal. To put it in the terms of this book, the practice might transfuse life force into you in the short term— and this can help you cope and give you a boost—but it won't plug the leaks, no matter how many hours per day you meditate.

It's not easy to be a sincere spiritual practitioner and avoid spiritual bypassing. Some of the most famous spiritual teachers in the world actively promote and glorify it. Entire New Age movements and mega-churches are devoted to preaching and practicing it. We tend to exalt those who seem to have transcended natural human emotions such as anger, jealousy, or grief, as if achieving a state of dispassionate equanimity is evidence of enlightenment or holiness. We even deify them or call them saints.

This reveals one of those paradoxes of healing. It's true that we can get so enmeshed in our painful emotions that we lose touch with our spiritual essence and the potential peace we can experience when we remember our true nature. It's true that there is a spiritual dimension where we are not our bodies, we are not our emotions, we are not our egos or identities—we are far more expansive than these earthly realities. It's true that transcending our earthly reality and visiting this spiritual dimension can provide a rest from the suffering of the human experience and offer temporary pain relief. It's true that contacting the unconditional love of the ground of being, which we can experience in deep levels of meditation, might help us heal and aid healers in transfusing energy into us. However, it is also true that bypassing certain emotions can put us at risk of abuse, interfere with our self-care and protection, and predispose us to illness. It's true that all human emotions are valid, necessary, and potentially helpful when we know how to translate them into emotional intelligence.

Welwood sums up this paradox of spiritual bypassing: "Absolute truth is favored over relative truth, the impersonal over the personal, emptiness over form, transcendence over embodiment, and detachment over feeling."[4] He also says, "When we are spiritually bypassing, we often use the goal of awakening or liberation to rationalize what I call *premature transcendence*: trying to rise above the raw and messy side of our humanness before we have fully faced and made peace with it."[5]

Favoring the "absolute" over the relative is the primary problem. The truth that we are not our bodies and we are not our emotions—we are more than these small human personalities—is free from stain. It does not mean there is no relative truth. The bliss-hunting spiritual bypasser risks getting hooked on the absolute view the spiritual teacher is peddling. It's not that the absolute truth isn't true; it's just not the *only* truth. But absolute truth is so seductive, and relative truth is so messy. It's tempting to buy into half of the paradox, which feeds the healer or teacher's ego even as the unhealed wound in the student festers.

People good at spiritual bypassing might come across as calm, kind, helpful, and peacemaking types. They tend to be docile and people pleasing, cooperative and gentle, easygoing and mellow. They also tend to get chronic illnesses that don't respond to conventional medicine, and they're more likely to die young—the reason I address this practice in the context of becoming miracle prone.[6]

THE 2017 WAKE-UP CALL

All that spiritual bypassing stopped working for me (and many others) in 2017. On January 21, the day after Trump's inauguration, my daughter and I marched with millions of women around the world to protest Trump's abusive "pussy-grabbing" treatment of women. A week later, a doctor in an urgent-care facility in Ohio called to tell me my mother had been there after noticing her heart rate was 140. Her hemoglobin was half what it should be (7.0, instead of about 14.0). Even worse, her blood count showed what looked like cancer cells. In February, a bone-marrow biopsy confirmed my mother's leukemia. In April, I was attacked by the dog and took my mother to Africa and Italy on our messy pilgrimage as part of my mother's "bucket list." In August, unhooded "Unite the Right" torch-bearing white supremacists marched in Charlottesville, Virginia, further fueling the anger, terror, and grief of the Black Lives Matter movement, founded in 2013 by Alicia Garza, Patrisse Cullors, and Opal Tometi in response to the acquittal of Trayvon Martin's murderer, George Zimmerman.[7] In October, Alyssa Milano ignited a firestorm by tweeting the story of her sexual assault and adding the hashtag Tarana Burke coined in 2006, #MeToo, amplifying the fury so many women felt toward the men who harassed and harmed us while expecting us to stay silent.

On October 30, just before midnight, I phoned my mentor, Rachel Naomi Remen, and put her on speaker as I stood over the body of my mother, who had just exhaled her final agonizing breath. My sister, my mom's two sisters, and my daughter (via phone) were all with my mother in her last moments—all women, although my mother also had a son, three brothers, and two grandsons. Apparently, death was women's work.

Rachel said, "There is a profound silence in the room. Don't miss it." She was right. The noisy death rattle had ended, and the bustle of the hospice nurses and funeral home attendants hadn't begun. I was grateful she directed our attention to that holy silence.

The next morning, on Halloween, I woke up *enraged*. But riding shotgun with my rage was guilt, shame, and sadness. I loved my mother, so why was I so furious? I called Rachel, who said, "Good, Lissa. Your mother messed up your anger mechanism, and she's left you a precious inheritance. Claim it."

In 2017, I began the slow process of reclaiming my healthy, boundary-protecting anger. With it, I saw how I'd been using my spiritual practices to cover up a boiling fury and a deep well of sadness. My spiritual bypassing tendencies kept me blindly on the ascension path, but life caught up with me. Now I was plummeting down to the holy ground of darkness. I tried to outrun my pain, but that persistent suitor I had rejected again and again finally caught up with me. So I said, "Come, enter, show me what you've got." Without enough strength left to resist the centrifugal pull into soul work, I let go . . .

Spiritual Bypassing Tendencies

Do you recognize these spiritual bypassing tendencies in yourself?

Aversion to any emotion not deemed "spiritual"

Anger-phobia that resists calling for a clear and firm intolerance of hurtful behavior

Difficulty expressing a firm, clear "no"

Toxic positivity to the point of fakeness in situations where grief, anger, sadness, jealousy, or disappointment would be natural

Premature forgiveness rather than expecting others to be held accountable for harmful behaviors with a healthy process of making apologies, amends, or other measures to ensure that harmful behavior ceases

Exaggerated tolerance of abusive people and behaviors

Weak or porous boundaries

Spiritualizing "boundarylessness," mistaking unhealthy fusion as a mystical experience

Excessive niceness to the point of being unable to take a firm stand or protect oneself from abusive relationships

Trouble staying firmly grounded in earthly reality (tending to prefer mystical experiences like meditation visions, astral travel, spirit guides, channeled beings, medicine journeys, and other multidimensional experiences to the exclusion of being fully present in this dimension)

Avoidance of all judgment to the point of being unable to discern abuse

Exaggerated acceptance of situations in which a clear stand and a firm "no" are necessary

Failure to extend compassionate care to people suffering from legitimate victimhood, bypassing with aphorisms like "Get out of your victim story" or "Your soul is growing" or "Everything happens for a reason"

Emotional numbing and repression

Tendency to lose empathy in the face of other people's legitimate distress if others are expressing emotions the spiritual bypasser has repressed

Prioritizing transcendence over presence and feeling normal emotions—responding to painful life experiences with aphorisms like "We are not our bodies; we are not our emotions" or "We are beyond this reality"

Immersing oneself in spiritual practices while ignoring social justice issues or even practicalities such as earning a living or parenting

After examining your tendencies, notice how you're feeling. Take a moment to extend compassion to yourself, patting yourself on the back for your courage, strength, and willingness to be humble and curious. Remind yourself that there's nothing wrong with you. If you've been spiritually bypassing, it was a necessary strategy—and you can still use it when you're having trouble coping. Remember to stay attuned to your body, try to notice how your nervous system is handling these insights, and stay as embodied as you can, titrating your awareness to make sure you don't hit a threshold that takes you faster than you can handle. If you feel yourself dissociating, ground yourself with slow, deep breaths. Remember to go only as fast as the slowest part of you can go without causing yourself harm. Slow and steady always beats out pushing or bullying yourself to speed up the process. If you feel at all wobbly, put on some music, hug yourself or ask someone you trust to do so, pet an animal, dance, sit on the sand and imagine a grounding cord connecting you to the earth, or try out any of the part one practices your Whole Health Intelligences guide you to do. If you find yourself flooded with more pain than you know how to handle, please reach out for help from a trauma-informed therapist or a trusted friend or mentor. Moving beyond spiritual bypassing can be uncomfortable, and you deserve the support you need.

WHEN THE BODY SAYS NO

Although spiritual bypassing is an understandable way to suffer less, hard-to-treat illnesses can be an unwelcome side effect of this tendency. When we're practicing blind compassion—out of touch with the healthy, boundary-protecting anger that helps us find and enforce our firm "no"—consequences might show up in our bodies. When a child's core needs for connection are not met, the resulting nervous system dysregulation can manifest later in life as migraines, digestive problems such as irritable bowel syndrome, allergies and environmental sensitivities, asthma, fibromyalgia, chronic fatigue and other autoimmune disorders, anxiety disorders, ADHD, and even scoliosis.[8]

Gabor Maté caught on to this when observing chronically ill patients in his family practice. In his book *When the Body Says No*, Maté suggests, "When we have been prevented from learning how to say no . . . our bodies may end up saying it for us."[9] Referencing a plethora of studies linking disease to emotional repression, Maté explains that it is often the safest choice for a child who isn't given permission or support with handling painful emotions. That child might grow up with spiritual bypassing tendencies, having spiritualized the emotional repression and justified the reasons for doing so. Sadly, this tendency might set you up for bodily disease later in life.

Lydia Temoshok and Henry Dreher extensively researched emotional repression and its link to cancer for their book *The Type C Connection*.

According to the authors, the psychological profile of cancer patients is diametrically opposed to the hard-driving, ambitious, quick-to-anger, explosive Type As, who are at greater risk of heart disease. After an exhaustive psychological study of patients in a melanoma clinic, Temoshok defined the Type C personality as "a person who exhibits compulsive, unyielding niceness in any situation—no matter how stressful, insulting, or dangerous. Such a person has a sizable gap in his emotional repertoire . . . it has a forced, unnatural quality."[10]

Whether you tend to emotionally repress like a Type C personality or explode like a Type A, it's important to keep returning to the awareness that these coping styles were once an intelligent defense strategy that might have saved your life or at least protected you from abandonment, rejection, or withheld affection. If this sounds like you, remember, such tendencies are *in no way* a reflection of something being wrong with you. These strategies are the result of having been hurt, although they might have overstayed their usefulness.

Keep in mind that *you are not your personality*. Although Maté and Temoshok point out certain personality characteristics that might be risk factors for certain diseases like autoimmune disorders or cancer, such as emotional overdependence on other people; expending tremendous effort to please others, willingness to tolerate mistreatment and abuse, avoidance of conflict, oversensitivity to criticism, and placing the needs of people upon which one is emotionally dependent upon above one's own, these tendencies are not fixed. They are the result of trauma, and as such, they can be treated. In other words, your personality can *change* as part of your healing in ways that allow you to be even more of who you *really* are.

As radical remission researcher Jeffrey Rediger explains in *CURED: The Life-Changing Science of Spontaneous Healing*, those who became "health outliers," having better-than-expected recoveries from seemingly "incurable" health conditions, often had a complete transformation of identity and personality. One health outlier Rediger studied, a woman with breast cancer, spent most of her life being a bit of a doormat. She let her husband trample all over her and didn't speak up about her many resentments. But after she got cancer, she changed into someone saucy, racy, and irreverent. She started telling it like it was and didn't put up with his shit anymore. *And* she overcame the odds into recovery.

Rediger writes, "If you can die to an old version of yourself in such a way that a new, truer version of yourself can be born, maybe you don't need to die physically yet. If you are reborn in a way that allows you to experience the world and yourself differently, you are a different you, and your body might reflect that." In other words, if who you think you are and how this distorted perception causes you to behave in the world is a risk factor for disease, you can change who you are in ways that make you not less yourself but more of your true essence. This might or might not make you the next health outlier Rediger studies, but it is likely to heal you and help restore wholeness.

YOU HAVE TO FEEL TO HEAL

What's the antidote to spiritual bypassing? I'd like to say that it's simply to *feel your emotions*. But something that glib would be bypassing the undeniable fact that almost *nobody* in Western culture knows how to do this. I'll go as far as to say that most people are poorly equipped to even *know* our feelings, much less feel them in a healthy, skillful way without numbing, repressing, or getting so carried away by our emotions that we either explode or fall apart and can't function. It's not our fault. We are experts at bypassing our feelings, and the ways we've been taught to do so would fill an entire book. In short, our culture conditions us to do everything *but* feel our feelings.

Through the growing field of psychoneuroimmunology, best described in Candace Pert's *The Molecules of Emotion*, we now understand scientifically how your emotions are linked to your physical health. But all the science in the world doesn't change the fact that almost everything in our culture shames emotions. Although it's a sweeping stereotype, in general, people who identify as male are shamed out of feeling their sadness, and those who identify as female are conditioned to tamp down their anger. If you start paying attention, you'll see that emotion-shaming messages are everywhere. *Don't worry; be happy. If you don't have anything nice to say, don't say anything at all. Focus on the positive. You're being emotional. Big boys don't cry. Stay strong. That's not ladylike. Don't cry because it's over; smile because it happened. You're so much prettier when you smile. Don't play the victim. Simmer down. Take a chill pill. Get a grip. Suck it up, buttercup.*

A multibillion-dollar self-help industry—and most organized religions—encourage us not to feel our feelings, especially those we label "negative."

Conventional religions, New Age spiritual circles, and some positive psychology advocates tend to promote a bias toward emotions we deem "positive" and shy away from the "negative." Teachings such as the "law of attraction" are even more damaging in this way because "your thoughts create your reality" implies that your negative thoughts and emotions will manifest a negative reality for you, which is terrifying—and fundamentally untrue. It's also untrue that advanced spiritual development means being blissed out all the time, though many understandably cling to this attractive fantasy.

Although it's an easy sell to promise that working with a particular healer, religion, spiritual practice, or teacher will take away your pain and suffering forever and grant you some kind of pain-free enlightenment, and although it can be shattering for some spiritual seekers to learn otherwise, such teachings do not necessarily promote wholeness and healing. Instead, they often glorify dissociation, repression, and spiritual bypassing and can put you at risk of disease rather than doing the opposite, as these teachers claim.

This isn't to suggest that there aren't valuable, peace-inducing, transformational teachings in positive psychology, conventional religions, Eastern philosophies, yoga, and New Age spirituality. We need not throw out the baby with the bathwater. Instead, it behooves us to hold more paradoxes. Yes, it can be helpful to resist running away with unbridled emotions and getting caught up in reactivity, aggressive behavior, hostility, paralyzing fear, nonstop crying, looping self-pity and regret, feelings of helplessness, disempowered victimization, blaming and shaming judgment, and other emotions that can rob us of our inner peace. It's also true that bullying yourself into staying positive when you're hurting, scared, angry, jealous, disappointed, or sad does more harm than good.

I once sat at a round table at a spiritual conference where I had just given a talk. I was surrounded by mostly senior, white men who were also presenters at the conference. Huddling together like fraternity brothers, they spoke with contempt about the increasing number of women who presented at the conference. With a mocking eye roll and tone of voice usually reserved for talking to children, one of them looked at me and said, "Well, go ahead and feel all your emotions if you want to. We'll be here for you when you *transcend* that phase."

I wanted to let one of those emotions rip, but instead, I felt it and tuned in to it: anger. I'd been insulted and infantilized. These aloof, detached guys thought they were better than me and the other women teaching about feminine spirituality, which includes emotional intelligence. I scanned my memory to recall how Karla McLaren, in *The Language of Emotions*, recommends dealing with anger. Anger arises when your self-image, behaviors, or interpersonal boundaries are challenged—or when you see them challenged in someone else. Anger comes bearing gifts, like the healthy protection of your boundary when someone has overstepped it. Anger begs the question, "What do I value? What must be protected and restored?"[11]

If I indulged my anger, I might have laid into them, violating their boundaries and embarrassing myself—or shaming them. If I repressed my anger, I'd have bitten my tongue, stayed silent, felt resentful, and broken our connection. Instead, I said, "It makes me angry when you undermine the importance of healthy emotions in ways that can make people sick."

One of them shook his head. "You women, with all your coddling of the ego, all your emotions run amok. Ego is ego. If you want to wake up, you gotta get rid of it."

Something softened in me when I heard him say that. If he was bullying me about my emotions and his students about theirs, chances are he was also bullying himself about his own. I confessed to him that I had just lost five loved ones in six weeks, and I was grieving, so it was hard to be around all these nondual teachers telling me that my emotions weren't real—that it was all an illusion.

His expression shifted from contempt to compassion, with empathy replacing righteousness. He put his hand on mine and said, "I'm so sorry for your losses." *There it was.* A moment of connection arose like a blessing.

Even the Pixar movie *Inside Out* recognizes the healing value of feeling all your emotions. The protagonist, a little girl whose parents move her from the Midwest home she loves to San Francisco, experiences a jumble of emotions managed by a control center in her mind, where Joy, Anger, Sadness, Disgust, and Fear battle it out to take the reins of her behaviors. Although Joy bullies all the other emotions, trying to keep the little girl bubbly and cheerful 24/7, Sadness finally takes over the whole system and lets her grieve the loss. Only then do her tears invite the connections from others who help her feel, heal, and let go. Then, after Anger gets to vent and the pain of Sadness flows, Joy returns naturally.

THE ART OF EMPATHY

Good healers, whether they're doctors, energy healers, or therapists, know you can't heal unless you can feel. The best ones do not foster bypassing emotions, even temporarily. Instead, they create the conditions for their movement and flow. Skillful healers are comfortable with intense emotions in others because they know how to handle those emotions in themselves. Good healers who foster wholeness can hold safe, brave space, bolstering your ability to express sadness, anger, disappointment, fear, shame, jealousy, or whatever else arises. Good healers are experts at healthy empathy.

What is healthy empathy? In *The Art of Empathy*, McLaren unpacks the six aspects of empathy, which I've summarized:

1. **Emotional contagion:** the ability to sense that someone is having an emotion that might call for you to respond to it.

2. **Empathic accuracy:** the ability to accurately identify and understand emotions in yourself and in another.

3. **Emotional regulation:** the ability to work with your emotions without being overtaken or frozen by them.

4. **Perspective taking:** the ability to ask, "What's it like to be you?" and to see through someone else's eyes.

5. **Concern for others:** might seem obvious, but if you don't care what it's like to be someone else, you won't behave in ways that will be perceived by the other as empathetic.

6. **Perceptive engagement:** the PhD level of empathy. Perceptive engagement allows you to make decisions based upon your empathy and to respond to someone else's intense emotion in a way *they* perceive as care.[12]

Some healers are geniuses at perceptive engagement. I can't emphasize this enough—even people who might not be expert practitioners (e.g., they're not skilled at putting their acupuncture needles in the right place, or they're not the best surgeon on the planet, or they're not manipulating the energy fields quite right) can facilitate healing if they're good at perceptive engagement. That doesn't mean you won't want to pick doctors, acupuncturists, and healers who know what they're doing! By all means do your research, and make sure you choose to put your body in skillful hands. But understand that skill is only part of the package. If you can create a safe enough space for someone's suppressed emotions to arise; if you can respond in a way that feels empathetic to the one emoting; if you can create safe space when someone feels vulnerable, helpless, scared, and isolated, you're a healer—whether you're putting your hands on someone's body, making someone's cappuccino, or cutting their hair.

Unfortunately, many people who hang a shingle and call themselves healers do the opposite. Although this is not true for everyone, doctors can be *the worst* at creating safe space and practicing perceptive engagement, given the limitations of the system that creates so many barriers for doctors to intimate connection with their patients. This might be what drives the multibillion-dollar complementary and alternative medicine (CAM) business. At least when people are paying cash for healing services, they usually have more time with the practitioner, and empathetic connection rarely happens when we're rushed.

But it's not just doctors. Those who identify as energy healers, especially when they identify as "empaths" or "intuitives," might try to shut down your emotions before you can even pop out a tear or vent some anger—so they don't *feel* your pain so acutely. This can cause them to behave in ways that lack empathy and shut down your emotional release. Empaths might be good at emotional contagion or empathic accuracy, but because they don't know how to regulate emotion within themselves, they often can't get all the way to real empathy.

I once saw someone who claimed to be a healer, whose writing I admired but whose empathy was clearly wounded, bring a person with stage-four cancer up onstage in front of a large group. After he peppered her with penetrating, boundary-violating questions and allegedly used his intuitive empath skills to point out her core wound, she started to cry. When her healing emotions started to flow while she told him the details of how she got hurt, he—no joke—cut her off and pretended to play a mini-violin in the most condescending way as he mocked her, saying, "Whaddaya want me to do? Play you a widdle sob song?"

Her healing had started and stopped so abruptly that the audience was shocked, silenced in horror. Her shame spread through the room like motor oil on snow as our emotional contagion picked up on it. He was trying to "fix" her when what she needed was feeling and healing.

I had once been guilty of this same distorted attempt at healing, but I was lucky. Rachel taught me—and countless other doctors—the vital difference between helping, fixing, and serving. Rachel has had a lifelong chronic illness—Crohn's disease—which has given her great empathy for the suffering of others and makes her a phenomenal healer and teacher for doctors like me.

Helping, Fixing, and Serving

Rachel Naomi Remen, MD

Helping, fixing, and serving represent three different ways of seeing life. When you help, you see life as weak. When you fix, you see life as broken. When you serve, you see life as whole. Helping and fixing might be the work of the ego and service the work of the soul.

Service rests on the premise that the nature of life is sacred; life is a holy mystery that has an unknown purpose. When we serve, we know that we belong to life and to that purpose. From the perspective of service, we are all connected: All suffering is like my suffering, and all joy is like my joy. The impulse to serve emerges naturally and inevitably from this way of seeing.

Serving is different from helping. Helping is not a relationship between equals. A helper might see others as weaker than they are, needier than they are. People often feel this inequality. The danger in helping is that we might inadvertently take away from people more than we could ever give them; we might diminish their self-esteem, sense of worth, integrity, or even wholeness.

When we help, we become aware of our own strength. But when we serve, we don't serve with our strength; we serve with ourselves, and we draw from all of our experiences. Our limitations serve; our wounds serve; even our darkness can serve. My pain is the source of my compassion; my woundedness is the key to my empathy.

Serving makes us aware of our wholeness and its power. The wholeness in us serves the wholeness in others and the wholeness in life. The wholeness in you is the same as the wholeness in me.

Service is a relationship between equals: Our service strengthens us as well as others.

Helping and fixing are draining, and over time we might burn out, but service is renewing. When we serve, our work itself will renew us. In helping, we might find a sense of satisfaction; in serving we find a sense of gratitude . . .

What is most professional is not always what best serves and strengthens the wholeness in others. Helping and fixing create a distance between people, an experience of difference. We cannot serve at a distance. We can only serve that to which we are profoundly connected, that which we are willing to touch. Helping and fixing are strategies to repair life. We serve life not because it is broken but because it is holy. Serving requires us to know that our humanity is more powerful than our expertise.

In forty-five years of chronic illness, I have been helped by a great number of people and fixed by a great many others who did not recognize my wholeness. All that helping and fixing left me wounded in some important and fundamental ways. Only service heals. Service is not an experience of strength or expertise; service is an experience of mystery, surrender, and awe. Helpers and fixers feel causal. Servers might experience from time to time a sense of being used by larger unknown forces. Those who serve have traded a sense of mastery for an experience of mystery and, in doing so, have transformed their work and their lives into practice.[13]

EMPATHY VERSUS COMPASSION

Empathy is neurologically distinct from compassion. Empathy means we feel *with* people. This means that when someone is happy, excited, or joyful, our brains respond as if something wonderful has happened in *us*. Conversely, if we are empathizing with someone in pain, it lights up the pain centers in our brains. The more we lack the distinction of self/other, perhaps because of boundary wounding in childhood, the more someone else's pain feels like our own, which might cause people to withdraw when others are in pain. For those with the rare condition *mirror-touch synesthesia*, this tendency is exaggerated. For those with mirror-touch synesthesia, if you touch your cheek, they feel as if a hand is pressing against their own cheek, and if you get punched in the stomach, their own bellies might ache. At its most extreme, which has been observed in twins, when one twin is injured, the other twin might experience the exact same wound, even though that twin did not get directly injured.

As you can imagine, if you felt other people's emotional or physical pain as if it were your own, you might feel desperate to make their pain go away so you would feel better. Unfortunately, this is not an impulse that helps others heal; it's a self-protective impulse that can feel like the opposite of empathy to someone else in pain.

Compassion is not feeling *with* someone; it's feeling *for* someone. Neurologically, it lights up our love centers more than our pain centers, so you might say it's neurologically easier on us. In an article that distinguishes between the two neurologically, Tania Singer and Olga Klimecki report that compassion elicits feelings of warmth, concern, and care for others as well as a strong inclination to ease the suffering and improve the well-being of others, whereas empathy with someone in pain feels painful to the one empathizing.[14] Empathy can lead to burnout, especially among healers who spend their days with suffering people. Fortunately, the slight distance offered by compassion—and how it connects us to love—can help protect the health-care provider from emotional overwhelm and burnout.

Singer and Klimecki write,

> While empathy refers to our general capacity to resonate with others' emotional states irrespective of their valence—positive or negative—empathic distress refers to a strong aversive and self-oriented response to the suffering of others, accompanied by the desire to withdraw from a situation to protect oneself from excessive negative feelings. Compassion, on the other hand, is conceived as a feeling of concern for another person's suffering, which is accompanied by the motivation to help.[15]

When parts of the brain responsible for pain are stimulated through an empathetic response, how much someone is inclined to help people in pain depends on other social factors, such as whether they are perceived as part of an "in group." For example, if someone on your football team gets hurt, you're more likely to help them than if someone on the opposite team does.

Compassion, however, because it is rooted in love, is less likely to be reserved for people in your in group. Meditation practices, such as Buddhist lovingkindness, are teachable, and neuroscience proves that compassion can be learned, even for those who aren't in your in group.

Although we are wired to be compassionate, many have this capacity wounded. Caring about others means allowing their heartbreak to penetrate you, not by taking it on as your own but by being close to it, moved by it, touched by it, and broken open because of it. The open heart feels not only love but pain. You might notice that anything that touches your heart—whether because of beauty, horror, or kindness—also activates your tear ducts. It's as if we have this heart–tear duct highway that *feels* when the heart is open and can offer our presence to whatever shows up. If you're sick, and nothing has helped you so far, this kind of open-hearted presence with compassionate people can be immeasurably healing. It might not cure the cancer or paralyzed legs, but it can heal the loneliness.

Traumatized individuals might become so self-absorbed that they stop caring about how other people feel, which robs them of the love, belonging, and sense of connection that is their health-inducing birthright. Sadly, too many health-care providers are hurt in this way. They might have mad skills, but their hearts are closed.

LETTING PEOPLE OFF THE HOOK

Keep in mind that just as helping and fixing can be mistaken for service, empathy and compassion are often mistaken as letting others—or ourselves—off the hook. Widening the circle of your empathy or compassion to include not just the people you like but also those you might be tempted to demonize is another challenging skill set; however, it's a necessary one if we're ever going to heal, personally and collectively.

The ability to do this *does not* mean that by tuning in to how other people feel and extending ourselves to connect with them or feel warmth for them, we necessarily let them off the hook. If we are healthy and healing, we can absolutely extend compassion to someone while simultaneously setting boundaries and holding someone accountable.

If we're failing to set boundaries or hold someone accountable, we're back in the spiritual bypassing territory of *blind compassion* or *neurotic tolerance* or *premature forgiveness*. We don't have to agree with what people are saying or validate their actions to resonate empathetically with them or extend compassion to them. Empathy is what allows us to resist demonizing or dehumanizing people just because we don't like what they've done. Sociopathic behavior is defined by lack of empathy. If we can't feel what the other feels (empathy), and we lack care for their suffering (compassion), we can inflict horrific atrocities and not feel anything. So, empathy and compassion are crucial to the healing process, not just on the personal level but on the planetary scale.

After you have access to your emotions and the gifts they bring, you can extend compassion to people you don't like, but that doesn't mean you won't hold them accountable for their behaviors. Empathy and compassion do not mean we give anyone a pass for abuse or avoid imposing consequences. It means we can see them as human beings, flawed though they might be, which protects us from exiling them from the wholeness of humanity or casting them off as monsters in ways that can be traumatizing.

We also need to do the same with ourselves when we've done something that might harm ourselves or inflict pain upon others. This isn't easy, because acknowledging that we've perpetrated harm elicits shame—as it should. In its healthy form, shame is intimately related to our morality, ethics, and integrity, so it helps us stay aligned with how we want to treat ourselves and others. But if we've been unfairly shamed in childhood, if we've taken on the shame our parents or others who perpetrated harm, abuse, or control over us should have kept to themselves, shame might send us into a spiral and overwhelm our circuits.

Shame is one of the most intensely painful emotions and can make us feel like we've fallen into a deep pit of isolation, despair, and exile. We might be tempted to hide or disappear, so it's hard to feel shame even when feeling its healthy form might help us engage in prosocial behavior by allowing it to motivate us to repair a relationship or stop us from doing something that harms ourselves or others. If shame overtakes you, you might need a healer or therapist who can hold compassionate space for you and love you where you hurt until you're strong enough to extend compassion to the parts of yourself that inflict harm. As Miami poet Rune Lazuli writes, "Crawl inside this body, find me where I am most ruined—love me there."

EMOTIONAL MASTERY

How might we work skillfully with our emotions—neither getting dangerously lost in them nor repressing or trying to transcend them—to potentially improve our health? Proficient emotional intelligence requires developing emotional understanding. If Type A personalities tend to emotionally explode and get heart disease, and Type Cs tend to repress and get cancer (and perhaps autoimmune diseases), what is the "just right" of emotional health? Emotions arise for a reason. They're not something we're meant to ignore, bypass, transcend, numb, obsess over, or let explode, but to complete the action each emotion calls forth from us so it can flow through and the next emotion can arise. Just as Sadness had to flow its tears in the little girl from *Inside Out* so Joy could flow back in, learning how to work with our emotions effectively helps heighten our emotional intelligence, making it one of our core Whole Health Intelligences.

If healing requires empathy, compassion, and service rather than helping and fixing—if emotions need to be contained but also expressed rather than exploded, repressed, or bypassed, how can we foster this in ourselves and in others when everything in our culture pressures us to do just the opposite? Boundaries are key, and this is where an energy-healing perspective comes in handy.

If we have no physical, emotional, sexual, or psychic boundaries, we are unprotected from being penetrated—not only physically but also emotionally or psychically—by those who might wish to cause us harm. We must learn how to feel our feelings not by vomiting them all over someone else; not by exploding in catharsis in ways that leave us flooded, drained, or otherwise unable to function; and not by letting our emotions run away with us in ways that might cause psychic or physical violence but by learning how to work with our emotions as a helpful guidance system—one of the most important aspects of our Whole Health Intelligences. If our boundaries are wounded and porous, as I discuss in more detail in chapter 7, they'll need to be treated and strengthened using advanced trauma-healing methods, which I discuss in part three. But if our boundaries are clear—and we use our emotions to help keep them and the boundaries of others safe, we can feel our emotions, spread empathy, and extend compassion, resting in one of the paradoxes of healing: We are One . . . *and* we are separate.

As McLaren describes in detail in *The Language of Emotions*, all emotions bring gifts and require us to implement the action-requiring neurological programs they signal. Anger signals you to protect your boundary. Shame helps you protect your integrity—with yourself and others. Fear arises to help you become hyperfocused, attuned to your instincts, and able to protect yourself and those you care about from undue harm. Anxiety arises to warn you to think about the future and complete the tasks necessary for keeping you safe, responsible, and able to meet your basic needs. Jealousy signals you to pay attention to mate retention, arising when the security of a relationship is threatened. Panic signals you to fight, flee, or freeze—evoking a necessary stress response in the face of danger. Sadness arises when it's time to let go of things that aren't working anymore. Grief comes when the loss is permanent and irretrievable. These emotions bring gifts with them. If we repress or bypass them, we're cut off from the wisdom of our emotional intelligence, which helps us heal and protects us in countless ways.

Five Tools to Help You Channel Emotions

What are the tools you need to handle staying with your intense emotions in skillful ways? I cannot recommend McLaren's *The Language of Emotions* enough. It provides step-by-step instructions for tuning in to the gifts of your emotions, implementing the programs they activate neurologically, and healing by feeling emotions in a healthy way. Until you get a chance to read it, I've summarized it here.

1. Get Grounded
Think of your entire system like an electrical system, with your emotions holding potential charge. If you're not grounded, your emotions can jolt you like an electric shock and flood you with too much current. But if you're truly grounded in your body, you can send any extra charge back into the earth. Different healing methods use a variety of grounding practices—yoga asanas, earth-connecting visualizations, eating

heavier foods, and conscious breathing as well as avoiding ungrounding practices such as astral travel, certain transcendent types of meditation, and kundalini yoga.

2. Define Your Boundaries

You can use the concept of an aura to create some personal space for yourself and others. If you don't do this, people are likely to trod all over your boundaries. If you give yourself too much space, you'll trod all over other people. But if you rely upon your "proprioceptive territory," the space around you created by specific neural and muscular networks that map your body and position you with relation to what's around you, you'll know how much space you're entitled to. When you can protect this space in yourself and others, you'll know where you begin and end—and where others begin and end. That way it's easier to differentiate between your emotions and someone else's emotions. Keep in mind that if your boundaries were wounded in childhood, the restoration of healthy boundaries generally requires healing the traumas that wounded your boundaries, as I discuss in part three.

3. Burn Contracts

The practice of burning contracts is intended to help you release trapped emotions and behaviors through guided visualization. It's a way to change your relationship with a belief, behavior, point of view, or relationship you've outgrown—maybe one that's engaging intense emotions. To burn a contract, you ground yourself, illuminate your boundary in your mind's eye with a bright color, and imagine unrolling a large piece of parchment in front of you. Keeping it inside your personal boundary, you can project, envision, write, speak, or think your distress onto it. Put all your emotional expectations on that parchment.

With the parchment safely distanced from you but still *inside* your boundary so you don't spew your difficulties all over someone else, you can work with whatever emotions are arising in a safe, healthy way. You can use fear like paint or rely on anger like confetti or darken the image with sadness or grief. You can cover it with words or colors or music lyrics, anything that helps you get the emotion moving. Safe inside your boundary, connected to your grounding so you can release anything that threatens to overwhelm you, you are protected here—and others are protected from the solar flares of any big bangs that might arise from your emotional intensity. This is what it means to *channel* your emotions, in the way you would direct water so it doesn't flow all over the place and flood things. By properly channeling your emotions, you can let go *and* contain them inside your boundary, which helps restore their natural watery flow. When you're done, you can roll up your parchment and toss it outside your boundary. When it lands, imagine burning it up with whatever emotion feels right—anger, sadness, grief, fear, gratitude, joy. Whatever arises is the right one to set you free from a contract that no longer serves you.

4. Complain Consciously

Some emotions need more than burning contracts to get them moving. Emotions such as anger can be so charged that sometimes we need to let loose. But how do we do so without hurting anyone? Conscious complaining, which you can do by yourself or with a willing partner resourced to hold space for you, is a way to discharge your emotions. Whereas unconscious complaining can drain you and the people who must listen to you whine, conscious complaining is an intentional healing practice. To practice conscious complaining, you can write or speak exactly what you're feeling until you feel done. When you feel clearer and finished for now, say thank you. Make sure your partner doesn't rile you up, though. This is not a conversation. If you do this with a partner, make sure that person simply holds silent space until the emotion is safely discharged.

5. Rejuvenate Yourself

When you burn contracts and clear a space in your psyche, you might feel a void. McLaren recommends filling it with something radiant and uplifting. For example, imagine your favorite nature scene, use guided meditation with breathwork to activate your imaginative senses—hear the roar of a waterfall or smell the scent of jasmine. If you're in a hurry because you've just burned a contract in the toilet stall at work because your boss is enraging you, you can fill your boundary with bright light.

Chapter 7

SHORING UP YOUR BOUNDARIES

I t was not my intention to study boundaries when I embarked upon my Sacred Medicine journey, but it didn't take me long to realize that healing and healthy boundaries (or lack thereof) are intimately entwined. In her research on what makes "wholehearted" people so *whole* of heart, Brené Brown bumped into one finding repeatedly: *The people with the clearest boundaries were the most wholehearted.* Why? Because they didn't have to fear they would be overrun if they kept their hearts open. Their boundaries protected the fragility of their open hearts. Because they didn't let just anybody close to that vulnerability, people with good boundaries were freer to love generously.[1]

Without healthy boundaries and emotional understanding, the permissive gap in our boundaries can put us at risk of parasitic relationships, narcissist/codependent pairings, exploitative dynamics, and spiritual cults that masquerade as intentional communities, transformational groups, congregations, or sanghas. Wounded boundaries can also create holes in our psychic boundaries, putting us at risk of what shamans call "entities," "dark energies," or even full-on "possessions"—something I didn't even believe in before my Sacred Medicine journey convinced me otherwise and left me stunned by what can happen when boundaries are violated in the spiritual realm.

The sun was setting as the circle of doctors from the Whole Health Medicine Institute stood on the beach at Monterey, California, watching the red-orange ball of fire paint a pastel watercolor over the ocean. We frolicked in the surf, dancing our mirrored footprints on the silvery sand. Although the program is not limited to females, this year's class was all women, so we were all relaxed and playful with each other at our annual retreat, shedding our white coats, laughing, and enjoying the bonding of women who usually take care of everybody but themselves. During our sunset reverie, a siren wailed . . . then another . . . and another. Within minutes, our peaceful beach in paradise had transformed into an emergency rescue site, teeming with ambulances, fire trucks, and police cars, followed by a helicopter, a Coast Guard boat, and jet skis. A huddle of surfers in wetsuits wept. When we asked what happened, they explained that two teenage brothers had been swept out in a riptide. One brother had been saved. The other had disappeared. A full rescue was under way as everyone prayed for a miracle.

The group of doctors I'd been dancing with moments earlier grew visibly agitated. One admitted she wanted to dive into the water and search for the boy along with the Coast Guard. Others shared the same reaction. I used it as a teaching moment, helping them notice how uncomfortable they felt if someone was in trouble and they were not in charge. Their addiction to rescuing was so unmistakable that nobody could deny it. This was a chance to discuss boundaries. They were off duty, on retreat. The paramedics were handling it. But the doctors weren't buying it. Peeling them away from the beach was like asking an addict to quit cold turkey. We were late for dinner, but keeping these doctors from a rescue in progress was like uprooting an entire aspen grove.

"*It's not your rescue.*" I reinforced. "It's being handled."

That's when I heard the howl.

One of the doctors came running toward me, looking ashen. "Come. *Quick.* It's Amy."

I followed her and found a member of our group, shaking and crying, her body trembling as if she were having a seizure. I tried to make eye contact with her, but her gaze was distant, glassy, and wide-eyed with terror.

In a strange voice, she screamed, "Where's my brother? Where's my mother?"

My colleague Anne, who was helping run the retreat, is a depth psychologist, trained in the practice and science of the unconscious. Anne stepped in and approached Amy with a firm but calm demeanor.

"Gather around, everyone," she announced, herding people into a circle. "We're going to do a STAT aura clearing."

These conventional medical doctors looked perplexed.

"I'll explain later, but it looks like Amy has been possessed by the boy who is dying."

Without wasting time to tend to her colleagues' bewildered intellects, Anne took charge, shouting at Amy with unusual ferocity, "Out! *Out!* Follow the light! Go to the light. Get out of Amy!"

Amy was bawling. "I don't want to die! Where's my brother? I want Mom."

"Your brother is okay. Your mother is okay. Go to the light."

Anne instructed us all to put our hands on Amy. We went around the circle, repeating after Anne the words she instructed us to say: "You are Amy."

She instructed Amy to repeat after her: "I am Amy."

Amy said, "I'm not Amy," her forehead wrinkled with confusion.

Anne looked fiercely into her eyes and said, "Yes. You are Amy." We all repeated, "You are Amy . . . you are Amy . . ."

She stopped trembling, and her gaze shifted. She looked baffled.

Anne said, "Repeat after me. I am Amy."

"I am Amy."

Amy looked at us huddled around, touching her body, and she asked, "Where am I?"

Amy was back.

Within a day of what happened with the drowning boy, Amy developed chest pain, shortness of breath, and extreme fatigue, which worsened over the next five days. By this time, she was back in her midwestern town, where she sought help from her doctor, who ordered a battery of tests. The results revealed the apparent cause of her symptoms. At the age of fifty, she had a newly diagnosed complex heart defect, which included an atrial septal defect and a patent foramen ovale, a large flaplike hole in her heart that was allowing deoxygenated as well as oxygenated blood to circulate throughout her body.

Heart defects like this are usually congenital. If they're severe enough to become symptomatic, they usually present as cardiac or pulmonary symptoms in early childhood. Yet, not only did Amy not have a childhood history of cardiopulmonary symptoms but also she previously had a normal echocardiogram—one of the gold standard cardiac tests—because of her many previous spinal surgeries. How was it possible she had developed a brand-new hole in her heart?

Amy consulted a cardiologist, who suggested that open-heart surgery would be necessary to repair the large hole. But Amy got an intuitive hit that caused her to press the "pause" button on emergency surgery. As bizarre as it sounded, she wondered if this new hole in her heart could have something to do with having been possessed by the dying boy.

She sought help from Anne and me. "Do you think I opened my heart *too* much this weekend? If so, can I reverse it without surgery?"

STUCK SOULS

Amy asked for referrals, so I helped arrange an emergency trip to meet some of the healers I'd studied with, one of whom was a Qigong healer from China. Although she had been told nothing about Amy's health issues, her intuitive diagnosis (via translator) was surprisingly accurate. She called out the hole in Amy's heart, told her that her liver had been weakened by all the antibiotics and pain medications she had taken, and assessed that her thyroid was not functioning optimally. She said the bones in Amy's back were crooked and overlapping and would likely be a chronic issue. She said she did not think Amy would need further surgery but warned her that she would have ongoing suffering.

The Qigong healer said that on the spiritual level, Amy had an energy drain from two souls stuck to her who were feeding off her life force. One was her godchild, who had died when he was four years old in a freak hayride accident. The other was her nephew, who suffered from addiction and mental health issues.

After her assessment of Amy, the Qigong healer chanted and performed mudras around Amy while going into what appeared to be a trance. Her translator explained that she was entering the "Buddha field," an ineffable dimension where time and matter cease, where the Medicine Buddha and Bodhisatva of Compassion can be accessed, where matter can be brought back to this dimension and manifested as medicinal granules from the other side. The healer then appeared to produce pungent Chinese herbs from the palms of her hands, as if out of thin air, gave Amy a handful of them, and instructed her how to take them.

The healer also impressed upon Amy the need to perform a "passport ceremony" to send away the two entities sucking on her life and help them cross over from this dimension into the next. She explained how to detach the stuck souls from Amy's energy field by burning a ceremonial piece of cloth Amy purchased for an additional $100, which would send her godson and nephew to the light. The healer warned that the cloth might spark or even explode, an indication that the souls had gone on their way to the other side. She recommended performing the ceremony outdoors.

After three solid days of Sacred Medicine healing work that included visiting two other healers, Amy and her friend Renee went to a beach to perform the passport ceremony as the Qigong healer had prescribed. By the end of her week with the healers, Amy's arrhythmias had resolved. She was free of chest and back pain; she felt expanded, amazed, and grateful for the support. She intended to return to her cardiologist's office to follow up.

The cardiologist wanted to perform a heart catheterization to make sure Amy didn't have pulmonary hypertension because the atrial septal defect had appeared so dangerously large on the initial echocardiogram. During the procedure, he was surprised to find that the opening in her heart had shrunk enough to be repaired through a catheter with small patches. Open-heart surgery was no longer necessary. Amy went home the next day with no pain, had a quick recovery, and has had no trouble with her heart since.

Amy's spine, however, continued to cause her problems. After initial relief, the back pain returned, and despite the Qigong master's prediction that she wouldn't need more surgery, in 2016, Amy decided on a twelfth treatment for her distorted spine. She underwent two days of surgery, and rods were inserted from the T4 vertebra to her pelvis. Her recovery was swift and the results so miraculous that she was walking more than two miles a day only two weeks after the surgery. Her outcome was so optimal that the orthopedic clinic wrote about her on its website as a testimonial of how miraculous surgery can be when it goes well.[2] Having given up her medical practice because of her disability, Amy now works at the Center for Courageous Kids as their camp physician, and she delights in her job with the medically fragile children.

What can we conclude about this outcome? Did these healers help Amy heal? She still needed repair of her heart, but the repair was performed with minimal intervention, without the trauma and risk of open-heart surgery. Although Amy still needed surgery on her spine, the twelfth surgery gave her relief after eleven failed attempts. From Amy's perspective, it was a miracle. She feels emotionally healed, spiritually connected, and pain-free for the first time in her memory.

Like Amy's, my worldview was unsettled by this experience. It's one thing to hear about entities; however, watching what happened to Amy shook my certainty that such things were the superstitious delusions of gullible or even psychotic people. As a physician and scientist, do I believe in stuck souls and vampiric entities causing illness? Through a literal scientific lens? *Not so much.* From a metaphorical, poetic, and trauma-informed point of view? *Maybe.*

NEOSHAMANISM

The idea that humans can become mentally or physically ill because of stuck souls or vampiric entities attached to their energy fields is common among many ancient and modern Indigenous healing traditions. Recently, Americans and other Westerners interested in this more mythic way of relating to the past traumas of patients have developed a way of practicing *neoshamanism*, something related to but distinct from traditional or Indigenous shamanism.

What is shamanism? How does neoshamanism differ from it? *Merriam Webster's* defines a shaman as "someone who is believed in some cultures to use magic to cure people who are sick, to control future events, etc." The *Oxford English Dictionary* defines a shaman as "a person regarded as having access to, and influence in, the world of good and evil spirits. . . Typically such people enter a trance state during a ritual and practice divination and healing."

The distinctions can be fuzzy and triggering for people understandably sensitive to issues such as cultural appropriation, but as I've come to understand it, shamanism refers to any tradition that involves a healer, maybe one with relatively porous psychic boundaries, who has the ability—either through natural gifts, heritage, rigorous training (often traumatic), or an unintentional side effect of boundary-violating trauma—to interact with the invisible realms and the spirit world. Trance states are commonly used to induce this ability to traverse dimensions of reality from the material plane to more subtle realms. A shaman's intent is to communicate with spirits or energies and to bring back knowledge, wisdom, gifts, or insights from the spiritual plane into the material plane, especially for the purpose of healing people, elements in nature, the community, or the culture. They also receive guidance about practical matters, such as when to plant crops.

Neoshamanism, however, refers to an eclectic range of beliefs, rituals, and practices that involve the attempts of people to mimic what traditional shamans might do but without having been raised within the traditional cultural framework, training, or tribe. Like traditional shamans, neoshamans attain altered states and communicate with the spirit world, and they also tend to share worldviews, philosophies, and activities that bind them to each other. Many neoshamans claim to have had a lifelong relationship with the spirit world that might have left them feeling on the fringes, especially in mostly white, science-dominated cultures that don't acknowledge such a world. They might pursue contact with the spirit world through a variety of techniques intended to induce altered states of consciousness, such as chanting, drumming, dancing, breathwork, or use of psychedelics.

Most neoshamans identify as animists who believe that nature is imbued with consciousness with which they can communicate, that matter (e.g., a mountain, a river, or a rock) is filled with spirit and Beingness, and that humans can interact with it as if it were sentient. Neoshamans might have been trained by traditional shamans, or they might self-identify as shamans because they've read books, taken an online course, participated in some sort of "shaman school," or otherwise developed these gifts naturally.

Both traditional shamans and neoshamans might describe themselves as "highly sensitive people" (HSPs, as identified by Elaine Aron in her book *The Highly Sensitive Person*), which tends to fall on the scale of neurodiversity. Most would identify as being an "empath." Many neoshamans have experienced one of the chronic illnesses considered "shaman sicknesses." In Indigenous cultures, shamans called to service who haven't yet said yes are often struck with physical ailments. In modern culture, these shamanic sicknesses might fall into difficult-to-treat categories such as chronic fatigue syndrome, fibromyalgia, chronic Lyme disease, chronic pain, and autoimmune disorders. Acceptance of the call to shamanic service often resolves the symptoms of shaman sicknesses.

Neoshamans might have certain gifts in their capacity to tune in to their Whole Health Intelligences. They might have heightened intuition, finely attuned somatic senses, and extremely accurate emotional intelligence. They might feel like outsiders, as traditional shamans typically are. Traditional shamans tend to live on the outskirts of a community for a reason. Community members might even fear the shamans because their spiritual power might be intimidating, and this is accepted. But in the modern world, it might leave those on a shamanic path feeling like they don't ever fit in—except with other shamanic types.

It's tricky if you identify with this shamanic archetype and grow up in a culture without traditional shamans. You might go to medical school or become a therapist or a life coach instead, but those conventional systems might not feel like your true calling. There's been a surge in interest among mostly white Westerners in learning to become neoshamans.

Understandably, some members of Indigenous cultures and religions are critical of neoshamanism, asserting that it represents an illegitimate form of cultural appropriation and that it is a ruse by fraudulent spiritual leaders to disguise or lend legitimacy to fabricated, ignorant, and/or unsafe practices in their ceremonies. Critics of neoshamanism, most of them of Indigenous origin, condemn such elements, especially the commoditization of shamanic rituals and trainings, as inauthentic at best and dangerous at worst. In response to the explosion of neoshamanic activity, a variety of Indigenous activist groups, such as New Age Frauds & Plastic Shamans, have arisen to call out what they consider unethical practices.

Given the sensitivity around cultural appropriation, my sincere desire to learn more about Indigenous healing methods as part of my Sacred Medicine research, the reality that—ethical or not—many non-Indigenous people are making a living from neoshamanic practices, and my hesitation to dabble in these realms as a privileged white woman, I knew I'd have to tread carefully, but I didn't want to neglect it in my research.

I started my self-education with books, websites, and the limited scientific data I could find. I read a book by a woman who said her breast cancer was cured by an Amazonian shaman who treated her with herbs, *ayahuasca* (a psychedelic tea), spiritual healing, and (red flag) a juicy erotic affair with the shaman. I read case studies online (with names conveniently changed for privacy so I couldn't track down the patients) of shamanic cures for diseases modern medicine often fails to cure, such as cancer, Parkinson's disease, deafness, diabetes, addiction, depression, and schizophrenia, but I was unable to verify these reports. I studied books by Americans who claim to have apprenticed under Indigenous healers and report witnessing miraculous cures. I watched documentaries such as Nick Polizzi's *The Sacred Science*, which follows several sick Americans into the Amazonian rain forest, where they undergo care by Indigenous shamans. I spoke with Polizzi over the course of several years to educate myself as best I could without going to the Amazonian jungle, and I learned a lot from him and was grateful for the gracious way he taught me about the herbal and spiritual medicines Indigenous shamans use.

I interviewed a neoshaman who leads training programs in the United States, claiming to have been trained by the Q'eros and authorized by the Indigenous healers there to share their knowledge with the white people of North America, but the Q'eros people I met said they felt betrayed by him and did not endorse what he was teaching. Other neoshamans claim to have been taught by Native American healers or Mayan healers and lead workshops for mostly privileged white people. I attended a workshop with a Colombian man of European descent who claims to have been trained by the Kogi *mamas* in Colombia and initiated as the first white mama given permission to share the teachings and practices of the Kogi with North America.

I met several neoshamans who seemed ethical and full of good intentions. I met others who lit up my red-flag intuition, which guided me to give them a wide berth. One white neoshaman I encountered made international headlines and served three years in jail because three people died when he wouldn't let them out of his sweat lodge. Another worked one-on-one with clients who reported being sexually molested during their sessions with him. Yet another was allegedly swindling his sick and vulnerable clients. Suffice it to say that the world of neoshamanism seemed filled with both light and shadow.

Although I learned a lot from these neoshamans, I also learned to tread lightly and keep my discernment attuned. That said, some I met seemed to be helping people conventional medicine wasn't sure how to treat, like Amy.

Clearing Negative/Dark Energies

Sonya Amrita Bibilos

Want to try a do-it-yourself exorcism? Here are some tips:

1. **Declare:** *"My body and my life are mine!"*

2. **Call in Divine support.**

3. **Use prayer and sacred chants as you like.**

4. **Expel negative interferences.** You might yell, "Get out," or you might declare something like, "I allow only highest vibration light energy in my body, my energy fields, and my life."

5. **Bless your being with a visualization of light.** Visualize the light coming down from the heavenly realms into the top of your head. Allow the light to flow through and bless every cell of your being until you reach your feet. Send the light down through your feet, visualizing golden roots into the earth.

6. **Bless and restore your energy fields.** Imagine a shower of light cleansing the space up to about three feet in circumference around your body. Seal your energy fields with golden light.

7. **Use tools that can raise vibration and resonate for you.** Experiment with ethically sourced sacred herbs, incense, essential oils, Epsom salt baths, amulets or crosses, and icons.

8. **Chant sacred songs or pray as you go through your space.**

9. **Go outside and bless the land.**

Bonus: Eat a celebratory snack or meal. Doing energy work is more intense than you might think. Food helps ground and restore you.

A SACRED MEDICINE PERSPECTIVE ON PSYCHOSIS

If you, someone you love, or a healer ventures into the territory of possessions, entities, stuck souls, and dark energies, you might wonder how you can tell the difference between multidimensional healing, mystical experiences, and psychosis. After all, if you go to typical psychiatrists and tell them you're channeling other beings, seeing Jesus, feeling threatened by dark spirits, or being haunted by people who have crossed over, they might label you psychotic. How would you know if you had a real problem or just needed to do a little shamanic exorcism? I wondered about this too.

In the realm of conventional medicine, some of the stuff that comes up when people have porous psychic boundaries blurs into the territory of what psychiatrists would pathologize. Yet many energy healers, shamans, and neoshamans view such openings through a spiritualized lens, coming to the defense of the psychotic patient to act as protection for the patient's porous boundaries. Whether you call them psychic lawyers, exorcists, or shamans, having a healer who's got your back in the psychic realm can calm and comfort paranoid, terrified patients who feel helpless in worlds they might have stumbled into unprepared. Are those healers really engaging in psychic warfare to fend off the dark energies on behalf of the one under psychic attack? I can't prove that they are or aren't, but certainly many believe that they have the skill to do so and that their interventions can protect patients—and many patients feel safer, more grounded, and better able to function afterward.

How can we distinguish between generally healthy people who just need to shore up their psychic defenses and people with schizophrenia, bipolar disorder, drug- or trauma-induced psychosis, or organic brain disease? The distinctions can be subtle, controversial, and hard to discern. In his book *Spiritual Emergency*, psychiatrist Stanislov Grof unpacks how spiritual openings can masquerade as psychosis but are best treated differently by transpersonal psychologists and psychiatrists trained to navigate those realms. Although most psychotic episodes can devolve over time, reducing healthy functioning, according to Grof, spiritual emergencies are often a doorway into awakening consciousness and improved functioning, if treated appropriately.

Trying to make sense of this realm, I asked a physician friend. Rooted in both allopathic medicine and alternative modalities with a longtime spiritual practice, he serves both as an ER physician and as an energy healer with a unique perspective on how to access psychosis. He starts by trying to assess whether the psychotic symptoms were the result of a real spiritual opening, drug-induced delusions, an organic condition, or a trauma-induced escape from reality. Did they have a legitimate mystical experience, as with countless Catholic saints such as St. Teresa of Avila or St. Francis? Did something happen that made them feel worthless and triggered a sort of trauma-induced narcissistic grandiosity (i.e., their ego grabbed hold of them to counter the pain of feeling not special or not good enough)? Are they high? Do they have Lewy Body Dementia (which causes hallucinations) or a brain tumor or a thyroid disorder? Depending on his assessment, the appropriate treatment would be quite different.

Using his own subtle awareness to assess the situation, he does his best to establish trust, become an ally, and show the patients that his intentions are benevolent. He grounds himself by visualizing a grounding cord and making sure he's in his body. This offers a solid presence to the patients and often helps them ground as well. Opening his heart just enough to establish safety for the patients, he lets his heart presence emanate so their nervous system can relax, and he can continue by making the following assessments:

- Is the patient embodied, and if so, how much are they in their body?

- Are they dissociated in another dimension, and if so, how much of them is dissociated?

- If they are dissociated and out of their bodies, are they stuck there?

- What is the status of their heart and their emotional landscape?

- Are they feeling tortured or safe?

After he has an initial sense of the answers to these questions, he uses his subtle awareness to get a feel for patients' nervous systems. Is it a chaotic pinball gallery in there? Is the brain confused, which can suggest methamphetamine use or dementia? If patients are really outside their body, the brain might not even feel like it's there. This assessment might lead to further diagnosis as needed.

Of course, after the patients are stabilized, my friend does a medical workup, screening for organic causes of psychosis or drug side effects. If need be, depending on the acuteness of the situation and the assessment of safety, he might or might not medicate the patients, recommend hospitalization, or refer them for outpatient trauma treatment and/or psychiatric consultation.

Sometimes, he explains, the patients just need to be met where they are. For example, one day he heard a dog barking in the ER. The nurse approached him and said they were about to sedate a child, the source of the barking. When he approached the barking boy, the boy proclaimed, "I am Matrinon! You are Zorr!"

He played along. "Yes, I am Zorr."

The boy became sad and explained that his children were upset and scared, and he was trying to protect them.

He went with it. "When you bark like a dog, it scares the children, so you need to stay really quiet so you can protect them."

The boy got onboard and quit barking, avoiding sedation and complying with the rest of the evaluation. It turned out he was deeply traumatized and didn't know how to cope with the overwhelming circumstances. He just needed reassurance his "children" were going to be safe. Of course, a good physician would know that he needed to be treated with cutting-edge trauma-informed therapies more so than he needed to be medicated. However, medication sometimes might be needed in the short term because therapy can be a slow, tedious process. As I discuss in part three, most likely, the "children" this boy was trying to protect were his own scared, wounded inner kids.

APPRECIATION VERSUS APPROPRIATION

Cultural sharing is common in our globalized world and generally considered positive, sometimes leading to tolerance and appreciation of differences. Americans share our culture with and bring back influences from many other countries. This can foster compassion and diversity, but sharing and stealing are not the same.

A dominant or privileged group can culturally steal from a marginalized, oppressed, or underprivileged group without consent. This is especially unethical if members of the privileged group then exploit what they've appropriated for personal or financial gain, inflating privilege and further securing their dominance over the marginalized group.

Appreciating another culture means you're interested in learning about it, and maybe you wish to respectfully adopt some elements of it into your life. This is lovely, assuming you share what you've learned from another culture only after you've received that culture's permission—and you credit and compensate them fairly. When you appreciate a culture, you buy products representing that culture only from the culture that creates those products and use cultural elements only with consent and as they were intended to be used (not in an inappropriate and possibly disrespectful manner). For example, using Hindu malas for chanting mantras would be different from wearing them as a necklace and never saying a prayer.

If you do speak, teach, or practice healing on behalf of another culture, it's crucial not to take work from people who might lose power or money because members of a dominant group have replaced them. Be clear that you're not an authority and remain cautious about taking space from members of that culture who might not otherwise be heard.

Given the plethora of opportunities in the West to mess this up, it's a tricky proposition—*and* a moving target. What is deemed ethical one day might change the next as the practice of diversity, equity, and inclusion (DEI) grows and surges.

Where do things get dicey? When white people dominate the yoga world or the martial arts world without acknowledging their appropriation of a Hindu or Asian tradition; when they dress in clothes signifying priesthood or tattoo sacred symbols without context; and when they practice Traditional Chinese Medicine (TCM) or neoshamanism, potentially taking jobs from Chinese or Indigenous healers, they travel in the fraught territory of cultural appropriation.

Why is it problematic if privileged white Americans wear clothes from other cultures? After all, other cultures copy American ways of dressing. Americans might win status points, especially in certain spiritual circles, if they wear another culture's traditional jewelry or ceremonial clothing, but when someone from that culture wears their traditional garb in the West, they might not get the same status boost. On the contrary, they might be targeted and oppressed, diminished for not being modern or harassed for not assimilating. Those clothes might even mark them for hate crimes.

Finding the culturally sensitive sweet spot between appreciation and respect can be confusing. I've been told by Indigenous people that I should perform a ceremony on land where I lead healing work, asking permission and honoring the original caregivers and ancestors.

But if I invite workshop students to join me in that ceremony, am I culturally appreciating or appropriating? It's hard to know how to handle it. I know I'll make mistakes, but I'm doing my best to be aware and sensitive.

Does this mean you shouldn't go to a yoga class with a white teacher, seek healing from a white TCM doctor, or consult with a white neoshaman? It depends on who you ask and how your Whole Health Intelligences respond to what might be new DEI education. Countless people have benefited from yoga, TCM, and shamanic practices. If the only practitioners you have access to are white, it would be foolish to omit any tool from the world's medicine bag from your Prescription for Healing if you sense it could be right for you. But if you have a choice, consider choosing the Indian yoga teacher, the Chinese TCM doctor, or the Indigenous shamanic healer, even if they grew up in the United States and have learned their healing art to reconnect to their culture of origin. If someone calls you out for cultural appropriation, resist becoming defensive. Instead, learn from them and modify your behavior.

Cultural Appropriation Checklist

People guilty of cultural appropriation:

> Choose treatment from a white neoshaman over an Indigenous one.

> Dress in "spiritual" clothes from another tradition, but don't practice that religion.

> Wear their hair in a style associated with another culture to benefit from association with that culture (e.g., dreadlocks when you're not Black).

> Gain status, money, or power from elements of another culture.

Mock another culture using their customs (e.g.,
   Halloween costumes or sports fans who use
   Indigenous war cries).

Romanticize, fetishize, or sexualize customs or people,
   perpetuating stereotypes, racism, and systems of
   dominance.

Casually use words possessing strong significance in
   another culture such as tribe, spirit animal, totem pole,
   powwow, woke, or enlightened.

Purchase products such as art, food, or music from
   white people who copy traditional cultures rather
   than from people of those cultures.

Learn about shamanic healing from white people rather
   than directly from Indigenous people.

Participate in ceremonies or other traditional medicine
   journeys facilitated by white, non-Indigenous people.

Chapter 8

SACRED MEDICINE DIAGNOSTICS

I f you spend enough time in the world of Sacred Medicine, you're bound to bump into some curious ways healers attempt to diagnose illness. Remember the Balinese healer poking me with sticks? I also had Peruvian healers scatter and "read" coca leaves to assess my body. Donna Eden uses her unusual vision to "see" dark spots or funky flow in the energy field. Others might "feel" those stuck areas when moving their hands over someone's body, something I experienced once when I was in an altered state after a lengthy meditation. Some people use muscle testing, also known as applied kinesiology or energy testing, and others rely on medical intuition, such as the kind popularized by Caroline Myss and Mona Lisa Schultz. Sacred Medicine diagnostics are all over the map, and every tradition seems to have its own way of "reading" the body's health.

Although I would never recommend using Sacred Medicine diagnostics *instead* of seeing a doctor to get a thorough medical work-up, sometimes traditional Western medical methods fail to find or solve a problem. Some patients and practitioners swear by Sacred Medicine diagnostics when everything else has failed, so I wanted to cover two of the most common forms—medical intuition and the muscle test. At least half of the Western-trained energy healers I met, including Donna, use muscle testing regularly. It's also commonly employed by chiropractors, herbalists, nutritionists, holistic health practitioners, functional medicine practitioners, and energy psychologists.

Medical intuition is used not just by healers but also by doctors on the sly. You can even get a degree in intuitive medicine these days. Several of my physician friends have graduated from an intuitive medicine school in Marin County, California, and use what they learned to complement traditional medical diagnostics. When my doctor friend Cynthia Li was suffering from a mystery illness, medical intuition helped her in such a startling way that she chose to get trained in it herself. I recommend reading her book *Brave New Medicine*, but I'll summarize her story here.

Until her early thirties, Cynthia considered herself healthy and thriving. She worked full-time as a doctor in a human immunodeficiency virus/acquired immune deficiency syndrome (HIV/AIDS) clinic, traveled with her husband, and exercised regularly until she had a baby and developed postpartum thyroiditis (inflammation of the thyroid gland). She was treated pharmacologically by a top-notch endocrinologist but was still plagued by dizziness and fatigue, even when her thyroid hormones were returning to normal. Her second pregnancy spiraled her into a vortex of debilitating diagnoses, including chronic fatigue syndrome and dysautonomia (a dysfunction of the autonomic nervous system, which regulates vital functions such as blood pressure, heart rate, digestion, and breathing). As a practicing physician, she had dismissed conditions such as this one, considering them pseudo or catch-all diagnoses to be used when nothing could be confirmed via diagnostic testing. But as a patient, she felt hopeless, frustrated, and despairing, longing to reclaim her previous vitality.

Leveled by her symptoms, she was housebound for two years and severely disabled for the better part of a decade. Yet, she held on to hope in those times of despair. She writes, "Hope is a deep orientation of the human soul that is held in the darkest of times."[1] This dark night of the soul thrust Cynthia onto a healing journey she'd never have chosen willingly.

She tried everything outside her area of expertise of conventional medicine: integrative medicine, acupuncture and herbs, and mind-body medicine. She focused on neuroplasticity-rehabilitation exercises to rewire the communication between her brain and hormonal pathways. She tried whole-foods-based ancestral diets, such as gut and psychology (GAPS) and paleo. Some things helped sometimes, but she couldn't return to her former self.

She wound up working with a medical intuitive, Martine Bloquiaux, who helped reveal some of the missing links in her diagnosis and guided the rest of her treatment. After a lengthy recovery, Cynthia's vitality finally returned, and she wound up learning medical intuition from Martine and now uses what she learned to help others find a way to return to their lives.

EXTRAORDINARY KNOWING

The way Martine and Cynthia work with medical intuition is unstructured yet systematized. In addition to thoroughly assessing a patient's history, reviewing traditional diagnostics from a patient's often extensive medical records, and closely observing a patient's body upon physical examination (using a physician's training and mental intelligence), Cynthia also finds it helpful to include her intuitive intelligence. Before she sees a new patient, Cynthia spends ten minutes meditating to empty her mind and prepare space for insights, images, and intuitions. She might see an image that gives her a clue, or she might realize something she couldn't glean from mental intelligence alone. Other times, she might consult a list of obscure diagnoses, and scroll through, checking in with her intuitive "yes" and "no." A yes might cause her to order a specific test for something obscure she might not have thought about. In this way, she won't waste a fortune testing every obscure condition. Her intuition helps her whittle down the potential diagnoses. For example, is there mold in the client's bedroom? Does this person have a magnesium deficiency?

Many healers have trained themselves to feel their "yes" or "no" using somatic intelligence. Perhaps a "yes" is a feeling of love or warmth in the chest, whereas a "no" is a contraction in the solar plexus. Some visualize images. Some hear a voice conveying information. Others *just know* something that helps the patient but don't know how they know.

When I've discussed medical intuition with other like-minded doctors, most have a remarkable story of knowing something they couldn't possibly know about a patient in a way that helped save a life—such as Rachel Naomi Remen, who during her pediatric residency days was the only woman at Cornell Medical School, and intuition was decades from entering the medical conversation. A distraught mother brought in her healthy-looking baby, crying "My baby is going to die!" A full work-up showed nothing, and the baby was sent home, but the mother returned, panicking and insisting something was terribly wrong.

In that moment Rachel knew she had to do a lumbar puncture, an invasive test that would not have been indicated in a baby with no other symptom or laboratory evidence of meningitis. As she performed the spinal tap, guided only by her intuition and the mother's certainty that something was wrong, the doctor responsible for overseeing Rachel called for her to stop. What was she thinking? The baby had been worked up and discharged! Resisting his orders, Rachel advanced the needle into the baby's back just in time to see a drop of pure pus secrete. The baby had a lethal case of meningitis and would have been dead by morning if they had gone home. The mother's intuition—and Rachel's—saved that child's life.

In University of California–Berkeley psychologist and "anomalous knowing" researcher Elizabeth Lloyd Mayer's book *Extraordinary Knowing*, she tells the story of one of her therapy clients, a neurosurgeon from a nearby university hospital who had been suffering from severe migraines that weren't responding to conventional medical treatment. His doctor referred him for therapy, hoping it might help. Upon interviewing him, Mayer discovered that his headaches had begun when he stopped teaching medical students and residents, which he loved. Why did he stop teaching, she asked? He reluctantly confessed that he quit because he couldn't answer the question all the residents wanted to know: Why did he never lose a patient on the operating table when his surgeries were so risky? The reason, he finally explained, was that when he felt that surgery was indicated, he camped out at the patient's bedside and waited . . . sometimes for thirty seconds, sometimes for hours. He waited however long it took to receive the sign he had come to interpret as the green light that the patient was safe for surgery—a distinctive white light that appeared around the patient's head. If the light didn't appear, he waited.

I spoke to an intensive-care unit (ICU) doctor who said that his patients sometimes communicate with him during a code blue, when they've stopped breathing and their hearts have stopped beating and the doctor is trying to resuscitate them. Sometimes he will hear a voice that says simply, "I'm already gone." It doesn't mean he doesn't continue to follow the code blue protocol; but he doesn't go to any extreme measures the way he might if a similar kind of otherworldly voice said, "Keep going! I'm coming back."

When you ask doctors who feel safe sitting in a circle at a retreat together whether they've had similar experiences, the way I do, it's stunning how frequent such stories are told. This has been true for me too. I was also guided by intelligences beyond the mental when I was seeing patients. As I described in

The Anatomy of a Calling, one such intuition led me to perform a healing that I later learned was similar to a classic exorcism. I had no clue what I was doing, but I had seen a movie-like flash in my mind's eye about a patient with a mystery illness that her doctors couldn't solve. Her condition caused her to be life-threateningly anemic and ultimately required weekly iron infusions that kept her tethered to an IV all day in the infusion center of the local hospital with all the chemotherapy patients. Her doctors told her she would need to get these infusions forever, but after the vision arrived, I shared what I had seen with my patient and asked her if she wanted me to try to re-create the specific vision I had seen. She said, "Yes," so I painstakingly reenacted what I had seen in the vision—how she'd lie down on the ground with her back to me and her head in my lap; where I'd put my hands, one on her forehead and one on her heart; the lit candle; the song I would play (Mumford & Sons' "Awake My Soul"); the exact crystal she would hold in her hand. Her body shook as if she were having a seizure, and it scared me, but a voice inside said, "Just love her. Ground and stay the course." I visualized a grounding cord, opened my heart, poured my love on her, and waited about half an hour until she stopped shaking. When she was still, I held her in silence for a long time. When she finally spoke, she said, "My mother came out of my belly." She slept for thirty hours in the bed where I saw clients. That was ten years ago, and she's never needed another infusion.

When I think back on that experience, I hear Bill Bengston's voice in my mind: "Be playful; avoid ritual." If I tried to re-create that same experience with a different patient, my guess is that nothing would happen. I would have turned the mystery into a ritual I tried to control, copy, and re-create. Perhaps the outcome was as it was because I had trusted the mystery without trying to control it or duplicate it. Aside from the story I told you about Hugo—and how I laid my hands on him and practiced Bill's "cycling" while we waited for the helicopter to take him to the ER after his horrible fall—nothing quite like that has happened to me since.

IS IT INTUITION OR IS IT YOUR AGENDA?

Just as I would not recommend relying on mental intelligence alone because it might lead you to make unbalanced choices, I also would not recommend relying on intuitive intelligence alone. That would be like using only one of our senses to interpret the world. I would hesitate to trust any healer who uses only one of the four Whole Health Intelligences. If somebody ever tells you they have a direct line to God—and that their intuition is 100 percent accurate—be wary. As you can imagine, those with easy access to intuitive intelligence might have wise insights—as long as they can stay open to the mystery from a place of humble curiosity. But it can be *very easy* to get seduced into grandiosity if any part of you needs to feel special enough to believe you have the Divine on speed dial. Especially if someone has a deep wound of unworthiness as the result of trauma that needs the balm of specialness to assuage the agony of unlovability, those hits of grandiosity can be inflating—and inflation can distort the accuracy of intuition.

Although learning to tap into and trust your intuition can help you make clear, balanced choices when rounded out with your other Whole Health Intelligences, intuition alone can get us into trouble, especially when we cut ourselves off from the critical thinking, common sense, and rationality of mental intelligence. Intuition is never 100 percent accurate, and as I discuss in more detail later in this chapter, scientists have proven that even the most gifted intuitives make big mistakes when guided by intuition alone.

As it turns out, we are all vulnerable to getting tricked by our inner agendas, which can masquerade as intuition. All humans, healers included, can conflate a sense of receiving guidance from our true inner knowing with that of our inner agendas, which want something, are attached to something, are engaging in wishful or magical thinking, or are afraid. The ability to distinguish between intuition and ego agendas takes considerable practice and mastery, so we'd all be well served to practice yet another paradox of healing: Trust our intuitive intelligence *and* maintain a healthy skepticism about our own knowing—be on the lookout for agendas dressed up in holy drag.

One would hope that a good healer would be relatively neutral, but even healers are human, so they, too, might have agendas, such as wanting to be right or to convince a patient to use their services or buy their supplements. They might be attached to a patient's health outcome to inflate their self-importance. Unfortunately, as I discuss in chapter 9, healers who claim to be following their intuition as a cover for unethical or manipulative practices (and even flat-out con artists) are frighteningly common in the Sacred Medicine world.

At one point in my professional journey, I partnered with one of the Sacred Medicine healers I'd been studying. We were going to coteach and had a successful $100,000 plus launch of our online program. After we had collected the money from our students but before the program started, he told me he had to pull out. Why? *Because God told him so.*

I called bullshit. God was not telling him to cancel a program we had been preparing to teach for more than six months. Something else was going on—and I wanted him to be straight with me. He stuck to his guns. God had given him the green light to teach the program, but now God was rescinding consent. "God can be fickle that way, you know? I don't question God. I just follow orders."

He asked me to lie to the students and tell them we were canceling the class because I was recovering from the dog-bite injury or because my mother was terminally ill. But that wasn't true. I was capable of keeping my commitment despite what was happening in my personal life. I refused to lie, but I did not tell the students the whole truth either because I was still in my conflict-avoidant, spiritual bypassing phase. Instead, I canceled the program with no explanation, apologized, and refunded their money, putting myself in debt to do so. I chalked it up to an expensive lesson in discernment, but I was hurt . . . and *pissed*.

It's hard to argue with someone who swears they're getting their guidance directly from God, so it can be a nonnegotiable tactic people employ to dominate a situation and leave you defenseless. Just keep that in mind when you're in Sacred Medicine territory. Be on the lookout for anyone who uses their intuition to justify dishonesty, harm, or agenda-driven actions.

There was a lot of this among alternative medicine types during the Covid pandemic, when people used "I'm following my intuition" to justify not wearing a mask, not social distancing, and not getting vaccinated, not to mention generally rejecting public health guidelines, especially when those guidelines affected their ability to make a living. Even some previously intelligent, high-profile doctors went as far as to claim, "My intuition says Covid is a hoax," and leveraged their social media platforms to influence public opinion to convince people not to listen to public health departments. *Was it their intuition?* Or were they justifying rebellious, antiauthoritarian, oppositional, or libertarian tendencies with nonfactual claims? When Sacred Medicine diagnostics are used to justify a lack of critical thinking or attention to science, not only is it troublesome but also it can be lethal.

SCIENCE AND INTUITION DON'T ALWAYS COOPERATE

Is medical intuition accurate? The few peer-reviewed studies performed on people who consider themselves medical intuitives show that medical intuition alone is disappointingly inaccurate. Although one qualitative study published in the obscure journal *Subtle Energies* showed promising results,[2] a quantitative study published in the more reputable *Journal of Alternative and Complementary Medicine* showed only 14 percent accuracy. Researchers concluded, "Results indicate some correspondence between the psychic diagnoses and the medical records, but the correspondence was not sufficiently impressive to warrant considering psychic diagnosis as a useful alternative method for diagnosing disease. It would appear that patients relying solely on psychic diagnosis as the basis for therapy are at risk of serious medical problems going undetected."[3]

Well . . . *duh*. I'm not suggesting using medical intuition instead of traditional medical diagnosis. Most of the patients who wind up seeing a medical intuitive do so as an adjunct to medical diagnostic testing—because conventional medical diagnosis and treatment have failed to help them.

But are medical intuitives reliable diagnosticians? A study examining whether they could accurately diagnose pregnancy showed they could not.[4] Another study correlating intuitive diagnosis of disc disease with magnetic resonance imaging (MRI) showed that the psychics were accurate 54 percent of the time, whereas the MRI was accurate 90 percent of the time.[5] A more recent study found that medical intuitives were 94 percent accurate in their ability to locate and evaluate the participant's primary physical issue (49 percent of participants had a known diagnosis).[6] Keep in mind this was based on the patient's self-reporting, not objective measures such as a laboratory test or radiology study. Also, one of the researchers is a medical intuitive and medical intuition teacher, so there's always a risk of bias when someone might have an agenda to prove or disprove what they personally teach and practice. Clearly, more research is needed.

We know science doesn't do a great job of measuring subjective things, such as whether someone can pray hard or whether they're good at medical intuition, especially in the sterile and high-pressure environment of a laboratory, which doesn't lend itself to conditions that foster good intuitive hits. But still, those aren't great odds.

Because she had benefited personally from the input of a medical intuitive in finding a cure for her own illness, I asked Cynthia her opinion of these studies. She made the valid point that one of these studies lacked power given the case size—a single healer—which makes the data not particularly trust-worthy. She told me, "Intuition is, of course, not 100 percent accurate, even for the best intuitives. Analytical data is never 100 percent accurate either. But we accept analytical data when it's far less than 100 percent, whereas we don't want to accept intuition unless it proves itself to be close to 100 percent. The latter is more susceptible to misguided error, though, and abuse. I understand the justified hesitation to trust it."

She's also uncertain her intuition would test well in a laboratory. She said,

> I've experienced challenges myself with intuition and "diagnosing" per medical diagnostics—because with intuition, we're tapping into subtle energies. We may well pick up imbalances or pathologies before diagnostics can pick them up. We also know this through integrative medicine and functional medicine, where the standard labs are classically within normal limits. But with subtler and more nuanced testing, we can detect abnormalities. So there's that piece too. A medical intuitive may pick up something before it becomes obvious on a standard diagnostic, for example.

She also admitted, "I know my intuitive capacity goes down when I'm being 'tested.' It puts me into my egoic mind. I imagine that for more seasoned intuitives, this is less a factor, but setting it up for empirical test-ing seems inherently to interfere with subtle energies." There's the same catch-22 when it comes to science and Sacred Medicine.

MUSCLE TESTING

Although medical intuition is commonly used in Sacred Medicine to diag-nose illness, it tends to be unreliable as a standalone test. It might, however, be more useful alongside other diagnostic tools—both conventional and alternative, such as muscle testing. Millions of practitioners use muscle test-ing to verify their intuition or check the body wisdom of the client.

When I started my Sacred Medicine journey, my only exposure to muscle testing was through a friend in New York City. We were in a bustling restaurant when one of her other friends said, "Let's muscle test the new boyfriend!" One of them pressed down my friend's arm while she said the guy's name. Her arm went down, which apparently meant he was a dud. There was a collective sigh. I didn't understand what was going on, and her friends explained that her mind might like this guy, but her body and intuition didn't. They described muscle testing as another type of knowing and used it for everything from dating to grocery shopping to health-care decisions. Everyone but me was a devotee, and they seemed bewildered I could manage to navigate life relatively successfully without it. They swore their muscle tests were less fickle and misguided than their minds.

My friend texted the poor guy and told him it was over. I felt sorry for him and wondered how I'd feel if I got dumped over a muscle test.

A year or two later, at the beginning of my Sacred Medicine research, I received a muscle test from an energy healer sitting next to me at a luau in Hawaii, after a conference where I'd just given a keynote speech. According to her, the handsome surfer sitting across from us had hinted he'd like to go paddleboarding with me, and I had completely missed it. Knowing I was recently divorced, the healer sensed there was chemistry between the surfer and me but that I might be clueless. Nudging me gently, she asked if I wanted to go to the bathroom. Because I didn't have to pee, I was confused until the healer glanced at the surfer. *Aha!*

Leading me to the lawn in front of the hotel, the healer asked me to put out my arm parallel to the ground. She instructed, "Say 'I want to go on a date with the hot surfer.'" I complied, and she told me to resist her pressure as she pushed down on my outstretched arm. My arm dropped to my side as if I had no muscle strength.

She nodded and explained that she had just performed a muscle test and that although my words were saying I wanted to go on a date with the surfer, my body was signaling otherwise. It was common in her practice, she explained, that many of her clients came to her for help because they weren't getting something they wanted—a cure for an illness, a romantic relationship, weight loss, money, or fulfillment of a creative dream. According to her interpretation of my muscle test, my conscious mind wanted the sexy surfer to ask me out, but the muscle test reflected an unconscious desire not to go on a date, probably because I was afraid of getting hurt because of my recent heartbreak.

She retested me with the phrase, "If it's safe, I want to go on a date with the sexy surfer." This time my arm stayed strong.

Nodding, the healer said, "Classic," explaining that often we want something, but we're simultaneously blocking it "energetically" because we're afraid it might not be safe to fulfill the desire for some reason. With a quick demonstration of the "energy-shifting" technique she uses to help people clear their unconscious blocks, she identified and then "treated" my core Daddy wound, helped me "shift my energy," then retested my arm strength.

"Again! 'I want to go on a date with the sexy surfer.'" I held out my arm and repeated the phrase. This time my arm stayed strong.

The healer said, "Good. You're ready, at least for now. But you'll need more work if you want to make it stick. This is a quick fix."

Five minutes later, the sexy surfer kissed me under a banyan tree, and we made a date to go paddleboarding. Was it mere coincidence or had "shifting my energy" somehow made me more available for a kiss?

The next day at lunch, the healer and I were sitting together discussing the menu, and she said, "Why don't you let your body decide?" Usually, I pick what I like. Just for fun, she muscle tested me for each menu item until we got a positive result. Apparently, my arm wanted the vegetarian Indian plate, although my tummy would have ordered the coconut shrimp. I ordered the shrimp anyway. I could get Indian food anywhere—but we were in Hawaii!

After that encounter, I was more attuned to how frequently people in my social circles seemed to be muscle testing situations. Was this a fad, or had they been doing it all along, and I just hadn't noticed? I observed laypeople using it to choose which apartment to move to, job to take, invitation from an online dating site to accept, or vacation to go on. They would make a statement that began with "It's aligned for me to . . . ," interpreting "yes" if the test was strong and "no" if it wasn't.

If a test like this has any efficacy, validity, and reproducible reliability, we could muscle test patients like this:

It's in my highest good to . . .

> get surgery for my cancer.
> get chemotherapy for my cancer.
> get radiation for my cancer.
> decline all conventional treatments for my cancer.
> find Sacred Medicine treatment for my cancer.

You get the gist. What if we could muscle test appropriate doses, frequency, and duration of treatment to customize care? Treatment protocols are standardized, so we can test them in scientific studies, but human beings are *not* standardized. An individual patient's needs might be unique and hard to individualize from the statistical model of evidence-based treatment. As unscientific as it is, maybe the more subjective muscle test could add another data point to medical decision making, creating space for subjectivity during our otherwise objective attempts to standardize treatment.

UNDERSTANDING MUSCLE TESTING

To make sense of this diagnostic practice, I interviewed dozens of healers who use muscle testing. I asked them about method, purpose, reliability, and how to troubleshoot confusing results. Finding consistent answers was as difficult as finding healers who use the same terminology to describe energy anatomy, but there was some overlap. Some proponents claim the muscle test uses the body to bypass the conscious mind. You might say it's testing somatic or intuitive intelligence to override mental intelligence. The test relies upon the body's muscle strength to determine what's good for the body, what's true or aligned, like a lie-detector test would. Essentially, muscle testing is based on the hypothesis that the body will not let you tell a lie. Therefore, if you hold a thought or question in your mind or a substance in your hand, your muscle will be strong if the thought is true or if the substance is beneficial, whereas your muscle will be weak if the thought is untrue or the substance is detrimental.

Family physician and energy psychologist Kristin Holthuis describes muscle testing as a bridge between the conscious and subconscious mind, a way to know something that helps circumvent analysis or logic (mental intelligence) and access other reliable ways of knowing. Especially for people whose intuitive intelligence is blocked or who have lost access to their somatic intelligence (often through trauma), muscle testing can be a portal to ways of knowing familiar to many Indigenous people but from which modernization has disconnected us.

Many practitioners allege that the conscious mind often wants something—such as being cured from an illness, earning more money, or meeting a soul mate—but a deep part of the unconscious doesn't, much as my muscle test responded to the surfer. It's as if we have one foot on the gas and one on the brake. Healers often use muscle testing to reveal this inner polarization. In other words, if you feel befuddled because you want to lose weight, yet you've tried every diet and exercise regimen and you're gaining weight with each attempt, muscle testing "I want to lose weight" might indicate that although the conscious mind might want to lose weight, some other aspect of you might not want that.

According to the neuroscientists at Cambridge University who developed the Passive Frame Theory, our conscious mind influences our thoughts only a small fraction of the time, whereas the unconscious affects our thinking and decision making the vast majority of the time (if not all the time).[7] As summarized in *Time*:

> Nearly all of your brain's work is conducted in different lobes and regions at the unconscious level, completely without your knowledge. When the processing is done and there is a decision to make or a physical act to perform, that very small job is served up to the conscious mind, which executes the work and then flatters itself that it was in charge all the time. The conscious you, in effect, is like a not terribly bright CEO whose subordinates do all of the research, draft all of the documents, then lay them out and say, "Sign here, sir." The CEO does—and takes the credit.[8]

According to this logic, if you're running on autopilot, not your Inner Pilot Light, and your autopilot wants to resist change, you might be unconsciously sabotaging your efforts at transformation—and the muscle test might reveal this. Upon further investigation of the person who wants to lose weight but can't, muscle testing might reveal that, because of childhood sexual abuse (for example), their unconscious might want them to stay overweight to protect themselves. The conscious mind might wish to weigh less, but a stronger part of the unconscious might prefer to avoid receiving sexual attention, and it might have assessed that obesity will keep the person from getting noticed. If they muscle test, "If it's safe, I want to lose weight," the muscle test might be positive. In other words, the unconscious wants to keep you safe, and that extra weight will protect you. The same might be true if you think you want to be free from physical symptoms, yet nothing seems to be working.

A WORD OF CAUTION

This is speculation, of course. It's a common belief among Sacred Medicine practitioners, but it's certainly not scientifically proven. I've found that it can be distressing to people if someone, perhaps with a self-interested agenda to prove how "right" they are, applies a muscle test to someone who has failed to fulfill a deep desire—such as losing weight or finding a soul mate or getting pregnant—to try to "prove" to them that they don't really want it. Especially when someone has a potentially life-threatening or chronic illness, if someone who lacks empathy uses a muscle test to suggest that they want to be sick or don't want to get well, it can feel like a shaming, blaming, boundary-violating trauma.

Because of this risk of harming the person being muscle tested, it's crucial to resist the temptation to go rooting around in the deep unconscious willy-nilly. This can do more damage than good. Because muscle testing is commonly used by energy psychologists, as I discuss in chapter 12, many healers who specialize in treating trauma caution against practicing muscle testing as a do-it-yourself practice at home to test for delicate results. It's one thing to test for whether your body prefers peaches or pears or for the energy medicine tool or supplement most conducive to your healing. It's another if you have no memory of childhood sexual abuse but muscle test "I was sexually abused" and get a "yes." If you muscle test "I want to be cured" and discover that your muscle test says no, or you test "I want to die" and get a yes, this could be dangerously unsettling if you're not in the presence of a good therapist who can help you get appropriate treatment immediately.

Unfortunately, many healers are not trauma informed, do not apply care and sensitivity to their use of muscle testing, and might use it in boundary-violating and retraumatizing ways. You might want to be careful about how you use muscle testing and how you let potentially unskillful healers use it on your behalf. Muscle testing can be so damaging in the wrong hands, applied in the wrong way, that I considered not even mentioning it. But it's so commonly used by healers—and so ubiquitously misused on the internet—that I wanted to caution you, dear reader, and teach you how ethical, trauma-informed therapists and doctors I trust use muscle testing so that you can spot those who might harm you and protect yourself.

How else might muscle testing harm you? I once watched a famous life coach use muscle testing to predict when an infertile woman would get pregnant. The suffering woman was elated to hear she would conceive in three months. I watched her heart get crushed when this coach's "prediction" proved inaccurate. Had she not been as strong and well supported as she was, this could have triggered a suicide attempt, overdose, or other potentially lethal backlash.

Although I believe ignorance rather than malice caused that situation, I've seen people use muscle testing to manipulate, coerce, and violate the boundaries of vulnerable, often traumatized people desperate for relief from suffering. I've seen practitioners desperate for money use the muscle test to convince clients to hire them: "Let's muscle test you to see if working with me will cure your cancer." When the arm is strong, what sick person wouldn't be influenced by that show of hope? I've seen practitioners who peddle supplements use the test to convince people to spend money they didn't have on supplements supposedly crucial to their recovery, even when much of the product had been proven ineffective in scientific studies. I've seen boundary-violating healers penetrate the energy field of someone—outside the scope of their practice, such as at a dinner party—and call out a core wound in public. They use the muscle test to prove they were "right," as a "gotcha" or display of power, perhaps as an attention-getting strategy meant to impress people. I've also seen countless inexperienced but well-intentioned healers simply perform the test incorrectly.

THE VALIDITY OF MUSCLE TESTING

Is it a *reliable* test? How could pushing someone's arm down serve as a lie detector, diagnostic assessment, or treatment decision maker? People who swear by muscle testing assert that the basic principle is that if something is unhealthy for the body or the mind is asserting something untrue, the nervous system experiences a subtle stress that weakens the muscles. This assertion led me to study how traditional lie-detector tests work. Might muscle testing be similar?

Lie-detector, or polygraph, testing measures three indicators of autonomic arousal—heart rate/blood pressure, respiration, and skin conductivity. This is based on the idea that telling a lie causes a physiological stress response that can be measured on a monitor. But stress responses cause your sympathetic nervous system to activate, releasing stress hormones such as epinephrine. If this is the case, shouldn't telling a lie make your muscle stronger, not weaker? Aren't we supposed to develop superhuman muscle strength that allows us to lift cars off people we love or flee the bad guy when we're in a fight-or-flight stress response? Why would a muscle grow weak when encountering the psychological and physiological stress of an untruth? I found conflicting evidence. Some studies suggest that stress hormones strengthen muscles.[9] Others dispute these findings.[10] As often happened during my Sacred Medicine research, science was failing to help me make sense of things.

Could science guide me in an assessment of the validity of muscle testing? If you ask believers, they'll laud the data of researcher, chiropractor, and muscle testing teacher Anne Jensen, who has published countless articles and did her graduate thesis at Oxford on the science of muscle testing. Her results were published in "The Accuracy and Precision of Kinesiology-Style Manual Muscle Testing (KMMT)" in *Complementary and Alternative Medicine*.[11] Study participants underwent muscle testing on verifiable, indisputable truths or lies. These results were compared with those of participants assessed by practitioners using intuition alone. Forty-eight muscle testing practitioners were partnered with forty-eight test patients. In another segment of the study, human muscle testers were compared with machines. The study found that muscle testing was significantly more accurate than intuition alone or chance (60 percent accurate in differentiating truth from lies). In the discussion, she poses the question, "Is 60 percent accurate good enough in a clinical context?" and concludes that more research is needed before we can validate this technique as a "good enough" test. Certainly, a conventional medical diagnostic test with only 60 percent accuracy would not be considered a reliable standalone test. That's why tests such as screening mammograms that might be accurate in diagnosing breast cancer only 50 percent of the time in women with dense breasts are always followed up with more accurate, but more potentially invasive or expensive, tests, if results are concerning.[12] What would be the follow-up test to validate something found in the deep unconscious on a muscle test?

On the flip side, German scientists studied four practitioners muscle testing seven patients to see if the methodology could differentiate water from wasp venom, and the muscle test didn't work at all. Advocates of muscle testing hypothesized that water would result in a strong muscle test and venom would weaken the muscle. Altogether, 140 muscle tests were performed, leading the researchers to conclude that muscle testing is hogwash.[13] Two more studies found that muscle testing nutritional deficiencies and their replacements was no more reliable than chance.[14]

The skeptics explain away the results of muscle testing as mere "ideomotor effect," a psychological phenomenon wherein someone makes motions unconsciously in a way that looks magical, as might happen with a Ouija board. Anne Jensen disputed such a notion in a study in *Energy Psychology*.[15]

Suffice it to say that muscle testing does not qualify as an evidence-based diagnostic test. Conventional medicine has rigorous standards regarding the sensitivity and specificity of a diagnostic test to which the protocol must be adhered to be used by mainstream doctors. Muscle testing doesn't even come close to reaching these standards.

So why even mention it? I have four reasons. The first is because millions of Sacred Medicine practitioners swear by it, so any book surveying the landscape of this territory would be incomplete without mentioning it. Second, I've benefited from working with an excellent energy psychotherapist who used it on me throughout my trauma treatment, which really helped, healed, and transformed me. Third, it's my professional opinion that when muscle testing is used safely and appropriately by ethical, agenda-free, trauma-informed healers, it might be a helpful diagnostic and therapeutic tool under the right circumstances. Last but most important, I'm covering muscle testing because I want to educate you, dear reader, not to scare the crap out of you but so you can have your eyes wide open, using your discernment to protect yourself from having it misused on you in ways that might hurt you or make you vulnerable to unskillful or even dangerously corrupt con artists disguising themselves as healers.

Before I share the best way to perform a muscle test, I'll review the factors experts in the field believe can make a muscle test inaccurate, so you'll understand why the protocol I'll share for performing an optimal muscle test is so fussy. Keep in mind that none of the scientific studies I read controlled for all these impossible-to-control variables; for example, how would a researcher test for whether the muscle tester had a hidden agenda?

Remember: I'm reporting what healers have told me about how to ensure an accurate muscle test, but I cannot confirm scientifically that this is the "correct" way to do a muscle test. I also cannot confirm that this is the *only* right way to do a muscle test, so take it with a grain of salt if your own healer is doing it differently and has been through your discernment process and earned your trust.

Also, because many healers practice remotely via internet or phone, they often learn to surrogate muscle test themselves on behalf of the testee, and this is standard practice for some advanced energy psychologists, such as those trained in Advanced Integrative Therapy (AIT). But be careful with someone who claims to be able to muscle test you accurately without touching you. Although my own therapist surrogate muscle tested me during my trauma treatment—and it helped me—I have seen others abuse surrogate muscle testing.

If you start playing around with muscle testing, you're likely to discover a curious side effect. The more you practice, the more you're likely to boost your own intuitive abilities. If you feel called to do so, approach it playfully. Try testing things you can easily prove or disprove, so you can get feedback on how you're doing, such as using muscle testing to figure out the age of someone whose age you don't know.

You'll have to decide for yourself, and please don't take my word for it, but I concluded that, for me, muscle testing is a useful way to access certain Whole Health Intelligences beyond mental intelligence. That doesn't mean mental intelligence isn't also valid—or that our intelligences might not sometimes contradict each other. But if we combine them, perhaps we can make wiser health decisions as both healers and seekers.

Factors That Can Affect a Muscle Test

1. Tester Bias or Agenda

The tester must be neutral and unattached to the outcome of the muscle test. If a skeptical researcher has a dogmatic belief that muscle testing is bogus and is trying to disprove muscle testing to get a hit of righteousness, the bias of the researcher might make the muscle test inaccurate. Similarly, if dogmatic healers or researchers are trying to prove that muscle testing works or that their intuition is accurate, this agenda can also make the test inaccurate.

2. Reversal of Electrical Polarity

Advocates of muscle testing say the human body is like a giant battery with a natural electromagnetic charge, including a positive and negative pole. If you put two similarly charged batteries head-to-head, they resist each other. If you put a positive and negative charge together, they do not resist. This kind of electrical polarity is supposed to run in a consistent direction in the human body and energy field. If the polarity of the testee is reversed, the muscle test might be inaccurate, so a good muscle test screens for this beforehand.

3. Dehydration

If the testee is dehydrated, it can alter the muscle test, so the tester should screen for this.

4. Psychological Reversals

Psychological reversal refers to unconscious ways we might sabotage ourselves, such as "upper limit syndromes," when just as something is starting to go well, we hit an unconscious threshold of how much good we can let in and wind up spoiling it. There are times when the muscle test is affected by these reversals, including any fears about the outcome of the test, feeling threatened by a deeply held core belief, worrying about any change that might be called for upon receiving the answer to a muscle test, attachment to a certain answer, or dissociation and lack of presence of the testee. For example, if you are testing someone about a trauma, and part of the unconscious does not want to even touch this painful realm, this might interfere with the muscle test. Such resistance can be screened for and treated if present.

5. Accuracy Requiring the Right Statement

Testing one clear binary statement at a time is essential. The phrase has to be a statement, not a question, and you should break it down into one thing you're testing at a time. For example, testing "It's in my highest good to move to California" might produce an equivocal result. Maybe it's aligned for you to move but not to California. It would be preferable to test those two aspects separately: "It's in my highest good to move" and "California is in my highest good as a new home."

6. You Can't Muscle Test the Future!
This is not a crystal ball. Muscle testing is measuring only what is true in this present moment. Because humans have free will and energy is shifting all the time, the future is untestable.

7. Injured Muscles
Obviously, if there's a shoulder injury, muscle testing the sore arm might not provide valid results. But any muscle group can be used for muscle testing, so just test a different, uninjured muscle group. If someone's muscles are all injured because of muscle illness or paralysis, surrogate muscle testing can be used (the healer tests herself or himself on your behalf, or another individual is used as a surrogate if you're not able to be in the physical presence of the tester). But surrogate muscle testing is an advanced skill that can only be trusted in expert hands, so keep your discernment in high gear if you're letting someone surrogate muscle test you.

Keep in mind that all diagnostic tests have risks, including screening tests such as mammography, which carries the risk both of missing a cancer when it's there and of overprescribing treatment for a cancer that might have gone away on its own. Muscle testing is no exception, but you can minimize potential risks by knowing how to spot a test performed according to the recommendations of those considered experts in the field. All muscle tests (and all muscle *testers*) are not created equal, although science has no standardized screening process. But if you know what's necessary to perform an accurate test and how *not* to use muscle testing, you can reap or share the benefits and minimize the risks.

The Optimal Way to Perform a Muscle Test

Adapted from Asha Clinton's Advanced Integrative Therapy and Kristin Holthuis's
Comprehensive Energy Psychology Muscle Testing protocols

Formulate the statement you wish to test. Choose a simple, binary, yes/no statement.

Stay neutral, ground yourself, ask your ego to relax and step aside, and center yourself.

Get consent. Say to the person you're testing something like, "We're going to use muscle testing to access your body's wisdom and bypass your mind. If that's okay with you, we'll do that now." If the person you're testing resists, stop, answer questions, and proceed only if consent is clearly given.

Check for injuries. Ask if the testee has shoulder injuries or weakness. Other muscle groups can be used if there are injuries to the deltoid.

Position yourself. Stand or sit close to the side of the testee, but do not face them directly or make eye contact because blending your energy field with theirs can muddy the results. Place two or three fingers on the testee's wrist bone.

Position the testee. Have the testee hold their arm straight out to the side at ninety degrees.

Cue the testee verbally. Say, "Meet my resistance when I say 'hold.'" Wait half a second after saying "hold" before pushing down.

Check for polarity. To test for whether the body's "polarity" is normal, have the testee put one hand a few inches above the head, palm down. Test the muscle strength of the arm. The arm should be strong if the polarity is normal. Have the testee flip the direction of the hand so the palm is facing upward. Retest the muscle strength. The arm should be weak when the palm faces up. If so, polarity is normal. If not, have the testee do Cook's Hookup. (Sit in a chair, cross the left leg over the right, put the left foot just above the right knee. Hold the bottom of the left foot with the left hand and the left ankle with the right hand. Breathe deeply for several breaths, then retest.)

Check for dehydration. If the testee is dehydrated, it can alter the muscle test. To assess whether the testee is dehydrated, ask them to pull on a few strands of hair and test muscle strength. If the testee is adequately hydrated, the arm should be strong. If the arm is weak, give them a glass of water and wait a few minutes to retest. If the testee is bald, use body hair.

Check for resistance or "psychological reversals." Have the testee say "I have reversals" as a muscle test is performed. If the muscle is strong, this means reversals are present and must be treated before proceeding. If no reversals are present, the muscle test will be weak. If psychological reversals are present, you can rub your neural-lymphatic reflex points, also known as your "sore spots," which are located on either side of the chest. Trace your hand three inches down from the base of the throat and three inches to each side of the sternum, then palpate with your fingertips until you find a spot about the size of a quarter that is tender or sore when you push on it. Gently rub those two spots for about ninety seconds to correct for reversals.

Do a test run. Have the testee say, "My name is . . ." The arm should lock. Have them say "My name is [something that is not their name.]" The arm should unlock. You can play with testing birthdays, age, and other known statements to ascertain what someone's "yes" and "no" feel like, and demonstrate to the testee how this will work.

Test the phrase. Have the testee state the statement you wish to test. Wait one to two seconds to let the statement land in the consciousness and body of the testee. Say, "Meet my pressure," and gently and steadily push down with two to three fingers in a gradually accelerating manner. Do not press for more than three seconds. Pressure should be light—enough to meet the resistance. Don't "floor it" or jerk the arm. Smoothly increase pressure until either a "lock" (strong/yes) or "unlock" (weak/no) is felt. If the tester presses down and the arm locks and is strong, it's a "yes." If the tester presses down and the arm unlocks or weakens, it's a "no."

Test the statement's opposite. If you're testing "It's aligned for me to take vitamin C" and it's strong, also test "It's not aligned for me to take vitamin C." The statement's opposite should be weak.

Chapter 9

FIRST, DO NO HARM

When we're in the territory of paradoxes, as we are when we're talking about Sacred Medicine, we'd be wise to remember that wherever there is light, there is shadow. Carl Jung might say that the more light there is, the more dominant the shadow—unless we reveal, examine, and integrate light and shadow into wholeness; that is, healing.

Many spiritual seekers, especially in the New Age, where there is no real lineage or system of institutional checks and balances that might protect people from this kind of misunderstanding, mistakenly think it's possible for humans to become pure light, free of shadow. You might even hear people refer to themselves as "light workers," and if so, watch out. Those who think they're full of light are often the ones most blind to their own darkness, not because they're bad people but because they are *hurt people*—and hurt people hurt people. In other words, unless you're able to do the deep dive of shadow work—to see, acknowledge, heal, and integrate your more shadowy, less rational, instinctive blind spots, they tend to come out unexpectedly.

I hadn't fully realized this paradoxical nature of Sacred Medicine—and the healers who practice it—until I encountered the corruption of some Sacred Medicine healers. I was shocked, then disillusioned and disappointed, but only because of my own unintegrated shadow and tendency to idealize spiritual types. I'd been naïve and idealistic, so I made the mistake many people do—assuming if someone has enough spiritual power to cure cancer, if someone can induce miracles that sound biblical, they must be like Jesus.

Bill Bengston tried to disavow me of this notion. He laughed aloud at the idea that healers should be placed on a spiritual pedestal. After all, he lovingly referred to his teacher, Ben Mayrick, as Asshole's Greatest Hits. Ben might have had many talents, including the ability to cure diseases others couldn't seem to, but Bill assured me Ben was anything but holy. Bill also didn't want to be saddled with weighty psychological messiah projections himself.

I now see my error and have a better understanding of why I once made that mistake. I share my insights as a way to help educate you so you can keep yourself safe. First, I offer a warning. This chapter touches on sexual and narcissistic abuse, spiritual cults, abuses of power, and the psychology of what might make healers vulnerable to abusing power and what might make those who seek them susceptible as prey for those tempted to abuse that power. Please be forewarned so that if this chapter brings up acute triggers, you have the support you need to deal with any issues that might flare up. If you don't have good support, feel free to skip ahead. If you choose to read on and start feeling wobbly, please take a break and get professional help if you need it.

I'll start by saying that virtuosity *in no way* equates to spiritual enlightenment, morality, ethical practices, benevolent intentions, or integrity. We wouldn't expect rock stars to be holy just because they can move us with what comes out of their guitars. Most know better than to assume movie stars are as sweet as the parts they play or they're deserving of savior status just because they can touch us with an Oscar-winning performance or give a convincing portrayal of a deity. We wouldn't compare Michael Jordan to Jesus, even though his three-point swooshes from the opposite side of the court might feel heaven-sent. Some people are skilled at moving energy with their music, some can touch us with their beauty and their acting, some might be said to move the Holy Spirit through them on a football field, and others can cure disease with their hands. No talent makes somebody a perfect, flawless human.

There are healers and gurus who want you to *believe* they're spiritually special, but that doesn't mean they are. Healers with the ability to move energy and affect disease remission are *no different* from other virtuosos. Some are kind, loving, ethical people who have gotten their traumas treated, integrated their shadows into their wholeness, and can be trusted. Others aren't. Usually, the ones who cannot be trusted cover up their shadow by spiritual bypassing and have been teaching others to do the same, light-washing their injurious behavior with "I'm waking you up" or "Your soul signed up to have me abuse you so you can develop spiritually through these triggers."

This realization can be especially painful for people with a history of childhood trauma, lacking "good enough" parents who nurtured and modeled healthy, secure attachment. It's as if many of us, myself included, have a strong impulse to idealize spiritualized parental figures, perhaps looking to replace unhealthy relationships with our parents with an enlightened, perfect one. We might be drawn to those with seemingly transcendent powers like moths to the flame, and we want to give *our* power away to these folks, as if to absolve ourselves of the responsibility to navigate an uncertain world. *If only Perfect Mommy or Perfect Daddy told me how to live and dictated how I can get a gold star in Life, I wouldn't feel so vulnerable, lonely, and threatened by often-harsh reality.* By abdicating personal responsibility and allowing oneself to be infantilized by that spiritualized parent, we hope that we can feel safe with someone we trust. In a therapeutic relationship, as with a skilled trauma therapist, this dynamic is expected, and therapists are trained to deal with those transference issues and projections. But in the world of spirituality, this dynamic goes awry. Unfortunately, this is how vulnerable people get seduced into cults.

The problem with pedestals is that if you put someone up that high and leave yourself defenseless, there's no place for that person you've deemed superhuman to go but down—and you're utterly unshielded from winding up gutted and retraumatized when they ultimately turn out to be imperfectly human, maybe even in ways that echo how your parents hurt you. Although reality can be hard to bear, there's no such thing as human perfection, and anyone who tries to convince you otherwise is probably exploiting you to feed their own trauma-induced need for worthiness, attention, specialness, and grandiosity.

When I began talking openly about the shadow of Sacred Medicine in my workshops, a surprising number of my students wept. This was before #MeToo, and I hadn't realized I was touching a personal and collective wound until hundreds of people told me stories of how they were raped by their shaman, molested by their guru, or swindled by their healer.

After one of those hurt people got therapeutic treatment, she tried to make sense of what had happened and wrote to me:

It's pretty basic snake oil salesmanship. Convince people they are special. Inflate their wounded self-worth by telling them they're the chosen one, here to do something grandiose in this lifetime. Convince them they're here from the Pleiades, on a rescue mission to save Planet Earth. Or tell them they're an old soul who has lived thousands of incarnations as someone gifted. Hook into their deepest childhood enmeshment, abandonment, or neglected wounds to make them dependent on the healer to get another fix of grandiosity and specialness. Tell them they'll never achieve their grand mission unless they keep getting the next round of treatment from the healer. Reveal to them that they have a glamorous past-life trauma that requires the healer's special form of expensive exorcism—for example. Just keep them coming back for more revelations of how special they are, as they parasitically feed the healer's sense of specialness. Now you've got them ensnared. If they tell you that you need to sleep with them to achieve that mission, or if they convince you to put yourself thousands of dollars in debt, you'll do it—because you've been groomed.

Our culture is in a massive reckoning with how we deal with influential people who abuse their power. From the #MeToo movement to #BlackLivesMatter, to two Trump impeachments and the investigation of an insurrection at the US Capitol, everyone in power—from Hollywood producers to yoga gurus to politicians to cops to billionaire pedophiles and wife cheaters to online messianic wellness influencers to famous healers—is being examined and called to accountability. It's about time! This behavior is nothing new; prominent people have been abusing power for millennia. But now a groundswell of public opinion has decided that nobody is free from inspection and consequences, neither presidents nor billionaires, gurus nor healers.

This shift is so fresh and abrupt that for many people, shining a light on so many cultural blind spots is difficult to do without feeling blinded. It hurts when vulnerable people who have been traveling on pilgrimages to Brazil find out a healer they trusted, such as so-called John of God, has been incarcerated as a serial sex offender. When countless yoga gurus who claimed to cure diseases were outed by devotees as being rapists, thieves, and abusers, those vulnerable to "perfect parent" projections were stunned and devastated. If you're one of those people, dear reader, and you found yourself wondering, "Who can I trust?" you're truly not alone—and I'm so sorry you got hurt.

WE ALL MIGHT BE VULNERABLE

People often feel foolish, humiliated, or stupid after they realize they've been conned or seduced by someone with shady ethics, but it can happen to anybody, including me. Maybe some people who experienced less trauma or have healed their trauma and honed their discernment more pointedly are less vulnerable. But given the number of people I've met harmed by spiritual leaders, gurus, shamans, priests, and healers, I want you to know you're not alone if you're among us. I know a trauma therapist and yoga teacher who specializes in guru abuse—and her practice is booked. I also know a lot of spiritual cult survivors, and the residue of pain this kind of trust betrayal and trauma can leave behind is tragic. If you've been vulnerable to this, I sincerely hope you have the access and resources to get the help you need to heal those traumas and integrate the experience.

I'll start by telling you my own story, though it might seem trivial compared with the kinds of abuse way too many people have experienced at the hands of healers and gurus. One of the healers whose work I studied for this book groomed me with the same tactics, convincing me he had been my teacher in an ancient Egyptian mystery school in a past life, which was why so many mysterious phenomena were happening. *I was spiritually special!* He sought my permission to ask the Divine Intelligence (DI) how far I'd advanced in the mystery school. I gave him consent, not knowing anything about ancient mystery schools or their levels.

Apparently, the DI told him I had advanced to the level of "adept," while he had advanced to the level of "mage" (whatever that means). When I told my housemate April, she informed me, based on her understanding of esoteric Egyptian mystery school history, that I was pretty high up there, although of course the healer was higher.

The inflation worked. I felt special, chosen even. Although he was married, he made some passes at me. When I didn't reciprocate, he explained away my rejection: "That's because we only have five of seven chakras in resonance. Our second chakras aren't aligned." I didn't get raped or molested like many women do in such situations. Instead, he cheated me out of a great deal of potential income and wound up owing me money he never paid back. After three years of almost daily contact, he disappeared without a trace. I felt gutted, humiliated, disposed of, and worthless, like I had no more value than a scrap of dirty toilet tissue. Of course, this activated my deepest core wound of never feeling good enough for my impossible-to-please perfectionist mother and flooded me with shame—the emotions frequently evoked when people experience such exploitation. As with my mother, I thought he loved me, but it turned out he was mostly using me.

How and why does this happen? How in heaven's name can we make sense of this without dehumanizing corrupt or exploitative healers and gurus, casting them out of our capacity for compassion by labeling them monsters and potentially dismissing the value of the legitimate gifts some have? How can such gifted people wind up so screwed up? I found some helpful insights in an animated film directed by Michel Ocelot based on elements from West African folktales—*Kirikou and the Sorceress*.

KIRIKOU AND THE SORCERESS

Kirikou was born in a West African village, mysteriously capable of speaking and walking immediately after birth. Kirikou's mother was overjoyed by her precocious baby, but she had bad news for him. Their village was in grave danger. An evil sorceress had dried up the fresh spring they relied on for water, and the villagers couldn't survive without it. Their strongest warriors had tried to stop the sorceress from destroying their village, but all but one was devoured by her. Only Kirikou's uncle remained, so Kirikou set out with him to conquer the sorceress.

Things weren't going well for the poor uncle, who was about to be the next devoured warrior. While Kirikou watched from where his uncle was hiding him, Kirikou braced himself. If the sorceress killed the last warrior—and Kirikou along with him—his beloved mother, and the rest of the village, was doomed.

Kirikou might have been small, but he was cunning. The smart baby tricked the sorceress and saved his uncle. But when she continued to tyrannize Kirikou's village, he devised a plan. Taking grave risks for his tiny baby self, he made a treacherous pilgrimage to a cave in a mountain—the home of his revered grandfather. Kirikou asked his grandfather to help protect the village from the sorceress. The wise man let his grandson in on a secret—the sorceress was only evil because she had a thorn in her back.

"It's that thorn that gives her all that evil magic," the sage said.

The sorceress didn't know she had a thorn in her back, he explained. So it wasn't going to be easy. She was in pain, but she was so used to the thorn that she might not recognize how much suffering it caused. Even if Kirikou told her she had a thorn in her back and offered to help remove it, she might still be reluctant to let him take it out. Because the thorn was the source of her magic, she might not want to let that power go, even if it meant she would hurt less.

If Kirikou wanted to save his village from the sorceress, he was going to have to do something risky and brave. To remove the thorn, he would have to sneak up behind her and pull it out before she could stop him. After the thorn was removed, she'd no longer have the power to cast spells and hurt Kirikou or the others.

This would be good news, the grandfather said, not just for the village but for the sorceress, who would return to being an ordinary villager, just like everyone else. Instead of being hated and feared, she could possibly be loved.

Kirikou did it! He tricked the sorceress into removing the thorn and recovered the villagers' stolen riches. As his grandfather predicted, free of her thorn, the sorceress transformed into a beautiful woman with no special powers who fit in with the others. The spring was restored, and the villagers cheered their good fortune. The former sorceress leaned down and kissed Kirikou, who instantly grew into a handsome adult. The villagers didn't recognize either of them and couldn't believe this beautiful woman had once been the evil witch. When the sorceress's enslaved guards turned back into villagers who had disappeared, they revealed she hadn't eaten them after all. She was welcomed into the village, no longer suffering with private, invisible pain from the thorn in her back and no longer needing to overpower and torment the villagers to compensate for that pain. Belonging and feeling loved by Kirikou and the villagers turned out to be a more healing balm than the cheap substitute of power.

HEALING OUR RELATIONSHIP TO POWER

When I heard the Kirikou parable, I realized we are all vulnerable to a sorceress's spell when we are sick—or when our loved ones are. We are such easy prey when we are suffering or feel helpless to aid a loved one in pain. It's easy to throw caution to the wind even for a glimmer of hope, especially if someone tempts us with an easy way out of our suffering.

When I look back on the beginning of my Sacred Medicine journey, especially the bliss-hunting years, I can see how those spells had been cast on me and on others who were vulnerable. I can't tell you how many healers, shamans, and gurus fed me lines about how special, powerful, and chosen I was—catnip for my inner child who felt so fundamentally worthless and unlovable.

I'm sure we each have an Achilles' heel, but mine was my fascination and thirst for power, born of having been *overpowered* by my domineering mother. It's as if my child self said, "Never again," and did what she could to try to collect power, perhaps to fend off ever being dominated and overpowered again. I realize now it's why I tried so hard as a child to develop certain gifts—to sing and dance so I could get the lead in the church musical and have power over the audience, to make straight As so I had the power of intelligence, to become a doctor who had the power to save lives, to cultivate my sensuality so I had that power over men, to write books and develop a social media following to have the power of influence, to meditate hours every day to ramp up my spiritual power. As it was for the sorceress, power was a cheap substitute for love and intimacy, not the cotton candy kind you get in memes but real heart connection, which I craved. Of course, defense strategies such as collecting power so you can avoid being overpowered, once so valuable because they helped us survive, outlive their usefulness and wind up causing more pain.

But it would take years of therapy for me to unpack all that. Before I had, if someone told me a magical story about how they could cure cancer with their hands, grow herbs out of their palms, perform surgery without anesthesia, or touch someone's forehead and grant them instant enlightenment, I was hooked, especially if they promised to teach me how to attain that magical power for myself.

In my social circles, calling a woman a witch was a compliment. Like the light workers who were blind to the shadow, we fancied ourselves Glendas, the good witches, not Elphabas, the bad witches. It wasn't until

I was in therapy years later that I learned that the "witch" and "wizard" archetypes from Jungian psychology represent the narcissist, the seductress, the spellcaster, whether the one casting that spell is Marilyn Monroe, Donald Trump, or John of God.

Although your own wounding and vulnerability to corrupt healers might be different from mine, dear reader, it's crucial to practice self-awareness and know your own potential hooks if you're going to stay safe in the spiritual candy shop. For people who felt disempowered in childhood like I did, it's easy to get seduced by power and hooked by fascination, intellectual curiosity, or a desire to acquire special power, whether it be athletic ability, intelligence, money, political might, fame, beauty, talent, or sex. If you're not a mighty athlete, amplifier-shaking guitar player, gifted actor, valedictorian, bombshell beauty, or class president, you might seek whatever power you are capable of cultivating—such as spiritual power or the power to cure disease—or the power by proxy that might come from proximity to someone we deem spiritually special, such as a guru with special healing abilities.

If healers with thorns in their backs spot us as potential easy prey, we might unintentionally allow them into our inner circle, re-creating our childhood traumas by letting ourselves be overpowered or abused, yet again, in a devastating kind of retraumatization. This can be dangerous for traumatized individuals, yet many of the people most likely to seek out spiritual circles carry the highest trauma burden. It makes sense that people who are hurting would want to do anything to try to transcend their pain, whether through meditation, yoga, energy healing, Tantric sex, breathwork, or other potential spiritual narcotics.

The Kirikou story left me with one unanswered question. If the sorceress's evil magic went away when her pain was gone, what would happen to wounded healers if *their* thorns were extracted? Would it be possible for healers to cure disease if they were no longer wounded? Would they stop being special and become ordinary villagers? If so, who would serve the sick?

THE PRINCIPLE OF HARMLESSNESS

I once took an oath to "first, do no harm." The ethical principle of harmlessness is hammered into medical students. We are taught that along with the power to save lives comes the burden of responsibility to protect the patient from the harm our power could cause. There are many ways to harm our patients: by overriding their free will and right to informed consent; through human error, given that the tools we wield can cure *and* kill; by abusing our power and using it for self-serving ends, such as financial gain, satisfying our lust, or taking advantage of a patient's vulnerability to inflate ourselves. Because patients tend to trust doctors with matters of life and death, it is our responsibility to be trustworthy with that power. If we are not—because we are mere mortals who make mistakes and might have trauma around our own relationship to power and control—a series of checks and balances exists. Patients have the right to report us anonymously to the medical board, sue for malpractice, or press charges in criminal court if necessary. Our medical boards can investigate us, suspend us, or take away our licenses to practice medicine if we fail to be trustworthy with right use of power.

Admittedly, modern medicine has lost touch with some of its pure commitment to harmlessness, as evidenced by the paradox of healing: conventional medicine saves lives, and it was the third highest cause of death in the United States, at least until it got outpaced by Covid in 2020.[1] We pay lip service to patient well-being—and most of the doctors I know care deeply about their patients. But far too often, patient well-being is in conflict with the financial bottom line, not set by doctors for the most part but by hospital administrators, CEOs of for-profit insurance companies and pharmaceutical and medical device companies.

Never was this paradox of healing more obvious than in 2020, when doctors during a pandemic, unclear how best to treat Covid-19, rushed people onto ventilators, thinking they were saving lives only to discover those who refused ventilator treatment often survived, whereas many put on ventilators never got off. Doctors try to "first, do no harm," but it doesn't always work that way.

Because of this conflict between our oath to uphold harmlessness and an imperfect system that sometimes makes it impossible, many doctors suffer from what burnout researchers call "moral injury"—mental, emotional, psychological, and spiritual distress after "perpetrating, failing to prevent, or bearing witness to acts that transgress deeply held moral beliefs and expectations."[2] Because of moral injury, physician suicide, addiction, and premature death rates are skyrocketing. When you are called to become a doctor the way priests are called to the priesthood, it can feel intolerably painful to realize that we might harm as much as we heal. Healing and harming might even be two sides of the same coin. Even if we do our own trauma work to heal and integrate our own shadow elements, potential side effects of medical intervention can sometimes have the power to cause harm, even when applied with extreme care and the best intentions.

Sacred Medicine practitioners are not immune. Like surgery, chemotherapy, and other powerful conventional medical interventions, Sacred Medicine can have the power to cure, but it also has the power to cause great harm. When you give consent to someone messing with your energy field or poking around in the depths of your core wounds and deep unconscious, you are taking a risk. I don't mean to frighten you or make you feel paranoid; I do, however, warn you to use the same caution in choosing a Sacred Medicine practitioner as you would when picking a surgeon. Your most powerful protection against being victimized by wounded healers with thorns in their backs who haven't done their shadow work is your connection to your Whole Health Intelligences, which can help you discern which healers you can trust and which you're better off steering away from. Asking people you trust for referrals will also help you screen those you should steer clear of. It's relatively easy to spot the troublemakers after you know what to look for and after you've opened your access to these ways of knowing. I'll give you some tips about what to watch for at the end of this chapter.

The problem is that most healers have neither accountability nor oversight. If a doctor, therapist, or priest abuses power, there is a system, albeit imperfect, for doling out consequences and holding them accountable. No such system exists for many kinds of healers. The lack of regulation in the field of healing will continue to leave us vulnerable until we find a way to regulate the field and provide more safety.

ALL POWER CAN BE ABUSED

The Marvel Comics character Doctor Strange is a neurosurgeon who injures his hands and seeks help from the Ancient One, who appears to be an all-powerful mystic with access to healing powers and eternal life. But in the end (spoiler alert!), Doctor Strange discovers the Ancient One is drawing power from the Dark Dimension. In other words, some alleged light workers seem to be sucking their power from the shadows. The saying

"Power corrupts" doesn't just apply to political, financial, sexual, or charismatic power; it can also apply to spiritual power.

This doesn't mean healers who abuse their power are evil; it means they're traumatized. Like the sorceress, they have a hidden thorn causing pain. If someone skilled at healing trauma doesn't help them remove the thorn, they can cause considerable damage. As Mariana Caplan wrote in *Eyes Wide Open*, "Those who possess spiritual discernment have learned this skill in relationship to spiritual matters, and they can consistently make intelligent, balanced, and excellent choices in their lives and in relationship to their spiritual development. Their eyes are wide open, and they see clearly."[3] Only when we face our shadows with sober humility and accept responsibility as conscious patients, clients, disciples, and students can we develop the spiritual discernment that helps us see the unconscious shadow motivations of others.

Paramahansa Yogananda's *Autobiography of a Yogi* begins when he is a young man searching for his spiritual master. He encounters many Indian spiritual teachers with superpowers, known as *siddhis* in the yogic texts. One swami showed off his power by taming tigers and levitating, another by curing fatal illnesses. There was one who could materialize perfume and make it exude any scent from the skin of his devotees.

When this Perfume Saint invited Yogananda to become a student and spend twelve years learning to materialize perfume out of thin air to demonstrate the power of God, Yogananda asked, "Sir, is it necessary to prove God? Isn't He performing miracles in everything, everywhere?"

The Perfume Saint replied, "Yes, but we, too, should manifest some of His infinite creative variety."

"It seems, my honored saint, you have been wasting a dozen years for fragrances which you can obtain with a few rupees from a florist's shop."

Yogananda goes on to discuss how the manifestation happens and explains that he, too, would eventually learn, through his spiritual disciplines, the "how" of materializing matter, using breathwork and a kind of hypnotic power. But he sees it as an arrogant abuse of power to show it off: "Wonder-workings such as those shown by the 'Perfume Saint' are spectacular but spiritually useless. Having little purpose beyond entertainment, they are digressions from a serious search for God. Ostentatious display of unusual powers is decried by masters."[4]

THE CAUTIONARY TALE OF A
WOUNDED HEALER

One healer, whom I'll call Aliyah, lived in Hollywood and was a favorite among wealthy celebrities. Her healing powers were legendary, and her practice was robust through word of mouth. However, I discovered over the years there was a dark side to her gift. Using her intuitive powers to psychically "read" some bad deed a client had committed in their past, she caused them to become defenseless through humiliation. Then she would explain that their illness was the resulting karma from their bad deed and that if they wanted to be cured, they would have to donate *millions* of dollars to the healer's mission as a good deed.

Sometimes they'd fork up the money and die soon afterward, allowing her to pocket it. Other times, they'd wind up cured, and then the healer *really* had them hooked. After they were cured, they'd credit her and pledge their eternal gratitude. She would then hook them into giving her *all* their money, allegedly so she could expand her spiritual teaching and healing practice. Threatening them by telling them that their illnesses would come back unless they gave away all their wealth as an offering to God as penance for their misdeeds, she was raking in the dough. She carried out the same con repeatedly. She even extended her con to other famous healers when they got sick and conventional medicine failed to cure them.

Her assistant, who had experienced what she considered a miraculous cure for her incurable illness as a result of the healer's gifts, volunteered her services to the healer's mission for more than a decade with no pay, as her way of saying thank you. But when the assistant realized how rich the healer was becoming off of terminally ill clients and uncovered how the scam worked, she just couldn't stomach it anymore. She insisted that the healings were real, that Aliyah wasn't a total charlatan. But she cried when she told me that she stayed too long and felt ashamed that she had been an unwitting accomplice to the crimes. Unwilling to go to the cops, she just slunk away.

Over time, it became clear to me that this healer was a traumatized woman whose heart was closed. Even if her powers were real, she had been cut off from empathy, compassion, integrity, and ethics. A healer who can't extend compassion ultimately can't be trusted to use such powers for the greater good. When I heard more about her history from her assistant, which was more dramatic than even the fictional evil sorceress's tale, it all made sense to me through a trauma-informed lens.

Aliyah, the daughter of a poor farmer, was born with intuitive gifts. Once as a young toddler in her bed, she cried out for her mother, telling her to run outside because a thief was stealing from them. Her mother thought she was crazy, but when she went outside, she found that Aliyah was right. One day, a neighbor came to visit her family with her teenage daughter. The psychic toddler said out loud, "I see a baby inside her tummy." The girl was not far enough along in the pregnancy to show, so the neighbor was shocked and horrified. It was supposed to be a secret because it was taboo in her culture to have sex out of wedlock. The pregnant girl's family became infuriated, telling Aliyah's parents that if their little girl ever opened her mouth, the whole family would be outcast.

Nevertheless, word got out about the little girl who could see things. The villagers started coming by the family's hut, seeking advice and psychic readings. Every time she would tell the villagers what she saw, her parents would beat her mercilessly. Someone reported the toddler to the totalitarian government, which frowned upon all things metaphysical. Officials further traumatized the little girl by making her walk around the village wearing a paper bag over her head, with her hands tied behind her back, wearing a wooden plaque around her neck, marking her as a witch. As she marched around the village, she was publicly shamed and traumatized. The humiliation and beatings caused her to lose her mind. She ran away from home, wandering off into a mountainous area, homeless in the wilderness, hunting and gathering or coming off the mountain to beg for food at the local street market.

She took shelter in a cave, but the neighbors who still wanted psychic readings from her sought her out. They would bring food to the cave in exchange for intuitive readings. Her family shunned her and never saw her again, but someone else showed up to care for her—the head nun in a far-off temple who offered her own healing gifts to her village for free. The nun had had a dream about a little girl living in a cave who would become her apprentice. The nun knew that the girl had abilities but that she was wild and untrained and didn't know how to use them. In the dream, the nun heard, "You have to teach her how to become a healer like yourself."

The following morning, the nun went to the street market and walked right to where the little girl was begging. She found her, covered with lice, eating scraps off the street. The nun approached, inviting her to come with her, promising food, shelter, and clean clothes. Reluctant but enticed by real food, the little girl followed the nun home to the temple.

Aliyah grew stronger while the nun cared for her and attended to her needs. She grew to love the nun and enjoyed following her around every day as she did her healing work.

One day, Aliyah said to the nun, "I want to do what you do."

The nun agreed to take her on as her apprentice under one condition. If she taught her how to heal people, the little girl would have to take over as the temple's healer, taking her vows as a nun and devoting her life to offering her services to the villagers for free. It would be a sacred pact, and she would be ethically bound by the terms of the agreement. If she didn't agree, the nun would not let her apprentice. The little girl eagerly agreed.

She took to the healing work naturally, following the nun's instructions carefully, praying for many hours and honing her skills. The villagers were impressed. People started coming from far away to receive healings from the young apprentice, who was growing into a woman and would soon take her vows as a nun.

But the seductions of the world were needling their hooks into Aliyah. She found herself having rebellious fantasies about life outside the temple. She dreamed of getting married, making money, and living a worldly life. Life at the temple was so *boring*, and she was turning into a sexy, vibrant woman who wanted to live it up a little. So the night before she was to be initiated into the lineage, when she was scheduled to take her vows, the young healer ran away.

The nun's predictions came true. One horrific trauma after another plagued Aliyah, but she refused to keep her promise to use her healing powers for good. Instead, she earned a living showing off and was ultimately wooed by a prominent man who had seen her performances and was impressed with her abilities. He promised her that if she married him, he would help her get a green card and move to the United States. After they made it to Hollywood, they had to make a living. California was expensive, so the scam began.

Hearing the healer's history broke my heart. No wonder someone with that depth of trauma might grow up in such survival mode that conning vulnerable people might seem like the only option. Given how much trauma that little girl went through and how much power she ultimately developed, it would have been hard for her not to wind up troubled and abuse it, unless she got a lot of professional help. That doesn't mean she shouldn't be held accountable and that those conned shouldn't press charges. But it's difficult to write healers off as monsters when you can see the thorns in their backs.

TRUSTING YOUR WHOLE HEALTH INTELLIGENCES

When you're working with Sacred Medicine practitioners, it's helpful to learn to identify your own vulnerabilities, dear reader, so you can notice when you get hooked and use that to cue critical thinking, common sense, emotions, body awareness, and intuitive senses, calling your Whole Health Intelligences onboard.

Although I had hunches I had previously overridden, I was lured into the web of several American neoshamans who were powerful but corrupt. One of them was sexually molesting his clients, but they weren't going to the authorities and refused to press charges. Instead, they were coming to me to report the traumas. When I confronted the neoshaman and told him what I'd heard, he defended himself, saying he was in a trance when he did his healing work, and if he was engaging with a client sexually, it must have been because they needed sexual healing. He's not the first—and won't be the last—healer who might try to cause someone to abandon mental intelligence and trust his alleged intuitive intelligence instead. As I've said, you want to keep an open mind but not so open that your brains fall out.

I met another famous energy healer with a full schedule and many international requests for his allegedly miraculous treatments. As a screening interview, before I delved into studying his work or let him do a session on me, we went out to dinner, where he asked me to point out a woman, any woman. I didn't understand his request. For what?

"Just pick one," he said.

I pointed to a middle-aged woman with three kids eating pizza.

"Watch this," he said. "Keep your eye on her."

He then closed his eyes and did something with his hands, and I watched her. A minute later, she perfectly mimicked the famous scene in *When Harry Met Sally* when Sally fakes a loud orgasm to prove to Harry that women can effectively fake orgasms. Howling, writhing, and twisting in apparent ecstasy, the woman looked horrified when she saw her children's reaction and realized that the whole restaurant was staring at her. Grabbing her purse, she ran into the restroom with her hands covering her face, looking scared and humiliated.

The healer laughed as I asked, "What did you do?"

"I gave her an orgasm."

I hurried out of there. My emotional intelligence told me I didn't want to work with someone so unkind.

Another woman was referred to me by several people as a powerful priestess and healer able to cure long-standing chronic diseases that resisted conventional treatment. When I met her, I felt instantaneous and intense aversion. My solar plexus contracted, my chest hurt, I felt nauseated, and I experienced what I can only describe as a dark cloud cloaking me. She was pressing me hard to participate in a weekly invitation-only ceremony she was performing in secret. By this time, I had seen enough of the shadow side of Sacred Medicine to listen to my gut. I declined her offer and found out later that she had caught a celebrity transformational leader in her spell, exploiting her for her wealth and manipulating her for personal gain. Thank God my somatic intelligence protected me against that one.

I worked with yet another healer and planned to devote an entire chapter to her in this book, but I followed a hunch and looked at her social media feed. She had been seduced by Q-Anon conspiracy theories. I'm grateful my intuitive intelligence protected me from misleading *you*.

Some of the ethical breaches I witnessed were less obvious but still damaged people in the name of healing. I attended meditation retreats where participants were reputed to experience radical remissions and discovered that some modern-day meditation teachers are using ancient yogic practices meant to be shared only with advanced students who have been preparing for years—for their own safety. People who have hardly meditated before and have never been exposed to advanced pranayama breathwork were experiencing psychotic episodes, or what psychiatrist Stanislov Grof termed a "spiritual emergency." After opening these people up energetically, no integration support or follow-up was offered. Although some people felt they were helped by these advanced practices, others felt like their lives had been ruined. When I confronted these healers and suggested they might need to be more careful to avoid harming people, I was summarily dismissed. And why not? They were cashing in on those enormously profitable high-ticket retreats.

Other healers were obviously retraumatizing vulnerable clients in the name of healing them, especially in large-group contexts. Violating their psychic, physical, and psychological boundaries in egregious ways typically shown by abusive cult leaders, they spiritualized these boundary violations and blamed the clients for being triggered, using every spiritual bypassing trick in the book to shut down understandable resistance and anger. The alleged healers would inflate themselves, showing off how psychic they were to the other students, while the hurt students ran out the back door in humiliated tears, having had their core wound opened and left to bleed.

Witnessing such traumatic events disguised as healing broke my heart and inspired me to learn more and get more support to make sure I could lead my own workshops with safety, care, sensitivity, and support for those who might be triggered. Although it might be impossible to do certain healing work without eliciting intense emotions, I learned that there are kind, safe, and gentle ways to practice healing, like a careful dissection with teeny surgical scissors and effective anesthesia. There are also those who tear into someone with a psychic scalpel and no mitigation for the pain, who don't seem to care if someone hemorrhages or even dies by suicide. If you ever find yourself in a situation like that, dear reader, please be empowered to get up, walk out, and call a therapist—STAT.

LINES OF DEVELOPMENT

I was once told that discernment is one of the cornerstones of spiritual life. It requires us to deepen our awareness, strengthen our intuition, heal childhood trauma, open our hearts, be humble, and learn to see what *is* rather than what we project from our wounds because—*news flash!*— there is no perfect parent, no perfect human, no special enlightened being who will never let us down. Whether we like it or not, the world is populated by humans, full of sparkles and fog, compassion and deceit, talents and blind spots, love and pain. That said, we can educate ourselves so we are less naïve and more discerning.

It bears repeating that access to healing gifts has nothing to do with moral or psychological development. To help acknowledge these wide variations in human consciousness, Carole Griggs and Ted Strauss have developed the Griggs-Strauss Conscious Human Development Map.

According to this map, we develop in five areas:
- Awareness (consciousness)
- Design (uniqueness)
- Heart (emotion)
- Mind (thought)
- Body (physicality)[5]

This map helped me frame my understanding and apply more discernment and less hair-trigger judgment when I was interviewing healers. When you think about humans you know, you'll see that some are more developed in their embodiment (body)—think of elite athletes or yoga practitioners, or in the world of Sacred Medicine, Rolfing practitioners, craniosacral therapists, and acupuncturists. Others are intellectually developed (mind)—think of university professors and Nobel Prize winners—or perhaps they've developed certain mind control superpowers. Others are advanced in their spiritual development (awareness)—think of monks meditating ten hours a day for thirty years or the gurus in the *Autobiography of a Yogi*, who can cure their disciples from illness. Others have elevated levels of compassion, love, ethics, and an ardent desire to be a harmless, benevolent presence, devoted to kindness and service (heart), people such as American Civil Liberties Union (ACLU) lawyers, Mahatma Gandhi, and Mother Teresa. Some are developed in what the map calls "design," or a unique talent or expression. These people might be accomplished musicians, genius artists, skillful lovers, or unusually authentic, charismatic, humorous, or playful people. Some healers have tapped into a special method that sets them apart and might be effective at affecting the energy field of another person; however, these healers might not be kind or smart or grounded in their bodies.

Because many people do not realize that someone might be advanced in one line of development and immature in another, we might feel shocked and disillusioned to discover that someone who has a profound impact on our healing might be less developed in other areas. This might explain why Indian gurus who had lived in monastic male-only ashrams since they were children went off the rails when they came to the United States in the 1960s and had beautiful hippie women throwing themselves at them for the first time. They might have been spiritually developed, but sexually, developmentally, and morally, these gurus might have been infantile.

Recognizing that we are all on a spectrum in these lines of development—and that nobody is 100 percent developed in all areas—helps us manage our expectations of the healers we seek and work with.

FINDING AN ETHICAL HEALER

Some of the organizations in which healers congregate are finally engaging in the conversation about how to self-regulate their profession. After too many healers, nondual teachers, and yoga gurus wound up in the news with #MeToo accusations, and too many spiritual teachers and healers went the route of conspirituality, the Science and Non-Duality (SAND) community facilitated an ethics conversation spearheaded by Jac O'Keeffe and Rick Archer. This led to the formation of the Association for Spiritual Integrity (ASI), an organization of spiritual leaders who have voluntarily agreed to a code of ethics.

The Association for Comprehensive Energy Psychology (ACEP) also developed a code of ethics and an overseeing committee. Two excellent books have been published on the ethics of healing—Dorothea Hover-Kramer's *Creating Healing Relationships* and David Feinstein and Donna Eden's *Ethics Handbook for Energy Healing Practitioners*. Several training programs that teach Sacred Medicine healing methods assign these books as mandatory reading—and I recommend you use them to assess the ethics of any practitioner with whom you might work.

Despite the risks and shadows of Sacred Medicine, I don't want to discourage you from seeking skilled healers who can help you. If you feel called to find a Sacred Medicine practitioner to support you in your healing journey, always return to "Assess Your Whole Health Intelligences."

PLASTIC ANGELS

About halfway through my Sacred Medicine journey, I attended one of those big events led by a New Age healer where countless people claim to have radical remissions after they pay big money to travel to one of these mega-meditation retreats. We were on the second-to-last day, and we'd been prepared all week for the big shebang of the finale, the pinnacle of everything we'd worked for in our intense meditations. It was time for the 4:00 a.m. four-hour pineal gland meditation. We'd been told that mystical experiences and spiritual fireworks were commonplace and that some of us might experience a miracle cure or magical manifestation if we did this meditation right.

After easing our way into the breathwork, we were told to do what doctors call the *Valsalva maneuver*. You hold your breath and perform a forceful exhale against a closed airway, as if you're constipated and pushing out poop. The healer yelled at us like a football coach, "You can do it! Harder! Go for it—all the way!" This continued as we tried to push our breath from the base of the spine to the top of the head so we could coax our reluctant pineal glands into spitting out some "amrita," the famed DMT-laden "nectar of the gods" intended to open up our consciousness like a natural psychedelic. The healer warned us we might experience a hallucination, an inner world event as real as if it were happening in our outer world.

In the deepest part of my meditation, I experienced what felt like a real encounter at a discount store in a shopping mall. I was led to a room, crowded with what looked like junk, almost like a garage sale. At the center of a long plastic table stood a statue of a white angel, glowing as if it had a lightbulb inside. I couldn't resist the angel. I was drawn to it as if by a magnet. In the vision, I reached out to touch the angel, and when I did, I went down some sort of wormhole, traveling fast with stars and lights flashing on either side of an invisible tunnel. When the twisting and looping and spinning in space stopped, I was plunged abruptly into something that felt like a warm ocean of light, as if I were bathing in an illuminated hot spring. My whole being felt at peace, and I felt a rush of tenderness, as if Mother Earth were cradling me in her warm arms of unconditional love. I realized at some point that the angel was holding me.

The vision dissolved into pure feeling without imagery, just love, just peace. I have no idea how long I was held by that angel, but when the healer interrupted the meditation and told us it was time for breakfast, I felt jolted and disoriented. We were given only moments to feel our bodies and hug the person next to us before we were expected to get up and leave the room. I was not fully back from whatever journey I had been on, and I felt dizzy, ungrounded, and nauseated.

As I integrated the experience, I realized it was no accident that my "virtual reality" experience involved a plastic angel lost amid junk. Given how spirituality has been commoditized and turned into earth-killing, ocean-filling plastic junk you can buy at the countless gift shops at places such as Lourdes and Chimayo, some part of me remembered to focus on the direct experience of spirituality rather than getting distracted and seduced by plastic angels.

Paradoxically, in the vision, the false light of the plastic angel was a portal to a wormhole of direct experience, as if simultaneously drawing attention to the corruption implicit in commoditizing spirituality while compassionately acknowledging that it seems to be our human nature to commoditize the sacred. I didn't feel judged or judgmental after the meditation. I felt love for the part of myself guilty of commoditizing spirituality as well as compassion for others tempted to do the same.

How to Discern a Trustworthy Sacred Medicine Practitioner

To help you with the mental intelligence aspect of your discernment, here are a few tips.

1. **Ask for a screening interview.**

2. **Feel for the healer's heart.** Using your emotional intelligence, determine if you can feel your heart *and* the heart of the healer.

3. **Trust your gut.** Check in with your body. Is it tense or relaxed when you're with this practitioner?

4. **Check credentials.** Give your mental intelligence some assistance by asking your Sacred Medicine practitioner how they trained. In an unregulated field where anyone can hang a shingle or put up a website and claim to be a healer, it's worth checking credentials.

5. **Screen for ethics.** Look for practitioners who vow to abide by a transparent code of ethics you can ask to review.

6. **Look for healers who await your consent.** If a healer is reading your energy or starting to manipulate your field before you've agreed to a therapeutic relationship, get out.

7. **Ask to whom the healer is accountable.** Does the healer have their own professional board, therapist, or mentor who provides ongoing oversight, accountability, and consequences if power is abused? If they say they no longer need such help or feedback because their inner guidance is enough, be wary.

8. **Ask for referrals from people you trust.**

9. **Ask for permission to speak to clients who had good outcomes.** Although confidentiality must be respected, many patients who have experienced a radical remission at the hands of a healer are dying to tell their story and shout about it from the rooftops. If the healer doesn't have even one client who consents to discuss their experience, you should wonder whether they're telling the truth.

10. **Beware of exaggerated and unproven claims.** No medicine—sacred or not—works 100 percent of the time for 100 percent of cases. Ask the healer to discuss their treatment failures. If they say they haven't had any or blame the client, move on.

11. **Ask what their specialty is.** In addition to explaining what their method is not so good for, most honest healers will tell you which medical conditions their method treats best—and which they've had less success with.

12. **Avoid healers who create dependency.** True healers will empower you to strengthen your own self-healing power over time, making you less and less dependent on the healer.

Part Three

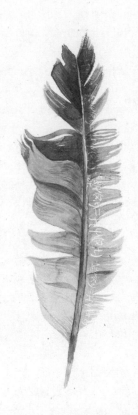

HEALING FROM
THE ROOT

was midway through my Sacred Medicine journey when I hit a critical turning point in my attempt to crack the code of healing. I certainly hadn't solved some of the great mysteries I set out to study, but pieces missing from conventional medicine were revealing themselves. A breakthrough came when I realized that many energy healers were spiritualizing trauma—and tending to it in their clients—but not always with the knowledge a cutting-edge trauma therapist might have. What might I discover if I leapt silos into the psychology department and started studying with experts who treated and saw trauma through the lens of Sacred Medicine?

Some energy healers didn't call it trauma. They called it blocked energy, stuck entities, or psychic attack, and they treated it by waving their hands around, removing daggers from the client's back, or repairing holes in the aura. Others believed that dark or stuck spots in someone's energy field were the result of trauma and the cause of disease. They also believed that unblocking them energetically and restoring flow could lead to a cure.

If that was true, was this the most effective way to treat trauma for medicinal purposes?

It made me pause and reconsider the mind-body connection, well studied but rarely practiced in mainstream medicine or psychiatry. Had the healers found a bridge that spanned the gap of mind-body dualism? I grew curious about what we mean when we talk about the "mind." Psychiatrist Daniel Siegel writes, "The mind is a relational and embodied process that regulates the flow of energy and information."[1] *Hmm . . .* doesn't that sound an awful lot like the way many healers describe energy medicine? If the mind is an emergent process in the body through which energy and information flow, might healing what got hurt in the mind simultaneously affect the body? That would make sense, at least for some kinds of physical symptoms and illnesses.

I had been orienting myself to think about the practices in part one as immediate interventions—energy transfusions meant to dose us with life force to relieve symptoms and help us function better. But are transfusions sufficient for permanent relief if the traumas that interrupt the flow of energy and information are left inadequately treated? The way I see it, if you're severely depleted, filling up your tank can give you a boost. But unless you invest in the more difficult work of diagnosing the reasons you might be leaking life force in the first place, energy transfusions might not be enough for a *cure*. If you're leaking life force because of inadequately treated traumatic energies stuck in the body, wouldn't neglecting those energy-depleting leaks be like pouring blood into your body while you were still hemorrhaging from an open wound? If we really want long-standing optimal health, wouldn't we need to stop the hemorrhage?

What drains your life force or causes it to leak, dear reader? Maybe it's a dysfunctional relationship or a soul-sucking job that requires you to violate your ethics. Maybe it's being unable to set boundaries, say no, and ask for what you need rather than caregiving for everyone else, causing your own exhaustion? Maybe it's exaggerated self-reliance that interferes with you getting help from your community when times are hard? Maybe it's feeling disconnected from Earth, nature, and the Divine? Maybe it's living in a white supremacist culture that overvalues consumption and undervalues social justice, equality, and genuine heart-opening intimacy?

What's at the root of all these life force leaks? What makes us tolerate abusive relationships and stay in jobs that deplete us? What wounds our boundary setting, interferes with our capacity for healthy interdependence, leaves us feeling spiritually disconnected, allows us to trash our planet, and affects the health and social justice of our culture?

Trauma.

This awareness was a hot track, a leopard's paw print in moist dirt, pointing me toward something that made my intuition tingle. After years of feeling lost and bewildered on my Sacred Medicine journey, I was on to something, and now, dear reader, I invite you to consider the holy grail I promised you at the beginning of the book.

Chapter 10

HEALING TRAUMA *IS* SACRED MEDICINE

* Trigger alert: The following chapter could be triggering for people with a traumatic history who struggle with mental or physical illness.

Afte years of working with healers, I realized that what ethical energy-transfusing Sacred Medicine practitioners do best is offer conditions that help people heal, feel, soften, relax, and hope. That's when I realized that good healers have one thing in common: *They offer an antidote to the traumatic aspects of traditional Western medicine.* Patients often perceive conventional medicine as frightening—cold, sterile, impersonal, chemically and technologically unnatural, rushed, disconnected, computerized, distracted, bureaucratic, distant, Godless, emotionally shallow, and prioritizing the financial bottom line over patients' well-being. After doctors have done all they can or moved on to the next patient, patients are left feeling hopeless and lonely.

What if some people with a significant trauma history have such fragile, sensitive systems that they need to be held especially tenderly when they get sick, which conventional medicine is not well equipped to deliver? All of us deserve this when we're frail and vulnerable, but perhaps some people literally *cannot tolerate* the blunt instrument of Western medicine. What if this is *not* because they're foolhardy or neurotic, as skeptics might unkindly assume? What if it's because they're our magnificent canaries in the coal mines—our tenderhearted empaths, multi-dimensional travelers, and thin-skinned love-o-meters who simply can't handle the way conventional medicine is usually delivered? It would make sense that some people might go wherever they're likely to find the gentler qualities of healing, even if it means turning away from a potential science-based cure. For those folks, when they get sick, it might be an energy healer or nothing.

At its best, Sacred Medicine offers patients the opposite of what they often find in a doctor's office or hospital—hope, safety, loving presence, personal touches, elements of nature, empathy, time and coregulation with the practitioner, warmth, a brave space for emotional expression, healing touch, ritual, and nurturing environments. Sometimes these Sacred Medicines also treat the social isolation and loneliness that can accompany illness, serving up intimate communion with others in need of healing and uplifting moments of connection with Spirit, as with pilgrimage sites, Indigenous offering rituals, meditation retreats, and communities of dance and creativity. No wonder energy healing, shamanism, spiritual pilgrimages, yoga and dance retreats, and other energy-transfusing Sacred Medicines are a multibillion-dollar industry! Who wouldn't want all those restorative blessings when you're suffering and traditional medicine has reached its limit?

Aren't these good healer qualities also what make a great psychotherapist? But therapists go to school to become experts in healing *the mind*. It makes sense that cutting-edge therapists have a leg up when it comes to skill and expertise in the realm of healing trauma, so if this form of healing is an embodied way to move energy and information throughout the nervous system and into the body—restoring flow to parts of the body where trauma might get stuck—could this make sick people miracle prone? Might we find medical miracles somewhere as mundane as the trauma therapist's office?

Although trauma as a cause of physical disease might be disputed by skeptics who resist information that contradicts their worldview, the body of scientific data linking psychological trauma and adult-onset disease is airtight. According to many sources in the mainstream medical literature, anywhere from 60–80 percent of illnesses have stress-related emotional underpinnings.[1] But what causes stress? *Trauma.*

ADVERSE CHILDHOOD EXPERIENCES (ACES) CAUSE DISEASE

If you doubt that trauma and disease are strongly linked, consider what California surgeon general and pediatrician Nadine Burke Harris said in her groundbreaking TEDMED Talk:

> In the mid-'90s, the CDC [Centers for Disease Control] and Kaiser Permanente discovered an exposure that dramatically increased the risk for seven out of ten of the leading causes of death in the United States. In high doses, it affects brain development, the immune system, hormonal systems, and even the way our DNA is read and transcribed. Folks who are exposed in very high doses have triple the lifetime risk of heart disease and lung cancer and a twenty-year difference in life expectancy. And yet, doctors today are not trained in routine screening or treatment. Now, the exposure I'm talking about is not a pesticide or a packaging chemical. It's childhood trauma.[2]

She's referring to the landmark 1990 study of ACEs in 17,421 patients conducted by Vince Felitti at Kaiser Permanente and Bob Anda at the CDC, which has resulted in more than seventy peer-reviewed scientific articles.[3] Patients were asked if they had experienced any of ten traumatizing childhood events:

1. Physical abuse
2. Sexual abuse
3. Emotional abuse
4. Physical neglect
5. Emotional neglect
6. Mother was treated violently
7. Household substance abuse
8. Household mental illness
9. Parental separation or divorce
10. Incarcerated household member

Each kind of trauma was given one point, and participants received an ACEs score based on a questionnaire.[4] Subsequent to this study, ACEs questionnaires continue to be revised and expanded to include racism, gender discrimination, witnessing a sibling being abused, witnessing violence outside the home, witnessing a father being abused by a mother, being bullied by a peer or adult, involvement with the foster-care system, living in a war zone, living in an unsafe neighborhood, losing a family member to deportation, and more.[5]

Even as the original ACEs questionnaire vastly underrepresents the scope of potentially traumatic events, sadly, the study revealed that trauma from ACEs is commonplace. Researchers discovered a striking relationship between trauma and disease: the higher the ACEs score, the sicker the patients—and the greater their resistance to treatment. Of the population studied, 67 percent had at least one ACEs, and ACEs don't typically occur alone. If you have one, there's an 87 percent chance you have two or more, and 12.6 percent of those studied had four or more. They also found there was a relationship between ACEs and health outcomes: For a person with an ACEs score of four or more, their relative risk of chronic obstructive pulmonary disease (COPD) or hepatitis was two and a half times higher than someone with an ACEs score of zero. The rate of depression was four and a half times higher. Suicidal depression was twelve times greater. A person with seven or more of the ten ACEs had three and a half times the risk of coronary artery disease, the number one killer in the United States, which often leads to heart attacks. They also had triple the lifetime risk of lung cancer.

ACEs have been well studied by scientists, and there are rigorous scientific data linking exposure to ACEs to autoimmune disease, cancer, COPD, frequent headaches, ischemic heart disease, liver disease, and health-related quality of life.[6] Even the most mainstream cancer centers are examining the link between trauma and disease. Researchers from Harvard University and Moffitt Cancer Center studied 55,000 people and found that those who had six or seven symptoms of posttraumatic stress disorder (PTSD) at some point in their lives have double the lifetime risk of ovarian cancer.[7] If you're curious about your ACEs score and what it means, you can take an ACEs quiz at ACEsTooHigh.com.[8]

Traumatizing events in childhood were linked to adult disease in all categories—including cancer, heart disease, chronic pain, autoimmune diseases, bone fractures, high blood pressure, obesity, and diabetes. The average age of patients in this study was fifty-seven years old, which means that childhood trauma can have a delayed effect on the body, making it entirely possible that something that happened fifty years ago might be predisposing someone to illness in the here and now. What's particularly startling is that the 17,421 ACEs study participants should have been among the world's healthiest, based on their demographics. They were mostly white, middle- and upper-middle class, and college educated; they all had good jobs and access to health care as members of Kaiser Permanente. What if the researchers had studied people in war zones or poverty-stricken areas? These numbers might have been even higher.

If you have a high ACEs score and you're not sick, don't worry. ACEs scores are not good predictors of future health outcomes in individual patients.[9] But they do signal a general risk at the population level, so it's worth getting your trauma treated as preventative medicine, even if you're not sick. Just because you have a high ACEs score doesn't mean you will get heart disease or lung cancer; it means you're at statistically higher risk than someone with an ACEs score of one.

THE NEUROSCIENCE AND PHYSIOLOGY OF TRAUMA

ACEs don't just harm the body; they also harm the nervous system and can lead to mental illness. The higher your ACEs score, the higher your risk for every possible kind of mental health issue, including suicide. Neuroscience shows that the toxic, unrelenting stress of ACEs damages children's developing brains. Some stressors are good for a child's brain development—being challenged by the first day of a new school, preparing for an exam, playing sports, or otherwise being pushed slightly beyond their comfort zone. Mild stressors such as these build resilience, encourage healthy risk-taking, and facilitate brain development. But when kids face adversity on a regular basis, the way those with high ACEs scores do, brain development gets interrupted, and this can lead to a lifetime of struggle, including physical illnesses that result from the nervous system's chronic dysregulation and endocrine and immune system changes that accompany repetitive trauma. Exposure to ACEs affects the developing brains of children, having impacts on the pleasure and reward center (related to addictive behaviors) and the prefrontal cortex (which modulates impulse control and executive function). This can impair learning and lead to reckless behaviors. Magnetic resonance imaging (MRI) scans of people with high ACEs scores measure changes in the amygdala, the sentry of the limbic brain, which looks out for danger, affects the fight-or-flight response, and responds to fear-inducing stimuli. So yes, people with high ACEs scores engage in risky behaviors that affect their health.

Even if you screen and control for high-risk behaviors such as substance abuse, ACEs still increase your risk for the two greatest killers—heart disease and cancer. Children who experience a lot of trauma develop maladaptive responses to adversity and overactive fight-or-flight reactions—inducing stress responses that release cortisol, epinephrine, and other stress hormones that predispose the body to illness. As I describe in detail in *Mind Over Medicine*, chronic repetitive stress responses shut down the body's natural self-healing mechanisms and make us vulnerable to almost every kind of disease.

But it's not just sympathetic nervous system hyperarousal as a side effect of trauma that can make you sick. Recent discoveries in neuroscience, including Stephen Porges's polyvagal theory, now show us that trauma also impairs the development of the vagus nerve, the longest nerve of the autonomic nervous system in the human body, running from the skull through the heart, lungs, and digestive system, and modulating the parasympathetic nervous system.[10] The vagus nerve has two branches—the ventral vagus and the dorsal vagus. A healthy nervous system is regulated by the ventral vagus in times of safety during wakefulness. When the ventral vagus is healthy, the body rests and repairs, seeks connection with others socially, and heals what is chronically breaking down and getting fixed in the body, as when we make and clean up cancer cells or fight off infections. When we are firmly grounded in our ventral vagal pathway, we feel safe, calm, connected, and social—*and* the body is optimized to heal itself.

The dorsal vagus, in contrast, leads us out of connection, which is fine when we're going to sleep or otherwise "checking out" during rest. The body can self-heal when we sleep and rest as well. The problems come when traumatized individuals default to the dorsal vagus during times of wakefulness, when a higher level of energy and arousal would be more appropriate. This leads to the "freeze" strategy of the fight-flight-or-freeze stress response. It's the "playing dead" collapse that can occur under extreme threat, as when a gazelle drops when being chased by a leopard.

The problem for those with high ACEs scores is that the dorsal vagus might get stimulated in response to even the slightest unconscious trigger—a smell that reminds them of a trauma, a color, someone's tone of voice—anything that makes them feel unsafe. Less traumatized people respond to feeling unsafe by reaching out and bonding with others, coregulating until their nervous systems calm down. Those with high ACEs scores often do the opposite. They shut down, retreat, withdraw, avoid connection, and maybe even go to sleep. Their nervous systems might deplete them energetically, causing them to experience chronic fatigue, brain fog, or even passing out—which can land them at the doctor's office.

HOW DOES THIS CAUSE DISEASE?

Researchers have sought an explanation for how an experience occurring in childhood can affect adult-onset disease. What are the mediating factors? Although psychoneuroimmunology explains this in part, and although our growing understanding of how trauma affects the nervous system helps us make sense of this, new data are giving us a better understanding of how childhood trauma might impair the self-healing mechanisms of the adult body and alter the biochemistry of the bloodstream and cellular makeup in a way that has grave consequences. Over time, these neurological changes also affect the child's developing immune and hormonal systems and even how DNA is translated and transcribed through epigenetic influences, making children more susceptible to diseases toward which they might have a genetic predisposition but from which they might never suffer were there no trauma.

In a meta-analysis in *Molecular Psychiatry*, researchers found a significant association between childhood trauma and inflammatory markers, providing strong evidence that childhood trauma significantly alters the immune system and leads to chronic inflammation, implicated as a risk factor for most physical disease as well as mental health disorders such as chronic depression.[11] As explained in *Inflammation: A Unifying Theory of Disease*, chronic inflammation might be the common factor in many diseases. Researchers conclude:

> Mounting evidence suggests a common underlying
> cause of major degenerative diseases. The four horsemen
> of the medical apocalypse—coronary artery disease,
> diabetes, cancer, and Alzheimer's—may be riding the
> same steed: inflammation. Research on inflammation
> has created a shift in medical thinking. For two
> millennia it has been viewed mainly as a necessary,
> even beneficial, response to illness or injury. But for
> many people persistent inflammation can be the most
> significant causative factor in many diseases.[12]

Such a link between childhood trauma, chronic inflammation in adulthood, and adult onset of body or mind diseases is a popular topic in scientific research these days because it offers a potential avenue of treatment that could bandage the destructive physiological impact caused by trauma without treating the trauma directly. Herein lies the crux of the problematic disease management medical model: We are always looking for the quick fix so someone can profit from it!

Yet even if it were possible, finding a pill to treat the impact of trauma will never be the whole solution. This is one of the fundamental differences between conventional medicine and Sacred Medicine. Although most Sacred Medicine practitioners are onboard to treat current symptoms pharmaceutically to ease suffering in the present or save lives, the healers I resonate with the most never dismiss the need to identify, treat, and clear the root blocks of life force caused by the traumas that predispose the body to disease. As much as I wish otherwise, I have no choice but to conclude that an allopathic approach, even one that acknowledges the link between childhood trauma, chronic inflammation, and disease, will be unlikely to make the body optimally ripe for the miraculous healings some people report, at least in the long term. I am becoming convinced that we need to treat not just the *symptoms* that arise from the biochemical disruptions in the body that result from trauma; we also need to find and clear the *traumatic blocks* that impede full mobilization of the life-force energy, which leads to vitality and disability-free longevity.

WHAT IS TRAUMA?

Energy psychotherapist and founder of Advanced Integrative Therapy (AIT) Asha Clinton defines trauma as:

> The combination of an occurrence that causes suffering and the body's and nervous system's reaction to that occurrence, which, when we think back to the occurrence or when it is triggered by some present event, produces difficult emotions and/or physical symptoms or sensations, gives rise to negative beliefs, desires, illnesses, fantasies, compulsions, obsessions, addictions, or dissociation and blocks the development of positive qualities and spiritual connection and fractures human wholeness.

In *Psychological Trauma*, Dawson Church defines a traumatizing event as:

1. Perceived as a threat to the person's physical survival
2. Overwhelms their coping capacity, producing a sense of powerlessness
3. Produces a feeling of isolation and aloneness
4. Violates their expectations

Church provides an example of a traumatizing event that could have lasting consequences but might be overlooked if you were not attuned to what traumatizes a child.

> When I was growing up, I idolized my older brother Gary. But he was pretty rough with me. He was six years older than I was. One day when I was three and he was nine, he wanted to have a "wrestling match." He "won" by lying on top of me. I couldn't breathe, and I began to panic. Gary just laughed when he saw me struggling. I almost passed out. When he rolled off of me, I began to cry uncontrollably. My mother came in, and I tried to explain what happened. He told her it was nothing. I was just being a crybaby. Mom told me, "Big girls don't cry."[13]

Although this example might be dismissed as children tussling, it meets all four criteria for a traumatizing event. The narrator thought she was going to die when Gary laid on top of her, so she *perceived a threat to her survival*. She tried to cope by pushing him off, but he was too big, so *her coping attempt failed, and she felt powerless*. Being smothered by her brother *violated her expectation* that her family would keep her safe. When her mother failed to support and comfort her by dismissing her emotions with "Big girls don't cry," she was left *feeling isolated and alone*.

Psychiatrist Bruce Perry, who cowrote *What Happened to You?* with Oprah Winfrey, points out that trauma is not so much the event that happened to you but the experience emotionally, neurologically, and somatically of that event *inside* your body.[14] As such, trauma is not so much a mental event as a whole-body cascade of neuronal impulses, hormones, and the physiological, neurological, and energetic processes it triggers.

But what if your ACEs score is zero? What if you're wrestling with a chronic or life-threatening illness and you can't remember anything traumatic happening in childhood? Does this mean there's no reason to treat trauma if you're sick or interested in disease prevention? First, it's important to understand that the ACEs scoring system in the CDC-Kaiser study measured only a small number of potentially traumatizing events. Second, I'll take a moment to further define trauma so we can take stock of how likely it is that we're all affected by it, at least to some degree.

THE TRAUMA OF EVERYDAY LIFE: DEVELOPMENTAL TRAUMA

Because so much of our culture is not trauma informed, many kinds are overlooked, especially developmental trauma. Researchers are discovering that although traumatic occurrences are dangerous for long-term health, even potentially riskier is what Buddhist psychiatrist Mark Epstein calls "the trauma of everyday life."[15] The absence of adequate childhood nurturing and the chronic heartbreak and neurological changes caused by developmental trauma might predispose you to chronic illness even more than growing up in a war zone where you were well supported by your family. Although discrete situational traumas, such as wartime events or genocide, horrific violence such as a terrorist attack, death of or abandonment by a parent, or sexual assault, can clearly cause trauma-related mental and physical health struggles, researchers are now finding that long-term, repetitive traumas, such as ongoing parental neglect or lack of unconditional love and emotional safety in the home, can be even more devastating to the nervous system and subsequently the body.

According to the NeuroAffective Relational Model™ (NARM) for healing developmental trauma, trauma happens anytime our core developmental needs for connection, attunement, trust, autonomy, and love/sexuality get interrupted.[16] Kids need grownups to help them tolerate and learn to feel intense emotions; establish a sense of safety in their bodies; regulate their nervous systems; manage connection and disconnection without freaking out; feel themselves as independent, separate beings who can also lean in to and trust others and receive love and help; feel a sense of agency, assertiveness, and empowerment to make good decisions and affect their environment without dominating others; and enjoy the pleasure of their budding sexuality while keeping their hearts open in an embodied way. Sadly, a huge percentage of us, myself included, did not get these core developmental needs met, and this affects us for life unless we get treatment.

We are traumatized anytime we lose our capacity to:

- be in touch with our bodies, emotions, and each other;

- attune to our needs and emotions;

- recognize, reach out for, and take in physical and emotional nourishment;

- trust healthy dependence and interdependence rather than solely practicing self-reliance;

- set appropriate boundaries, say no, and speak our minds without guilt or fear;

- live with an open heart, integrating a loving relationship with a vital sexuality.

This constellation of unmet core developmental needs can cause complex PTSD (C-PTSD). Whereas classic PTSD is often accompanied by visual flashbacks, C-PTSD tends to arise as emotional flashbacks, subtler and more difficult to recognize. As a result, those afflicted tend to experience severe anxiety and/or depression, irritability, fear, emotional or physical aggression, emotional numbness, irrational hostility, poor impulse control, and addictive and reckless behaviors. They also show signs of attachment wounding, such as emotional detachment, distrust even in safe situations, clinginess or avoidance during triggers, and social isolation.[17]

Also called "reactive attachment disorder," developmental trauma happens in the first years of life, when errors in how we were parented prevent us from developing psychologically, spiritually, and physiologically into healthy, whole adults. Little ones need safe, reliable, present, developmentally appropriate, loving caregivers capable of giving them a keen sense of self and helping them individuate as healthy, autonomous, well-boundaried beings in the world. When this "good enough" parenting is available, the young brain develops in a healthy way from the bottom upward. The most primitive aspects of neural development, which regulate survival and response to threat, happen first. More advanced neural development happens later, helping you make good decisions, evaluate experiences, exercise moral judgment, and participate in contributing to the world in a meaningful way. Because the brain develops in this stepwise fashion, more advanced neural functioning depends on the more primitive development happening as it should.

Because a child in an ongoing traumatic situation has to face the formidable challenge of adapting to an intolerable situation, repetitive childhood trauma distorts the child's developing personality structure. To get through life, the child must find a way to feel safe when safety is absent, to trust when their caregivers are untrustworthy, to develop a sense of control when life is out of control, and to feel some sense of power when actually powerless. This is a double-edged sword because on the one hand, it allows the child to survive intolerable conditions, but on the other hand, the price for survival is a devil's bargain.

Because children have no other choice, the only way they can do this is to use immature psychological defenses that tend to stay into adulthood unless the past is treated and healed. They survive, but at the price of their birthright to embody and live in alignment with their true nature.

What endures is a distortion that requires deep healing to untwist and unveil their wholeness. By adulthood, these children are no longer a pure embodiment of an authentic soul but a constellation of personality traits not aligned to who they originally were.

As described in Laurence Heller's *Healing Developmental Trauma*, when early needs for connection are interrupted, children might develop certain defense mechanisms such as feeling pride in being a loner, not needing others, or being unemotional.[18] If their needs for attunement go unmet, they might grow into caretakers, being the shoulder everyone cries on, making themselves indispensable and needed, and feeling pride in not having needs themselves. If their needs for trust go unmet, they might seek power—putting on an appearance of being strong and in control, successful, and larger than life—while tending to exploit and use people. If parents squelch the natural need for autonomy, children might twist themselves into nice, sweet, compliant, good boys or girls who fear disappointing others but secretly feel angry, resentful, and rebellious. If healthy intimacy and sexual development are not fostered, they might grow up perfectionistic, putting forth a mistake-free image, and be quick to reject others before they get rejected. All these tendencies protect the child from feeling the intolerable overwhelm of underlying shame-based emotions—feeling worthless, needy, unfulfilled, empty, burdensome, hurt, small, powerless, fundamentally flawed, unlovable, rejected, and betrayed by their caregivers. As I discussed earlier in this chapter, some of those trauma-induced personality traits have been linked to diseases such as heart disease, autoimmune disease, and cancer.

Going back to the mid-1950s in the Harvard Mastery of Stress Study, thirty-five years of follow-up with college students shows that in the absence of closely attuned parental caring, 87 percent have a disease of some kind versus 28 percent of those who felt well cared for by their parents.[19] What we're now learning is that *the absence of the positive can traumatize children more than the presence of the negative*. When safe, consistent, attuned, loving, nurturing relationships are absent, disease in adulthood is practically inevitable unless the traumas get treated. Considering how many parents are emotionally checked out because of *their* traumas, we're talking about epidemic levels of trauma in countless individuals worldwide.

Yet traditional ACEs scores do not measure these kinds of trauma, so they typically go undiagnosed and untreated. Because developmental trauma messes with our narratives about our families and the world, survivors of it often think they had an easy childhood and don't understand why life feels so hard. Their ACEs scores might be zero. Yet life feels chronically difficult, especially when it comes to navigating healthy relationships with good boundaries. Because relationships are so vital to optimal longevity and health (as I describe in detail in *Mind Over Medicine* and as Surgeon General Vivek Murthy discusses in *Together: The Healing Power of Human Connection in a Sometimes Lonely World*), impairments in relational connection become a huge health risk for those with developmental trauma, which often lands these folks at a physician's office with mystery illnesses and cancer recurrences rather than at a therapist's office.[20] By these definitions of trauma, most of us have experienced multiple, if not chronic, traumatizing events in our lifetimes. A complete trauma history, including screening for developmental trauma, should be part of any medical evaluation, especially when patients fail to meet criteria for a typical diagnosis or do not respond to currently available conventional treatments.

Have You Been Affected by Developmental Trauma?

Although there is no well-studied, universal measure like the ACEs score to assess risk for developmental trauma, *The Body Keeps the Score* author Bessel van der Kolk has suggested adding developmental trauma disorder to the *Diagnostic and Statistical Manual of Mental Disorders* (DSM-5).[21] Even so, his proposed description does not include a way to diagnose, calculate, and study risk in the way the ACEs score does. In the absence of a well-studied developmental trauma–informed way to test yourself, you might ask yourself the following questions to get a sense of your own developmental trauma burden.

Before your eighteenth birthday:

1. Did you often feel that at least one of your parents wasn't capable of connecting with you in a loving and bonding way, leaving you with poor self-esteem, chronic shame, or the feeling that you're somehow damaged?

2. Did you often feel like you could not trust one or both of your parents to attune to you, protect you, and meet your needs?

3. Did you often feel like you had to be the grown up or caregiver in the family when you were still the child?

4. Did you often feel like one or both of your parents smothered you, engulfed you, dominated you, or wouldn't let you individuate, make your own choices, and become your own person?

5. Did you often feel like you were expected to be a perfect, high-achieving, good girl or boy who made your parents proud or you'd be severely judged, rejected, punished, shamed, or abandoned?

6. Do you live with a persistent feeling of nameless dread or terror without understanding why?

7. Do you prefer being alone to being around people, fear and avoid closeness with people, or struggle to maintain intimate relationships?

8. Were you raised without good boundaries or the ability to say no, set limits, or protect yourself?

9. Did you grow up feeling like you were an imposition or burden to one or both parents?

10. Do you seek out spirituality or have frequent mystical or esoteric "out-of-body" kinds of experiences?

11. Do you struggle to know what you need or ask others to help you get your needs met?

12. Do you frequently feel overwhelmed, struggle with adult responsibilities, or fixate on your one big problem, assuming that if it could only be solved, everything would be fine?

13. Did your mother have a difficult pregnancy or trauma giving birth to you? Were you born prematurely or hospitalized at an early age?

14. Did one or both parents fail to help you normalize, feel, process, and handle difficult emotions?

15. Did one or both parents feel hurt or rejected when you tried to pull away, rebel, or become your own person?

16. Were one or both parents self-absorbed, narcissistic, or unable to see you as separate from them?

17. Do you tend to stay "in your head" or overintellectualize, rather than being in your body or your emotions?

18. Is it hard for you to manage conflict, express displeasure, or stand up for yourself?

19. Do you try to stay below the radar, make yourself invisible, or otherwise keep yourself small and safe?

20. Would you identify as highly sensitive, an empath, or neurodiverse?

21. Do you struggle with low energy; diminished life force; lack of motivation; and/or difficulty staying focused, achieving tasks, feeling pleasure, or following your dreams?

Because so many people with a heavy developmental trauma load are unaware of their trauma, answering questions like this can be distressing. Be gentle with yourself and give your body, your emotions, and your nervous system a chance to calm down before moving on. Try the Settle Your Nervous System with Somatic Experiencing exercise on page 248.

WHAT HAPPENED TO YOU?

If any of this sounds familiar, and especially if it is news to you that you might carry these kinds of traumas in ways that could make you sick and impair recovery, please be gentle with yourself. If need be, return to part one and tend to yourself with energy-transfusion practices as needed. Remember, when it comes to healing trauma, the slow path is the most direct. As Peter Levine teaches in his Somatic Experiencing modality, titrating the amount of discomfort your nervous system and body hold at any one time is key to recognizing the feeling of safety and orienting back to it. Allowing these smaller bits of discomfort to arise but not overwhelm you provides the nervous system the space it needs to let feelings of safety emerge to help you heal.

As Perry and Winfrey suggest, it can help to reframe the question, "What's wrong with you?" to "What happened to you?"[22] This acknowledges that childhood trauma is not your fault—and it doesn't make you damaged. It just means you were hurt, and sometimes, when we heal what hurts, the body responds with better health.

The good news is that we now know trauma is treatable and better understand the physiology that explains why treating trauma might relieve suffering in those whose diseases might have their roots in trauma. What has to happen to heal trauma? The ability to establish a sense of safety, regulate the nervous system, and engage in self-care are the first priority. Diving into traumatic memories if someone's dorsal vagus nerve causes them to collapse isn't helpful. Somatic psychotherapists like those trained in Levine's Somatic Experiencing focus first on establishing safety, orientation to the surroundings, embodiment, awareness of inner sensation (interoception), and trust in a coregulation partner such as a therapist. Those with a significant trauma burden often struggle to find a window of tolerance that allows their nervous system to stay regulated. As Kathy

Kain and Stephen Terrell describe in *Nurturing Resilience*, trauma survivors often develop a "faux window" of tolerance and accommodate to a dysregulated nervous system.[23] Although their nervous system is jacked up almost all the time, they might have adapted to this dysregulation through a series of defensive accommodations.

For example, if someone is typically hyperaroused, as when the fight-or-flight sympathetic stress response becomes the norm, they might compensate for this hyperarousal through self-soothing behaviors such as dissociation, compulsive eating, or drinking alcohol. Because they get flooded with too much energy, they learn ways to calm down. In contrast, if someone is hypoaroused, as happens when the dorsal vagus pathway becomes a more dominant kind of freeze response, they might overuse stimulants such as caffeine to perk up or engage in hypersexual behavior to try to get social connection to fend off the numbing, lethargy, hopelessness, and depression that can accompany the dorsal vagal state.

The first order of business when healing trauma is to help clients widen their window of tolerance so they're resourced, oriented, present, and embodied enough to move deeper into the healing process, which usually requires facing the traumatic memories head-on, but only when the timing is right. Somatic Experiencing and other similar therapies use a variety of exercises to achieve this goal; in general, those with severely dysregulated nervous systems tend to need to build a sense of safety, somatic support, and relational support with a skilled somatically oriented therapist before being capable of cognitive support or too much emotional intensity, which can lead to dissociation. Somatic therapies such as Somatic Experiencing and NARM support clients through grounding, orientation to surroundings and the present moment, tracking and reflecting when clients disconnect and dissociate, use of positive resourcing (such as remembering a safe person), titration of how much emotion the client can tolerate without dissociating, pendulation between expansion and the inevitable contraction that follows moments of greater connection, leaning in and leaning out of discomfort safely, mirroring what the body is doing, facilitating somatic discharge of hyperaroused energies that can get stuck in the body, and gently challenging distorted identifications and beliefs. Safe touch, gentle eye contact, and sometimes bodywork might be used by somatic therapists to help coregulate the body and heal attachment wounding.

After the client is better able to self-regulate a dysregulated nervous system and expand the window of tolerance of body sensations, emotions, and challenging of cognitive distortions and core negative beliefs, many cutting-edge therapies focus on facilitating *memory reconsolidation*, as described by Bruce Ecker, Robin Ticic, and Laurel Hulley in *Unlocking the Emotional Brain*.[24] Therapists know the tenacity with which emotional memories can "stick" in the brain, and we used to believe that these memories might be indelible and ultimately incurable. Fortunately, we now know this is untrue because of a process called memory reconsolidation, which allows the brain to learn new neural pathways and erase old pathways, not just suppressing the deep, unconscious, intensely problematic emotional lessons that result from trauma but also developing healthier pathways into those old grooves in the brain. In their research Ecker, Ticic, and Hulley found three things necessary to create radical and permanent long-term change:

1. **Exposure to vividly reimagining and revisiting the traumatic event (with care not to overwhelm the system).** Expecting severely dysregulated clients to recall their memories too soon can be retraumatizing, but neuroscientists seem to think some degree of this is necessary to remodel neural pathways caused by trauma. There seems to be some controversy among the therapists and healers I interviewed regarding whether this is necessary in *all* cases, but most agree upon this necessary aspect of healing trauma.

2. **A juxtaposition experience.** To create new neural pathways, you must juxtapose a neutral or pleasant cue with the traumatic memory or belief. In other words, you're now thinking and reliving that old painful memory—with all its relevant emotions and limiting beliefs, only now you're with a therapist—as your mature adult self so you can have a different experience of the same memory. You return to the event and create a new experience that contradicts the old because now there's a loving presence and you are not alone, isolated, powerless, and helpless.

3. **You retravel this new neural pathway enough to solidify it.** Repetition allows you to experience this new emotional state often enough that it overrides the old neural pathway. The memory is still there. You haven't forgotten it, but it's neutralized.[25]

Essentially, when old trauma is brought to the surface, a "recon-solidation window" opens for healing and repatterning. After you evoke the memory and emotions, you're in the thick of the traumatic memory, as if you've traveled back in time to the original experience. All the synapses become labile, so this is the window during which memory reconsolidation must happen. If you just review old trauma with talk therapy, you might experience catharsis or comfort from having your story witnessed, but if you don't override neural path-ways, you might strengthen the problematic one by retelling your traumatic story. Treatment that helps remove traumatic energy and integrate fragmented aspects of the psyche has to be delivered during that labile reconsolidation window. Many healers will try to sell you the "quick fix" that you can get your trauma exorcised without any painful feelings, but from my research of neuroscience, this assertion does not seem to be true.

Can a healer override that neurological process by moving your en-ergies around? Probably not, according to the majority of therapists I queried. Someone might feel like they've gotten relief from trauma or from a trauma-induced illness through hands-on or spiritual heal-ing, but unless the traumatized individual catalyzes a true and lasting change of consciousness, the old neurological grooves are still there. It's more like a bandage that, although offering temporary relief, might still leave someone vulnerable to being retraumatized the next time something in the environment or an experience retriggers the original neural pathway. The good news is that innovative trauma therapies al-low traumatized individuals to engage in those three factors necessary for memory reconsolidation.

It seems clear there is no "one-size-fits-all" solution to treating trauma. The best therapists are gifted in many trauma-healing tools and are flexi-ble, labile, and creative, able to customize the approach to each individual client depending on what arises in the moment. Although mastery is always important, the method itself might be far less important than the attunement, care, open heart, loving awareness, and degree to which a therapist has treated her own trauma and can be present for the cli-ent, especially for those with developmental trauma and the attachment wounding that accompanies it.

FRAGILE, HANDLE WITH CARE

When we discuss the link between trauma and disease, it's essential to normalize and destigmatize trauma, remember that it's not the traumatized person's fault, and acknowledge that humans are sensitive creatures who deserve to be treated with dignity. Again, when we're looking at the aftermath of trauma and how it affects disease, behavior, relationships, and so many other aspects of the lives of trauma survivors, "What happened to you?" is a more helpful orientation than "What's wrong with you?"

Donna Hicks, in *Dignity: The Essential Role It Plays in Resolving Conflict*, points out that when someone gets roughed up, they deserve to have their suffering acknowledged. Human beings should wear a warning label that says: "Fragile, handle with care." Yet trauma also leads to the opposite of acknowledgment. Trauma often leads to silencing; denial; gaslighting; trivializing someone's suffering; or judging, imprisoning, shaming, and casting them as a monster rather than witnessing, acknowledgment, and validation, which help heal trauma. The people who traumatize us are usually traumatized themselves and pass these burdens from generation to generation.

Mainstream medicine and even traditional psychotherapy rarely support the recognition, normalization, and healing of trauma. Doctors rarely screen for ACEs scores or developmental trauma when evaluating someone with a chronic or life-threatening disease. Ignoring the impact of trauma on the body can be retraumatizing rather than healing.

Even some psychiatrists, whom you might expect to know better, tend to lack a trauma-informed education. Instead of recognizing the link between trauma and mental illness, they parse out mental illness symptoms, labeling and diagnosing them via the *DSM-5* and medicating them accordingly (so they can get paid by insurance companies). But cutting-edge trauma experts claim that all mental health issues—and many physical health issues—are the direct by-product of untreated trauma. Although medicating such trauma might be helpful in reducing symptoms temporarily, and although common therapies taught in mainstream psychology graduate programs might teach life skills that improve functioning, only treating it with advanced trauma therapies treats its symptoms so effectively that it might affect disease remission and reverse mental illness permanently.

Unfortunately, just as medical schools do not train doctors to have a trauma-informed approach to physical illness, few, if any, of the current cutting-edge trauma therapies are regularly taught in academia yet. Most psychotherapists, even those with advanced degrees, are not trained to effectively treat trauma. The ones who do receive training have to pursue continuing education outside graduate school and figure out how to integrate what they learn with their academic training.

Especially after the collective traumatic devastation of 2020, it is my sincere prayer that our institutions wake up and prioritize including an integrated, trauma-informed approach to all our systems in medicine, psychology, education, law enforcement, finance, government, environmentalism, and social justice activism.

Although it might feel overwhelming to consider the massive impact trauma might have on your body, I hope it helps you feel more empowered to consider letting yourself be the one who breaks the chain of patterns of trauma that get passed down virally in families. I once attended a Dia de los Muertos (Day of the Dead) ceremony in my hometown's community center. The woman leading the ceremony to honor ancestors told me about a vision she'd received: Behind each of us is a long line of ancestors, most of whom have traumatized us in some way and who were traumatized by their ancestors before them. When they are in human form, they might not realize they've hurt us and might be defensive if we suggest it, but after they have insight from the other side of the veil, they stand behind us with so much love in their hearts, cheering us on with, "Let this be the one! Let it end with this one!"

Settle Your Nervous System with Somatic Experiencing

If you're a trauma survivor, it's highly likely that reading this chapter has left you with some nervous-system dysregulation. Before we go further, see if you can tune in and settle yourself by turning inward.

How comfortable are you in your body?

> Can you adjust yourself to make yourself more physically comfortable?
>
> Move your feet on the floor, adjusting and shifting until you feel connected to it.
>
> Pay attention to your bottom and notice how supported you are by whatever you're sitting on.
>
> Can you rest more fully into that support of the ground and whatever you're sitting on?
>
> Take a few moments to enjoy the comfort of being supported and stabilized.
>
> Look around and notice something that helps you feel more resourced. Maybe there's something beautiful outside your window, a piece of art on the wall, or a color you love. Savor the resourceful feelings.
>
> Now try a breathing exercise, comparable to chanting "Om" in yoga as you imitate a deep, vibrating foghorn with your voice by projecting the sound "voo . . ."
>
> Engage the entire length of your exhale to give your vagus nerve a gentle massage, restoring flow and calming your system.
>
> Now check again. Do you feel more settled?

If not, try the butterfly hug. Cross your arms over your chest at the wrist and interlace your thumbs, with your thumbs pointing up to make butterfly wings with your fingers (your thumbs make up the body).

Begin gently wiggling your fingers, touching your chest first on one side, then on the other, simulating the flapping wings of a butterfly.

Breathe slowly and play with pressure to see what you like—gentle fluttering or deeper pressure.

Continue the flapping until you feel more settled.

Chapter 11

ILLNESS AS A TRAILHEAD

had not intended to study trauma-healing psychotherapies as part of my investigation into Sacred Medicine, but after it became clear that effective trauma treatments might be a form of energy healing and could be a missing link for chronically ill people who fail to respond to other treatments, I figured I'd better seek the cutting-edge trauma therapists who have developed the latest and greatest models in treating trauma.

Reading books, attending workshops, and interviewing therapists, I asked cutting-edge trauma therapists whether they ever saw remission from physical illness as a side effect of trauma treatment. Many said they never asked their clients about their medical problems unless the clients brought it up, which further revealed to me the problem with fragmenting health issues into silos. It's problematic that we have three different professionals caring for different aspects of sick patients—the physician tending the body, the therapist focusing on the psyche, and the chaplain ministering to the soul. At least most energy healers try to consider all three in a more holistic way.

Among the therapists who bothered to track whether their clients were having improvements in their medical issues, their responses were surprisingly affirmative. Yet few therapists considered their trauma treatments any kind of medicine for the body, reserving that label for what doctors do.

Patients, however, told me otherwise. Among the radical remission survivors I interviewed, getting help dealing with traumas they had not yet touched—and feeling and moving through the stuck emotions related to those traumas—emerged as one of the most frequent commonalities among outliers who had better-than-expected outcomes. To even attempt to do justice to this thread in the tapestry of unraveling the mysteries of healing, I did my homework.

I surveyed eye-movement desensitization and reprocessing (EMDR); Internal Family Systems (IFS); NeuroAffective Relational Model™ (NARM); Hakomi; Havening; Brainspotting; Accelerated Experiential Dynamic Psychotherapy; neurofeedback; archetypal work; Gestalt therapy; Inner Bonding; the Resilience Toolkit; Family Constellations; enneagram work; psychodrama; Dynamic Attachment Repatterning experience; hypnotherapy; and several energy psychology methods, including Advanced Integrative Therapy (AIT), Emotional Freedom Technique/s (EFT), Thought Field Therapy (TFT), and Psych-K.

I also looked at treatments more mental in nature—cognitive-behavioral therapy (CBT), Compassionate Inquiry, the Diamond Approach, and the Work. Some, like Dynamic Emotional Integration (DEI) focus on the emotional aspects of healing trauma. Others focus on the somatic aspects, such as Somatic Experiencing, Sensorimotor Psychotherapy, Somatic Resilience and Regulation, Feldenkrais, craniosacral therapy, Myofascial Release, Trauma Releasing Exercises, Holotropic Breathwork, Rolfing, and various schools of yoga. Some of these treatments I assessed as healing and effective; others seemed like spiritual, emotional, or cognitive bypasses and didn't make my discernment cut.

Although I am not trained as a trauma therapist, and it would be beyond the scope of my expertise to give you a detailed assessment of which therapies are most effective for treating trauma—and which might be poison—I used my Whole Health Intelligences to dive deep into two trauma therapies with self-help practices that might help you heal— Richard "Dick" Schwartz's IFS and Asha Clinton's AIT. By no means are these the only effective therapies out there. I'm also a huge fan of Peter Levine's Somatic Experiencing and some of the spinoff somatic therapies that have evolved around that model. But for the sake of brevity, I've chosen to share with you the basics of IFS and AIT so you can try the self-help practices at home if you feel strong enough to do so. Although obviously no "cure-all" panacea that works for every medical condition exists, if you've tried everything else and nothing is working, it is my opinion that experimenting with some form of cutting-edge trauma treatment as part of your Whole Health Prescription can do nothing but help.

In case you're rolling your eyes, thinking, "Ugh, yet another doctor is telling me my illness might be all in my head," please understand that's not what I'm saying. As I describe in chapter 10, I have no doubt that your suffering is physiological. A chronically dysregulated nervous system—and the resultant hormonal, inflammatory, immune system, and epigenetic changes that accompany it—are all your body needs to make the breeding ground for chronic or life-threatening illness. I'm also not saying that there might not be some physical condition you just haven't found yet, such as a rare food allergy or heavy metals in your home or a virus that hasn't been detected. All I'm saying is that treating your traumas can heal you, and when healing happens, it just might make you miracle prone. If not, you will at least have more energy liberated in your system to help you live your best life, even if that means learning to accept and make peace with a permanent disability.

Before we proceed, just one word of caution. Depending on the kind of trauma you might have experienced and how early it happened, you might not be ready for the exercises I share in the next two chapters. Diving into healing trauma prematurely could even harm you and lead to what therapists call *backlash*. Before trauma survivors are ready to dig deep into the recesses of the unconscious, basic safety, ego strengthening, nervous system regulation, and embodiment practices might be prerequisites. Teaching these tools is beyond the scope of this book, but suffice it to say that if you notice yourself feeling disembodied, dissociated, or dysregulated, or if you find yourself ramping up addictive behaviors, indulging an eating disorder, becoming accident prone, having suicidal thoughts, or otherwise harming yourself or others, please stop reading, and if you can afford it, get a therapist to support your journey. You won't want to bully yourself into moving faster than your nervous system is ready to handle.

One more suggestion: Although self-help tools might support your healing journey, healing trauma is a necessarily relational activity. Even the tendency to be overly reliant on self-help is a trauma symptom, so make sure you are well supported. Even if you are strong enough to experiment with the practices in this book, you will need trusted loved ones to help you stay safe and coregulated.

AN IFS-INFORMED APPROACH TO DISEASE

Avery was a young mother and physician diagnosed with a recurrence of breast cancer a year after undergoing treatment. She planned to undergo surgery and possibly chemotherapy and/or radiation, but she was open to exploring the underlying roots of what might have caused her immune system to weaken enough to let a cancer grow, not just once but twice. As part of the Whole Health Medicine Institute I lead for health-care providers, Dick, the IFS founder and a family therapist, had come to work with our cohort. When he heard that one of the doctors had cancer, he offered to demonstrate how IFS can be used to work with people living with illness.

According to the IFS model, we all have multiple personalities, or what Dick calls *parts*. As Walt Whitman wrote, "Do I contradict myself? Very well then I contradict myself, (I am large, I contain multitudes)."

In other words, you are not just one unified being; you (and me and all of us) are a multiplicity of parts, which is why we so often feel conflicted inside. It might sound strange to discuss having multiple parts, yet IFS therapists believe the idea of a unified self is misguided, and we all, even the most mentally healthy folks, have lots of parts. The main difference between most people and the ones the psychiatric community labels with dissociative identity disorder (DID, formerly known as multiple personality disorder, portrayed in the 1976 movie *Sybil*) is that most people have at least some "Self-leadership"—a wise Self guiding the behavior of the parts. Without treatment, people with DID behave as if they have no leader guiding and negotiating with the parts, but even people with DID have a Self that can be accessed with IFS treatment.

What is the Self that's not a mere part? Poet Mark Nepo describes it best:

> Each person is born with an unencumbered spot,
> free of expectation and regret, free of ambition and
> embarrassment, free of fear and worry; an umbilical spot
> of grace where we were each first touched by God. It is this
> spot of grace that issues peace. . . . Regardless of subject
> matter, this is the only thing worth teaching: how to
> uncover that original center and how to live there once it
> is restored. We call the filming over a deadening of heart,
> and the process of return, whether brought about through
> suffering or love, is how we unlearn our way back to God.[1]

In other words, your "internal family" is populated with a whole busload of inner children with varying degrees of defensive and survival strategies. If you're reasonably healthy, your wise, grounded, loving, "good enough" parent Self is driving the bus the majority of the time, keeping the adorable, sometimes naughty, but always valuable and loveable parts from grabbing the wheel and hijacking the bus. These parts fall into one of two protector categories—managers and firefighters—and the parts they protect are the vulnerable and tenderhearted exiles. Managers are preemptive and try to head off danger by making plans and trying to control life. Firefighters tend to be a bit more unruly and get us into trouble with behaviors our managers might not like—such as addictions, physical symptoms, and suicidal thoughts—but they're still there for a good reason and think they're protecting us from feeling the pain of the hurting exiles. Both managers and firefighters look after the sensitive inner kids—the exiles—but instead of letting those exiles get healing, they tend to lock them up so that their pain gets buried, until something happens, and their emotional burdens flare up, leaking painful exile feelings through the cracks. The goal of IFS is to let Self heal the exiles so the protectors don't have to work so hard. When this happens, spiritual awakening might go hand in hand, tying trauma healing and spiritual development together in ways that were a surprise to Dick, who was raised by skeptical atheists.

I was particularly attracted to IFS over some of the other trauma healing methods because the model not only treats every mental illness in the *DSM-5* but also can be used to treat physical illness. The IFS model invites people struggling with a physical ailment to approach the illness as a "trailhead," a signpost for a trail you might hike to explore deeper. In IFS, a trailhead might be a physical sensation; an emotion; a painful thought; or an image that, if you stay focused on it, will lead you to the part from which it emanates. Trailheads are an invitation to enter your inner world and learn more about the parts that might be causing you physical or emotional pain or illness.

After introducing the idea that cancer can sometimes be related to a traumatized part trying to protect you by keeping you sick, Dick explored some of the circumstances of Avery's life when her cancer was first diagnosed. Avery shared how overextended she had been—sometimes on call for three days in a row for the hospital's trauma center without even a few hours of sleep. She was often stretched thin not just at work but also as the mother of young kids. She had always considered herself strong, capable, able to "force function" even when the going got rough. That's what got her through her general surgery residency training as one of the few women. When Dick invited her to explore this "force functioning" part, she revealed it was what got her through childhood.

Dick's approach to a sick person is gentle and empathetic. He does not suggest, as some of the healers I interviewed do, that all illness is the result of psychospiritual trauma, nor does he promise that treating trauma will cure the body. Coming from a family of physicians, he knows the dangers of overpromising or ignoring evidence-based medical treatments. But he also believes that too often medicine tries to kill the messenger without helping the patient learn the meaning of the message.

Dick explained that he has asthma, which has afflicted him since he was a child. He said that if he walks into a dusty room and has an asthma attack, it's usually not the result of trauma—it's the dust. But if he's about to give a presentation about something that scares him, the part of him that's afraid he might be humiliated might pull out the "asthma card" to protect him from embarrassment.

Dick asserts that parts of us trying to protect us might use extreme measures, including physical illness, to get our attention and try to keep us safe from feeling emotions we might fear we can't handle. These parts can act autonomously without realizing that something like cancer could be fatal. They think they're trying to help us, not understanding that this "protection" can also kill us. Usually, these parts are trying their darndest to keep us from being overwhelmed by intense, seemingly unbearable feelings erupting from vulnerable, traumatized parts from childhood. Rather than letting you be flooded with emotions such as shame, terror, grief, worthlessness, or helplessness stemming from beliefs that you are unworthy or undeserving of love, protector parts might try hard by using the body to make sure you don't get too close to the pain of those extreme emotions. Many people's bodies are like that, Dick explained to Avery. They might have a physical or genetic susceptibility, and if their parts are triggered, they might use the body to "take you out," or, if they feel shut out, get your attention or punish you.

Dick asked for Avery's permission to explore whether her cancer might think it was protecting her. If so, what was it protecting? He suggested to Avery that if a traumatized exile is discovered underneath a protector part that might be using an illness to avoid feeling intensely painful emotions, it might be possible that the illness would be willing to back off if that exile got relieved of its painful burdens. Avery had no conscious awareness of whether she had a traumatized part underlying her cancer, but she was game to explore, considering it might help her survive.

Dick asked Avery to close her eyes and guided her gently into her "inner world." When Avery was face-to-face with her cancer, Dick said, "Ask your cancer if it will let us talk to it."

The cancer said it was okay.

Dick said, "Can you ask it why it's here? What is it afraid would happen if it quit trying to protect you by showing up in your body?"

Without missing a beat, Avery said, "It says Avery will throw herself under the bus if I go away. She used to throw herself under the bus, and then when I came the first time, she quit throwing herself under the bus and took better care of herself. As soon as I went away, Avery started throwing herself under the bus again. So I'm back, and I'm not going anywhere unless Avery stops throwing herself under the bus."

Avery was shocked. She said to Dick, "I do that! I prioritize everyone's needs over mine." She admitted she had not told her colleagues, patients, or even her children that she had cancer. She didn't want anyone else to worry. She snuck around during her first series of treatments, not taking time off work or asking the kids to help out more so she could rest.

"What is the cancer afraid will happen if it stops doing its job?" Dick asked.

"Well," the cancer said, "Avery is going to keep throwing herself under the bus, so I'm here to help her take better care of herself."

Avery seemed dismayed.

Dick asked, "What if Avery was willing to quit throwing herself under the bus? Would you be willing to go away?"

The part trying to protect her said, "She won't do that. She's a hopeless case. She always says she's going to slow down and take better care of herself, but she's all talk. She needs to have the cancer as an excuse to take care of herself."

Dick said, "I get that. Makes sense. But what if she was willing to make some changes and stop throwing herself under the bus? Would you be willing to find a job you might like better?"

The part said, "I don't trust her. She might say she'll do that, but she won't. If I go away, she'll go right back to her old tricks and make everybody else more important."

Avery got defensive. "No, I won't! I would stop throwing myself under the bus if you would please go away. You're not helping me. You're killing me."

Dick jumped in. "What part is that? The part that doesn't like the can-cer part? Who's that?"

"That's my 'scared to die' part. It doesn't like the cancer part."

"Okay, can we ask it to give us space so we can keep talking to the part that's trying to use cancer to protect you?"

"It doesn't want to go away. It wants to make sure the cancer leaves me alone so I can take care of my children." Avery started to cry.

Dick said, "I get that. It makes sense that it would be scared Avery might die from the cancer. But if it will give us space and let me try to find out why some other part throws Avery under the bus, maybe the cancer will be willing to go away and let Avery live. I'm here to help the part the cancer protects, so maybe the part that uses the cancer won't have to work so hard. Would you give me a chance to help so the cancer might be able to go away?"

Dick describes IFS therapists as "hope merchants for hopeless parts." I could see that he was selling himself as a hope merchant here, trying to gently coax the part afraid of the cancer to relax. The rest of the session was tender. Dick facilitated what he calls an "unburdening of the exile." We discovered that, as a child, little Avery had to throw herself under the bus and prioritize everybody else's needs before her own because nobody else was there to take care of her sick mom and her younger brother. The developmental trauma of having a mother not attuned to her needs caused her to develop a core fear that if she expressed her own needs, she would be rejected, abandoned, and ultimately disappointed. As a result of her mother's illness, Avery became competent at a young age, the paren-tified child, overfunctioning to survive. Nobody taught her that she had as much right to get her needs met as anyone else.

Avery's beautiful process was extremely emotional and tender for those of us who witnessed it. There wasn't a dry eye in the room afterward. We felt so much compassion for Avery, and we celebrated her bravery to al-low her parts to be witnessed by us.

After gaining insight into the wound that might lie beneath her cancer diagnosis, Avery wound up calling a therapist trained to work with cancer patients. When I checked in with her while writing this book, more than two years had passed, and she was doing well in remission after conventional oncologic treatment, a variety of other interventions guided by her Whole Health Intelligences, and two years of trauma therapy. She says she has never been happier and considers herself healed, whether or not her cancer comes back.

UNPACKING INTERNAL FAMILY SYSTEMS

What happened between Dick, Avery, and all those parts? I'll break it down and explain the Internal Family Systems (IFS) model, starting with how the parts are forced out of their naturally valuable states into extreme roles by trauma—roles Schwartz labels as managers, firefighters, and exiles—as well as the Self, who can lead these parts in a well-functioning internal family system. Managers and firefighters are both protector parts, designed to prevent you from feeling the burdens your exiles carry—the intense feelings, sensations, and beliefs that result from trauma, which can get locked away in the basement of your psyche.

Managers

These parts are like busy micromanagers, frantically trying to avert danger. They tend to be the endlessly spinning voices of the "monkey mind" Buddhists discuss in meditation teaching, prattling on and keeping you from being fully present in the now. They're like those little meerkats that stand sentry on top of the mound, scouting out potential risks. Managers can be inner-critic parts, to-do-list parts, financial planner parts, timekeeper parts, stay-busy-so-you-can't-feel parts, and so forth. Although manager parts can be annoying, they seldom get us in trouble, but their jobs are important because underneath those busy managers are the firefighter parts. Managers try to make sure flames of emotions from the vulnerable exiles don't flare; if they do, in come the firefighters.

Firefighters

Although managers can be like busybody helicopter parents, trying to control you and keep you on the straight and narrow, firefighter parts can be more like reckless teenagers. They tend to act out when the managers fail to protect you from those hard-to-feel emotions. If those flames of emotion—intense shame, sadness, worthlessness, helplessness, powerlessness, unlovableness, emptiness, loneliness, lack of fulfillment, neediness, or feeling like a burden or not good enough—flare up, the firefighters will come out with hoses blaring, and they'll do anything to keep you from feeling pain, including risk-taking behaviors that might hurt you or someone else. Firefighters tend to be the parts we might pathologize, medicate, hospitalize, put on a diet, send to rehab, imprison, or otherwise demonize. Firefighters might run from intimacy, become addicts, behave narcissistically, harm others, try to convince you to commit suicide, make you psychotic, cause you to binge or purge, and yes . . . maybe make you sick.

Firefighters can use the body and act out as physical illnesses—or other parts can use some physical vulnerability in your system to take you out. Think: migraine part, back pain part, asthma part, accident-prone part, or even a cancer part like Avery had. Especially given that trauma survivors tend to have nervous-system dysregulation, common physical symptoms related to a chronically hyperaroused (fight-or-flight) or a hypoaroused (freeze) state include migraines, asthma, gastrointestinal distress, chronic pain, environmental or food allergies, fibromyalgia, high blood pressure, arrhythmias, anxiety disorders, and chronic fatigue.[2] Because chronic post-traumatic stress disorder (PTSD)/developmental trauma dysregulates the nervous system for such a long time, this type of trauma increases the risk of almost all diseases, including the two most common killers, heart disease and cancer.

Neither Dick nor I are suggesting that these are purely trauma-induced illnesses or that all illness is the result of psychological trauma. But according to the IFS model, your protector parts might make every effort to use your physical body to protect you from getting too close to your traumatized exiles. So . . . as a physician interested in interdisciplinary healing, this is where IFS made me take notice, especially after I saw Dick using IFS with a woman who received instantaneous relief from her migraine after healing the exile it was protecting.

Exiles

The whole goal of managers and firefighters is to protect you from feeling the agony of your exiles, who tend to carry intense burdens— painful emotions, sensations, memories, and beliefs about yourself and the world. We exile away these traumatized parts, and the protectors serve as the wardens for these parts we have imprisoned inside ourselves; the inner children locked away; the tender, despairing, vulnerable parts who didn't get their needs met at critical times in your development—or sometimes also later in life. As Dick described in the *Internal Family Systems Skills Training Manual*:

> When children feel shamed (often but not exclusively interpersonally), vulnerable young parts are particularly

liable to develop overwhelmingly threatening beliefs like "I'm unlovable" and "I'm worthless." Equally, when experience is terrifying and beyond our capacity to tolerate, our most vulnerable parts feel stripped of significance. Protectors step in to keep their toxic beliefs out of consciousness, and, as a result, vulnerable parts end up permanently alone, forgotten, and often trapped in the past. They long for help, but when they push into consciousness with negative feelings, beliefs, sensations, and memories, protectors again experience them as a hazard.[3]

No matter how idyllic you think your childhood was, we all have exiles who might arrive at conclusions such as "I'm not good enough." Managers come in to develop strategies like Avery had—"I'll throw myself under the bus to prioritize everyone else's needs so I don't get abandoned." Avery most likely did not have her developmental need for attunement met by a "good enough" parent, which likely caused her to develop exiles who felt needy, unfulfilled, empty, and full of inner longing. As an adaption, she then developed caregiving protectors who prided themselves on being the shoulder everyone else cries on, the one others rely on, the one with no needs of her own. It's no wonder some firefighter part might use her body by making her sick so she was forced to prioritize getting her own needs met.

Even if by some miracle you escaped all situational and developmental childhood trauma, most of us exile parts of ourselves even in adulthood. For example, if you get married and have children, you might develop "neoexiles," locking away parts you think don't belong, such as your slutty, potty-mouth, carousing, or daredevil parts.

Few among us are exempt from the burdens these exiles carry. Our exiles might have diverse stories and different wounding, but they tend to have the same painful feelings. Because your protector parts don't like the feelings these exiled parts evoke, they unwittingly exacerbate the problems, locking these exiles in an inner prison, so they're crying and screaming and begging for your attention all the time. The more traumatic the wounding, the more the exiles will make every effort to get your attention, so the more powerful the protectors must become, ramping up their extreme behaviors over time.

The managers might keep things under control for a while, but over time, as the exiles get more unruly and the managers fail to keep them under wraps, the firefighters might need to work harder to protect you from feeling when these exiles' feelings leak through. Often, you'll feel these exiles most painfully in your most intimate relationships, where they will tend to attach to a spouse or best friend to get their needs met the way they didn't at some point, usually early in childhood. You might seek that perfect partner or perfect spiritual teacher or perfect whoever so that person can function as your "redeemer," the one who will tend to all your vulnerabilities and take away your pain forever. If this happens, these exiles might choose your partners and close friends, then burden them with the pressure to make those parts feel better.

If exiles choose your partner, they can become excessively needy, which might cause your partner's protectors to run in the other direction because the desperation of these wounded parts is overwhelming, causing those parts to cry even harder in their inner prisons. Or you might activate a caretaker part (a protector) in your partner, who will soothe those exiled parts until your partner ultimately gets depleted and resentful from too much caregiving, and another protector might cause your partner to pull away or abandon you, causing more hurt for your exiles. Because only you can heal your exiles, this search for a redeemer can lead to agonizing disappointment, betrayal, or abandonment. This vigilance drains you energetically, dysregulates your nervous system, activates your chronic stress responses, and interferes with your body's capacity to heal, impeding the flow of energy through your physical, mental, emotional, and spiritual bodies, causing you to leak life force and putting your health at risk.

NO BAD PARTS

None of us is perfect, and there are no bad parts. But we all—even the Sacred Medicine practitioners we admire—"blend" with parts from time to time. Even those we might be tempted to idealize sometimes wind up with an inner child driving the bus, careening around steep turns, and making us act like we're not the wise, mature adults we are when the Self is driving. IFS is about developing a relationship with all our parts, becoming intimate with them, and earning their trust so they learn to let our Self lead rather than hijacking us.

Most of us have parts polarized with other parts, which allows "angel on one shoulder and devil on the other" inner wars to rage. If you've felt crazy because one part of you tells you to make a New Year's resolution to break a bad habit, but another part breaks the resolution days later, you already understand polarized parts. Polarized parts are at the root of all addictions, for example, because we tend to have manager parts who try to keep us out of trouble, but we also have firefighter parts who will do anything, even if it hurts us or others, to avoid feeling the deep pain of our exiles.

Although we might have parts who demonize other parts, such as the New Year's resolution part who hates the bad habit part, even the parts who get us in trouble think they're helping us. As Julie Holland says about bad habits in *Good Chemistry*, "You can never get enough of something that *almost* works." Although sugar, booze, sex, social media, workaholism, or codependent relationships might *almost* work to soothe our hurt parts, these solutions never fully satisfy us, leaving us starving for the nourishment our parts crave. The goal of IFS is to get those parts the substance of what they need—the unconditional love of Self, which many of us have trouble finding outside ourselves, given that other people have a hard time loving unconditionally when they blend with their own hurt parts.

What's the solution? What heals the exiles so the protectors can quit working so hard and the exiles can get their needs met in a healthy way rather than burdening other people with excessive neediness? The good news is that although humans need others, you are ultimately the best healer, caregiver, parent, teacher, and redeemer for your exiles, which can free up your protectors from all their excessive vigilance. Mostly what the exiles want is your love, attentiveness, care, nurturing, understanding, and compassionate witnessing. They want you to listen to how much pain they experience. They want you to remember what happened to them and acknowledge it rather than pushing their memories, feelings, and negative core beliefs away. They want an ally, not a warden. But they can't seem to get through to you because the two lines of protection (managers and firefighters) do their best to keep you from even remembering, feeling, or being present with these sweet, tender, hurting exiles. Fortunately, the solution is far simpler than anyone might imagine.

When exiles are healed and liberated from their prisons, they bring out your valuable qualities, which might have gotten exiled along with the part, such as the magical child or creative muse, with all their playful, curious vitality. Unburdening the exiles not only frees up stuck energy but also liberates sweet, exuberant qualities that make you attractive, magnetic, creative, energized, and sometimes healthier physically.

As Dick describes in *No Bad Parts*, in IFS, no parts are demonized or pathologized. The *DSM-5* is not used, and nobody gets diagnosed or labeled, even if they have dissociative parts, depressed parts, anxious parts, bipolar parts, addicted parts, eating disordered parts, cutting parts, enraged parts, suicidal parts, sex offender parts, personality disordered parts, or parts that use the body to make you sick. IFS is not just a psychotherapy model; for many who choose to travel it, it's a nonbypassing spiritual path. As it turns out, the only thing interfering with a natural spiritual connection is unresolved trauma. When parts get healed and integrated, spiritual development is a welcome and sometimes surprising by-product.

AVOIDING BACKLASH

IFS is a true path of nonrejection, like many paths of Tantra, because all parts are welcomed and none are demonized. The premise is that by demonizing and bullying these parts, we paradoxically make them more likely to act out. Even if we successfully bully one part into behaving better, other parts typically take over. Take 12-step programs—many addicts know that working the steps might help one kind of addiction but spawn a new one; for example, an alcoholic who gets sober and then overeats or takes up smoking, or a food addict who recovers and then becomes addicted to the spiritual bypassing highs of meditation. Only if they attend to and heal the exile the addict part might be protecting is someone likely to experience lasting recovery from all potential addictions. In my opinion, the reason 12-step programs aren't more effective is because most are not trauma informed.[4] Yet, when we approach healing our more challenging parts with IFS, even the most extreme firefighters no longer feel the impulse to act out because the traumatized exiles they protect have been healed, integrated, and reclaimed, which eases the burden on the firefighters of doing their song and dance.

Our manager parts (and our culture) tend to bully our firefighters, harping on them, criticizing them, trying to impose extreme discipline on them, and shaming them. Yet, when we demonize and bully our parts—or when therapists, doctors, spiritual teachers, priests, and transformational leaders demonize and bully our parts—we create *backlash*. Backlash can happen when one firefighter is bullied into submission by a manager part (or by someone else), but then another firefighter might show up and act out in even more destructive ways because the exile that firefighter protects has not yet been healed.

The awareness of backlash came to Dick when he was a young family therapist working with girls with anorexia. Because they were dying of starvation, he felt like it was his job to bully the anorexic part into eating, but one day, when he succeeded in bullying a client's part into behaving, she showed up with a gash on her cheek. Her anorexic part hadn't starved her that day, but a cutting part took over and left a permanent scar. This led Dick to conclude that most therapists were doing it all wrong by expecting clients to bully their own parts—or by pressuring a client's parts to do what we judge is best for them. Many recovery programs are run this way—by bullying the parts that get us in trouble and shaming or disciplining them into submission. But this is why so many people fall off the wagon. Whatever made someone start binge drinking or restricting food intake is still hurting, and until we treat the underlying wound, people continue to suffer and be at risk.

Facilitating transformation, whether through therapy, addiction recovery, life coaching, transformational programs, spirituality circles, plant medicine shamanic journeys, or self-help teachings can be risky business if those who facilitate it are not trauma informed and aware of the dangers of backlash. If you've been engaged in the world of transformation, spirituality, traditional psychotherapy, or even conventional medicine, you know that bullying people (including yourself) into transformation never works, certainly not in the long term. Sure, there's a fine line between healthy discipline and unhealthy bullying. But think about how effective it is to bully an overweight person into losing weight or an alcoholic into abstinence. How effective has it been to let your inner critic bully you into changing your behavior?

When inner or outer bullies pressure you to change, the exiled parts those behaviors might protect can get so lit up that other parts that might otherwise lie dormant, such as a suicidal part, psychotic part, self-injuring part, or binge-drinking part might act out and cause even more harm. This awareness of potentially dangerous backlash against bullying parts planted the seed for IFS in Dick.

At the root of IFS is the idea that we never try to heal exiles without getting consent from all protector parts. If the protectors don't consent, we keep getting to know the protectors until they relax, trust the client's Self, and allow us to proceed with healing deeper trauma. This is a more nuanced and trauma-informed approach than what tends to happen at big transformational events—or in many inpatient psychiatric wards, recovery programs, religious organizations, spiritual cults, and camps for troubled teens. There's a reason people often come out the other side of programs like this worse off than when they went in.

Backlash can show up in several ways, sometimes obvious and sometimes mysterious. From the IFS point of view, backlash can take the form of a suicide attempt; psychotic break; overdose; health crisis; self-harming behavior; worsening addiction; or even events that appear unrelated, such as a car crash or an injury that "takes you out" or distracts you so you don't have to feel what your exiles are feeling. Your parts might be so invested in protecting you that they'll do anything to protect you from feeling those unbearable feelings.

What's the alternative to bullying our parts or hiring someone else to do it for us: Violate our boundaries, penetrate our delicate systems, and exert authority over our parts? Resisting the temptation to let some parts bully others (or let some coach, doctor, spiritual leader, or sponsor bully you) doesn't mean it's a parts free-for-all with no discipline. Dick believes that when we become intimate with our parts, get to know them, earn their trust, and begin to understand why they do what they do, we can learn to negotiate with them, work with them, help them get their needs met, and gently but firmly discipline them when needed, the way we would a wayward child we love. The more we heal the exiled parts these extreme parts protect, the less they tend to act out. Instead, we can receive the gifts these parts offer us (they all come with gifts) without bypassing the pain, damage, and trauma these parts can cause. It's the ultimate path of self-love because all parts are welcome and worthy of love by the Self, even the parts we might find hard to love.

Although some might call these parts the *ego*, there's no demonizing of the ego or judging any part as "sinful" in the IFS model. Saying there are "no bad parts" is not an exaggeration—the parts that might do the most despicable things are approached with curiosity, respect, compassion, and a desire to help liberate them from their extreme roles. IFS has been successfully used to treat people with murderer, sex offender, addict, and child-abuser parts as well as narcissistic, dissociative, bipolar, schizophrenic, and suicidal parts. It's being used to treat parts that might weaken or cause illness in the body to motivate us to get help for our exiles so we can finally save our own lives.

THE "HOW" OF SELF-LOVE

At the most practical level, IFS is both the "how" of self-love and the connection to your inner guidance, and those change *everything*. Self-love is a popular buzz phrase these days, but how do you love the parts that might do destructive things, parts that hurt other people, parts that overpower and control, parts that break the law, parts that perpetrate abuse, or parts that might use your body to get your attention with potentially fatal illness?

Dick has discovered that every client has what he calls the eight Cs—a calm, curious, compassionate, clear, confident, courageous, creative, connected core shining from beneath the veil of the parts.[5] These don't show up in *some* of his clients—they are in *all* of them. Dick labeled this "part that's not a part" the Self with a capital *S*, the wholeness of one's being, where the ego-consciousness and the unconscious merge.

As Loch Kelly, a psychotherapist and consciousness teacher who incorporates IFS into his nondual spiritual teaching, explains,

> The goal in most meditation traditions from around the world is to awaken from the small separate self into what has been called our True Nature, ground of Being, unity consciousness, Heart Mind, or larger Self. In the IFS therapy model, this Self is the centerpiece and undamaged font that is the source of healing. Accessing this no-self Self, and welcoming all our parts, is the ultimate medicine.[6]

When the Self is caring for all the parts through "Self-leadership," the primary healer then becomes not the therapist or doctor facilitating the healing work but the Self of the person in need of healing. The therapist or doctor then becomes someone who might offer tools. A doctor might offer surgery or medication to relieve symptoms or save your life in the short run. A therapist might offer coregulation, presence, relational connection and resonance, somatic exercises intended to keep you in your body, and the Self in the therapist to entrain more Self in the client. All patients and clients need expert facilitation from time to time, including Dick, who seeks IFS therapists to help him unburden his own exiles. Even so, all good healers eventually give the power back to the patient—holding safe, sacred space and offering tools to facilitate healing—so the patient or client can become more independent in their self-healing over time. Even a broken bone put back together with surgery still needs to mend itself. Even a vaccination needs to activate the body's own immune system to mount a response to a virus. Even the best therapist can act only as a surrogate Self until your true Self bonds directly with your parts.

This becomes empowering for the patient and takes pressure off the therapist or doctor. It's also awe-inspiring to witness. People who have spent years in therapy without successfully liberating all that stuck traumatic energy shed decades of baggage, sometimes in short periods of time. TSW: This Shit Works has become a meme emblazoned on T-shirts in the IFS community. Even better, there's a growing body of scientific evidence to prove they're right because IFS is now registered with the National Registry for Evidence-Based Programs and Practices, not just for mental health disorders but also for medical treatment of rheumatoid arthritis.

As you become intimate with your manager and firefighter parts and earn their trust, as you keep demonstrating to them that your Self can take care of the exiles better than they can, they're likely to grant you access to the exiles they protect so those parts can get healing. When the trapped traumatic energy these protectors and exiles carry gets freed up, you're likely to feel reborn; full of energy; and emotionally, spiritually, and physically healthier than you've ever felt. You might uncover gifts you didn't know existed, such as sharpening your intuition, boosting your visionary skills, flowering of nondual awareness, greater ease of meditation, more compassion for the difficult people in your life, blossoming creativity or sexuality, and even the gift of healing yourself and others.

Keep in mind that your protectors do not always cause harm or engage in destructive behavior! As Dick admits, the protector obsessed with trying to impress his father fueled the creation of IFS. Many of us have protectors with great talent who help us, serve others, and create great acts of love, beauty, art, talent, visionary activism, and proficiency. This book wouldn't exist if my curious, intellectualizing protector wasn't constantly trying to hack healing to keep me from feeling lonely, scared, vulnerable, helpless, and worthless. So thank heavens for these parts, who do a world of good through their attempts to distract me from feeling.

When trauma therapist (and my cousin) Rebecca Ching introduced me to the IFS model, she said, "Lissa, this is a game changer." I had no idea how much I would come to agree with her.

Get to Know Your Protectors

Modified from the *Internal Family Systems Skills Training Manual*, by Frank Anderson, Martha Sweezy, and Richard Schwartz

Make a list of protectors you identified while reading the previous sections, or ask your protectors to introduce themselves to you. (They're usually dying to say hello once they realize you're listening.)

Close your eyes and go inside to see if there's a part that wants your attention. Explore where you feel that part in your body, and discover whether you feel a sensation or emotion. Or, perhaps, a part shows up in your inner world and reveals itself to you through pictures or words.

Find the protector part in, on, or around your body. This will be your "trailhead" to explore.

Focus on it. Inhabiting your Self energy, turn your attention to the part, and let it know you're with it.

Flesh it out. What does it look like, feel like, smell like, sound like? How close will it let you get?

Assess how you Feel toward it. This is your compass for assessing how much Self energy is present. If you don't like this part, find the part that doesn't like it and ask it to step aside. Your Self can be curious about any part without judgment, but some parts polarize with other parts, so make sure to protect the part revealing itself to you from other parts that might attack it. After any polarized part steps aside, check in with how you feel toward the part now. If all the parts are relaxed, you'll feel one or more of the eight Cs of Self—curiousity, compassion, clarity, calmness, confidence, connection, courage, and creativity.

Befriend the part by getting curious and finding out more about it. Engage in a series of inquiries:

How did it get this job?

How effective is the job?

If it didn't have to do this job, what would it do instead?

How old is this part?

How old does it think you are?

What else does it want you to know?

Ask this part what it Fears.

What does it want for you?

What is it afraid would happen if it stopped doing its job?

The answers to the last *F* will reveal either parts polarized with this part or the exile it is protecting. For example, it might say, "If the eating disorder part quits making me not eat, then I'm afraid the suicidal part will take over." Or it might say, "If I stop starving Liz, then I'm afraid she'll feel ashamed of how worthless and unlovable she is." The suicidal part would be another firefighter, and the part that feels shameful, worthless, and unlovable is probably an exile who needs to be unburdened.

Thank your part for revealing itself and giving you the chance to become intimate with it. See if it wants you to visit again, and if so, make an appointment to return. But don't make a promise you won't keep! Remember, you're building trust with your parts. If you bail on your promises, they won't trust you and are likely to punish you for your flakiness.

IFS MEDITATION

Dick is a longtime meditation practitioner, and IFS offers meditations that include healing trauma rather than bypassing it. *No Bad Parts* contains a variety of IFS meditations intended to help you get to know your parts. Keep in mind that all meditation can be contraindicated in the presence of certain types of trauma. If you have ungrounded parts or dissociative parts, you might be better off going for a silent hike than closing your eyes and meditating. Personally, I rotate between two types of closed-eyed IFS meditation. One is like sitting at a conference table conveniently situated in a beautiful spot in nature, where I can convene every morning with parts and do a "check in." Any part that wants my attention can chime in, and I listen, help them negotiate with each other, and try to parent them so everybody gets their needs met and feels seen and loved by my Self.

After your parts know you'll be checking in frequently, they're more likely to give you space for another kind of meditation that lets you access more of your Self with fewer intrusive thoughts or distractions. If you've had a meditation practice but you've been telling your parts to float on by like clouds or trying to ignore your "monkey mind," try this nonbypassing, IFS-inspired meditation.

IFS Self-Meditation

Close your eyes and drop into your body, focusing on your breath and allowing yourself to feel your body, your emotions, and any sensations that arise.

Notice if any parts are trying to get your attention—such as a thinking part, a remembering part, a planning part, or a part that doesn't want to meditate.

Acknowledge their presence and check in with them briefly, if necessary, using the Get to Know Your Protectors exercise on page 269.

When your parts seem relaxed, see if they'll let you go to the beginning of a hiking trail, either one you know or an imaginary one.

Let your parts know you'd like to go for a walk on the
trail without them, and ask if they'll stay together at
the home base of the trailhead.

Remind them that it's good for everyone if you get to refill
yourself with life-force-transfusing Self energy, and reassure
them you always return and you'll never abandon them.

If some of your parts get scared, see if parts who
aren't scared can look after them, like a teenage part
babysitting a younger part, for a while. Start walking
down the path and notice what happens in your mind,
your body, your emotions, your energy, and your spirit.

See if you can feel a vibrating energy filling you with life force.

Notice if you can feel your heart opening as you get space
from your parts. Allow yourself to rest in this expansive
space for a few moments.

If you notice parts who intrude, ask them to return to the
base of the trailhead. Start with five minutes, and return
and check to see how they responded. If they do well,
try ten, then twenty minutes, then extend up to an
hour if your parts handle it well.

If your parts get triggered that you left them alone, return
to the Get to Know Your Protectors exercise and invest
time in getting to know them better until they trust you
enough to spend more time in Self energy.

Some days your parts might not let you go down the path at
all. That's fine. Have a parts conference or do the Get to Know
Your Protectors exercise, one part at a time. Other days, your
parts might be chill and happy to give you a break. Be willing to
go with the flow of what your parts need, and resist the temptation to bully them if they won't let you do this. Over time, with
enough trust and healing of the exiles underneath, they will.

Chapter 12

ENERGY PSYCHOLOGY

Although I've been familiar with the more commonly known and heavily researched energy psychology Emotional Freedom Technique/s (EFT) for many years, I first learned about another energy psychotherapy—Advanced Integrative Therapy (AIT)—at an energy psychology conference where I'd been asked to speak. Duke radiologist Larry Burk, who researches how some women have precognitive dreams about breast cancer that help them save their own lives, said, "Come with me, Lissa. A trauma therapist, Asha Clinton, who developed AIT, is using energy psychology to cure cancer." My ears perked up.

Minutes later, I was in a plastic chair in a conference room, listening to Asha talk about energy psychology protocols, chakras, and how this trauma therapy was being used—at least with anecdotal success—to treat people with cancer. Asha explained that, after losing her husband to cancer, she became particularly passionate about finding a way to treat the psychospiritual factors that might predispose people to cancer. Although it's not the only physical illness AIT has been used to treat, given that cancer has been such a leading cause of death in the United States for years, second only to heart disease, any Sacred Medicine intervention that might be added to the cancer-healing medicine bag seemed worthy of further investigation.

Asha made it clear that psychospiritual trauma is not the only potential predisposing factor to cancer. Genetics can predispose people as well, but Asha believes AIT can help protect those with a genetic predisposition to illness through epigenetic intervention. Physical trauma also must be treated. If you smoke, drink too much, use street drugs, or eat junk food, treat the psychospiritual traumas that led to the nervous system dysregulation, causing you to downregulate hyperarousal with some addictions or upregulate hypoarousal with others. Of course, environmental traumas such as toxins in the home or water supply must be addressed externally. Cultural traumas such as systemic racism, financial inequity, and the aftermath of colonization and genocide must be rooted out systemically and treated individually *and* collectively, not just with trauma therapy but also with policy change. Without bypassing all those other potential influences, treating individual trauma energetically at the psychological, spiritual, ancestral, and past-life level seems to improve outcomes for AIT patients with cancer and other illnesses, by anecdotal testimony.

A former Princeton professor; a trained cultural anthropologist and psychotherapist with a master of arts, master of social work, and doctorate; a pioneer in the burgeoning field of energy psychology; and a practitioner of Buddhism and Sufism, Asha was far from the ungrounded realm of often self-taught energy healers I had been researching until that point in 2017. Not only had she developed an innovative healing method but also she had trained more than 2,000 psychotherapists to use it. Unlike some of the other healers I'd met, she was neither hoarding her wisdom nor creating dependency on her or her "specialness." She was not afraid to teach others how to do what she does. She also claimed that at least some of what AIT offered could be applied as a self-help healing treatment for patients and clients motivated to do their own work. This was part of what I was seeking—practical self-healing tools I could pass on to you, dear reader.

When I met Asha, I had the open wound on my leg from the dog attack, my mother had cancer, my mother and I had recently returned from our pilgrimages to Africa and Italy, and I needed healing myself. I invited Asha to what turned out to be a five-hour brain dump so I could share what I was learning and hear what she was practicing.

Fast forward two years, after I'd been trained in the basics of AIT, and I found myself pulling AIT out of my medicine bag to treat a distraught client at a workshop for therapists in Paris. I had been giving a relatively intellectual review of the Six Steps to Healing Yourself from my book *Mind Over Medicine*, talking about the role of treating trauma as part of any comprehensive medical treatment, especially for people with life-threatening conditions such as cancer.

One therapist asked, "What if your client or loved one is sick and not responding to medical treatment, but they're not willing to touch their traumas?"

I answered, "Then you comfort and treat the parts of yourself scared to lose someone you love and the parts who think you have any business interfering with the healing journey of someone else. Everyone is entitled to their own journey."

That's the moment one of the men in the group began to cry in wracked sobs. Everyone fell silent, and we all waited, holding safe space for him with open hearts and patience. When he was finally able to compose himself enough to speak, he explained:

> I'm a trauma therapist, and my wife, Sophie, who was the love of my life, had a significant trauma history. When she got cancer, I intuited that she'd have to deal with getting her trauma treated if she was going to have an optimal outcome from her cancer treatment. But Sophie had walled off that part of her life and wasn't willing to go anywhere near what happened in the past. I became increasingly panicked as her cancer got worse and pressured her to see a therapist, but the harder I pushed, the more she resisted. She died two years ago, and I've been blaming myself ever since. I just can't seem to move on. I'm a trauma therapist, but I wasn't even able to save my own wife.

He began sobbing again. The therapist seated next to him asked if he wanted a hug, and he nodded. She held him, rocking him while he wept.

There wasn't a dry eye in the room. A heaviness had spread over the space, and I asked if the man was willing to let me work with him in front of the group so I could demonstrate one of the simple tools of a cutting-edge energy psychotherapy—AIT. He agreed, settling himself up at the front of the room with a box of tissues and introducing himself as Philippe.

Philippe told a bit of his story, explaining how he had tried to convince Sophie to get trauma therapy alongside the chemotherapy and surgery her doctors recommended. No matter how he tried to explain how much unhealed trauma can make disease worse or interfere with the possibility of cure, and no matter how many studies he tried to get her to read about the impact of trauma on disease, Sophie wouldn't budge. Any suggestion that she go back into her childhood and get treatment for what happened cued her refrain: "*Not in this lifetime.*"

After Sophie died a slow, painful death attended to by palliative care nurses, Philippe explained how he got stuck in protracted grief. Every time he returned to memories of Sophie, he was flooded with unbearable feelings of helplessness, hopelessness, terror, shame, overwhelming sadness, and fury at himself for being such a loser and failure.

I asked Philippe to feel into the phrase: "Sophie wasn't willing to get treatment for her trauma, and she died of cancer, and I blame myself and feel like a loser and failure." I asked if this phrase resonated as true and invited him to customize the phrase and make it better if it wasn't quite right. Philippe said it felt right and rounded his shoulders as he repeated the phrase. I asked him where in his body he felt this phrase. He contracted around his chest and put his hand over his heart. I asked him to rate, on a scale of zero to ten, with ten being the most intense, how strongly he felt the sensations and feelings of this phrase. Philippe said it was a ten.

I instructed Philippe to keep one hand over his heart and move the other hand over thirteen energy centers (chakras) in his body while repeating the phrase. I demonstrated, putting my palm over the top of my head and saying, "Put your hand over the top of your head and repeat after me. 'Sophie wasn't willing to get treatment for her trauma, and she died of cancer, and I blame myself and feel like a loser and failure.'" He stammered through the phrase, crying in bursts between words, slowly making his way through the whole phrase with my prompting.

I waited a moment to let the energy move in Philippe before moving my hand to my forehead and instructing him to do the same. He mimicked my hand position. "Now repeat it again: 'Sophie wasn't willing to get treatment for her trauma, and she died of cancer, and I blame myself and feel like a loser and failure.'" Phillipe repeated the phrase with more ease this time around. Next, I moved my hand to a spot between my lower lip and my chin and instructed Philippe to repeat the phrase again. Philippe complied.

I walked him through all thirteen energy centers, moving down through the body and ending at the perineum, just between the genitals and the anus. By this point, Philippe was calmer and able to laugh at the awkwardness of the position as he put his hand under his buttocks. After he finished repeating the phrase for the thirteenth time, I asked him to rate the intensity of his sensations and feelings. He said he was down to a three.

Going back to the crown of the head, I led him through another round, repeating the phrase thirteen more times while touching each of the energy centers. By the time Philippe reached the perineum again, the emotional and physical charge had gone to a zero. The shift in Philippe's energy was visible to everyone in the room as he looked around and realized all eyes were on him, beaming with tenderness.

He let out another big exhale and smiled. Looking at me, he said, "You just freed me."

To which I replied, "*You* just freed you."

Philippe repeated what I had said: "Everyone is entitled to their own journey." He began to cry again softly. "Sophie was entitled to her own journey." He wrapped his arms around himself as if giving himself a hug. "It wasn't my fault."

I said what Asha teaches all AIT practitioners to say at the end of removing a particular traumatic energy—"Hallelujah!"

Philippe repeated, "Hallelujah!"

Philippe would need to follow up this quick fix with some deeper treatment for his sense of freedom to last. A sense of exaggerated responsibility for someone else's fate—and feeling like a loser and failure if he couldn't save that person—probably started much earlier in Philippe's life as a result of developmental trauma and would need to be treated. But to get him through the rest of the workshop, this application of a simplified version of AIT offered Philippe—and many others in the room who shared this tendency to take responsibility for other people's healing—some quick relief.

WHAT IS AIT?

AIT is a complete energy psychotherapy with Jungian roots, aspects of Gestalt therapy, some self-psychology, and influences from Buddhism and Sufism. AIT is based on a set of protocols and other methods with a psychodynamic, cognitive-behavioral, and transpersonal theoretical foundation that provides thorough, deep, and relatively painless treatment for trauma and its resultant mental, physical, emotional, and spiritual health challenges. As energy psychology was entering the therapy community, other therapists eager for an integrative way to add it to their practices jumped onboard and wanted to be trained in what Asha had created.

After being used by therapists to treat every psychiatric condition and many physical conditions, such as cancer and autoimmune disease, it has been used with great anecdotal success to provide treatment for depression, anxiety, post-traumatic stress disorder (PTSD), addictions, some chronic illnesses, and even hard-to-treat personality disorders and dissociative disorders. AIT treats the past trauma causing the present symptoms in the patient, along with traumatic underpinnings that might exaggerate and retrigger symptoms, thereby healing trauma more deeply and energetically.

EASY AIT CHAKRA POINTS

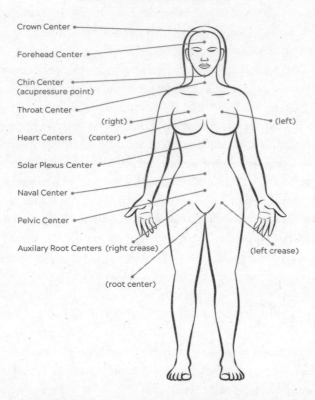

Crown Center
Forehead Center
Chin Center (acupressure point)
Throat Center
(right)   (left)
Heart Centers   (center)
Solar Plexus Center
Naval Center
Pelvic Center
Auxilary Root Centers   (right crease)   (left crease)
(root center)

Like Internal Family Systems (IFS), rather than pathologizing these conditions, AIT focuses on treating the traumas that cause them, the symptoms and beliefs arising from trauma, and the connections among them energetically so as to disrupt the traumatic patterns that predispose us to playing out our dramas in a seemingly endless succession of suffering.

AIT not only treats the psychological and somatic roots of trauma as well as its sequelae or long-term effects, such as the thoughts, beliefs, sensations, and feelings that scurry around your mind, land in your body, and cause emotional and physical pain, but also it includes protocols that focus on spiritual blockage along with methods for instilling positive qualities, centering, embodiment, grounding, and presence. AIT is not only a trauma-healing treatment but also a method that supports and makes possible spiritual opening. As AIT developed, Asha discovered that trauma blocks spiritual development, so that the more trauma gets healed, the more blocks to spiritual development are removed. As a result of healing trauma, it's natural for people who use AIT to open spiritually. Because of this, AIT provides protocols designed to create a bridge between the ego and the Center, the incorruptible Divine essence inside every human, which can be veiled by trauma but never lost.

AIT is based upon the well-accepted discovery in quantum physics that in the end, matter and energy are one phenomenon. Body, psyche, and spirit are profoundly linked, so that after a trauma has occurred the emotions caused by the trauma can dock in an organ or energy center, leading to traumatic blocks in the natural flow of life force, which might also be called qi (Traditional Chinese Medicine and Qigong), prana (Indian Ayurveda and yoga), or subtle energy (energy medicine), causing mental and physical illness to arise and leading to unnecessary but treatable pain and suffering. AIT is designed to remove these blockages so free-flowing life force can be restored, allowing emotions to flow so the body's and the psyche's natural self-healing properties can be restored.

When it comes to treatment, AIT does not distinguish between situational, developmental, generational, or collective traumas, although it does recognize "repetitive" trauma as AIT's way of diagnosing and treating what others might call developmental trauma. Although situational trauma might involve a single incident—a rape, an encounter at gunpoint, a car accident—other traumas are so repetitive and severe that they distort the basic character structures of the psyche and then rigidify them so that they become difficult to transform.

AIT AS MEDICAL TREATMENT

Asha believes trauma and cancer are often linked. Although science has yet to verify this assertion, treating the traumas of people who have cancer might well have the potential of helping reverse the disease and allowing the patient to stay in remission, at least for longer than expected. Some of the case studies AIT therapists have shared suggest that this method of treating cancer might indeed be worth further scientific exploration.

When Cal was sixty-eight, he had his cancer successfully treated with AIT. His doctors diagnosed him with stage-two prostate cancer and offered him surgical removal as well as radiation. Instead, he chose to be treated with AIT because his conscience told him that his cancer had psychological roots, and his wife, an AIT therapy client herself, insisted that any treatment that would destroy his sexual potency was unacceptable to her. When Asha sat down with Cal to take his medical and psychological history, she asked, among other things, about his sexual experiences because the cancer had taken root in his prostate gland, a sexual organ. AIT cancer treatment is based in part on the theory that illness, cancer included, is a symbolically meaningful message from a patient's Center and that understanding and energetically treating that message can help heal the cancer.

Unlike in some popular mind-body healing books that include tables of symptoms and the psychological or metaphorical meaning such symptoms might imply, AIT therapists do not have a list of symptoms and their metaphysical interpretations. Instead, they ask the patient. So Asha asked about Cal's sexual experiences.

Gentle prodding wasn't enough, though Cal was not at all a prudish man. Asha asked, "Are you feeling ashamed of something that has to do with your sex life?" Cal sat in silence while Asha watched his cheeks turn red. She felt bad about causing his discomfort. Finally, he said:

> I was a pretty wild teenager—lots of booze, dope, wild parties, and one-night stands. It was one thing when I slept with a girl who already had had sexual experiences. Those were pretty much times when the girl and I, as equals, agreed to use each other for our mutual pleasure. But it was another thing when I slept with a "nice girl" who had love fantasies rather than experience, one who was looking for her prince and expecting to live happily forever once she found him. When those girls realized, a day or two after we had sex, that they meant nothing to me but easy sex, and I never even bothered to call them, they were deeply hurt. All my life I've

thought of the two girls I hurt that way, but I've never
even tried to find them, let alone apologize to them.

Asha muscle tested these sexual experiences and determined that they
were related to Cal's prostate cancer and that it would be in his highest
interest to treat them as such. Asha also insisted on treating this prostate
cancer as an impulse to right the wrong of behaving so heartlessly. She
muscle tested that it was in Cal's highest interest to find the girls and
apologize. That is exactly what happened! Asha and Cal thoroughly treated the traumas related to Cal's sexual misuse of women, including how
he learned to think misogynistically from his dad and the guys in his
college fraternity.

The mass in Cal's prostate gland began shrinking soon after the first
trauma treatments. It disappeared after his visits and apologies to the two
women he had mistreated. Cal went into remission without conventional
medical treatment and stayed in remission for the rest of his life. He died
peacefully in his sleep some fifteen years later. Cal was one of a few AIT
clients whose early hurtful sexual behaviors seemed correlated with the
development of his prostate cancer.

Some years after Asha met Cal, she got a call from Amanda, who was
frightened by her cancer recurrence and sought immediate treatment.
Asha suggested to her that she have hour-and-a-half sessions daily for
four days, and they have normal weekly sessions after that if necessary.
Amanda agreed and was relieved that Asha understood her fear and her
consequent need for immediate, intensive treatment. During those four
days, they treated Amanda's tendency to care for and mother the people she loved, especially her sister, while neglecting to care for herself.
Amanda realized that even the timing of her recurrences made sense.
She'd had four so far, and each one had occurred after her sister, who had
been sexually abused by their selfish, psychopathic father, moved in with
Amanda. After Asha thoroughly treated Amanda's Type C cancer personality, Amanda experienced an immense inner shift and saw her whole
life through a new lens. The relief and understanding this brought was a
gift of grace. Less than one month later, a PET scan showed no cancer in
her body. Amanda remained cancer-free for four more unexpected years
but then developed cardiomyopathy, a known aftereffect of one of the
first chemotherapics she had received. Amanda died five years after Asha's
work with her, so she got to be alive when her grandchildren were born.

I asked Asha if, in her work with cancer patients, she had observed particular traumatic patterns that tended to be linked to cancer. She was familiar with Lydia Temoshok's work and agreed that the Type C personality could be a risk factor for cancer. Fortunately, she assured me, cancer patients need not be afraid if they recognize themselves in these personality traits. The psychological traumas that lead to the Type C personality, which manifests as emotional repression, denial as a coping strategy, excessive niceness, people pleasing, self-sacrifice, and martyrdom, can all be treated psychologically and energetically with AIT, effectively transforming the cancer patient's personality into a more life-renewing one.

In cancer patients, she also commonly observes repetitive early attachment trauma, especially the lack of unconditional love resulting in loss of self-value, the development of a false self, the tendency to obsessively strive to please others to be loved, and the retraumatization that can occur when childhood attachment wounds are retriggered by abandonment in adulthood such as a divorce or death of a loved one. Childhood abandonment traumas or attachment wounding do not have to mean Mom or Dad left. For many fetuses, babies, and children, abandonment is a heartbreaking everyday trauma occurring because of interruptions in healthy child development.

The developmentally traumatized child does not grow up feeling unconditionally loved, protected, nurtured, praised, encouraged, or appropriately tended—and this is its own devastating abandonment. Other abandonment wounds can arise in the form of being hated, betrayed, used, envied, abused, neglected, or deprived. These attachment traumas, especially when they are repetitive, can result in an adult who, consciously or unconsciously, loses touch with the will to live. Most cancer patients are not suicidal and might have no conscious awareness of a waning will to live. They might even be doing everything in their power to get better. But this decreased will to live, resulting from repetitive developmental trauma, can affect the body's ability to self-heal or adequately mount a response to the cancer via other conventional medical therapies. AIT protocols include using muscle testing to assess the conscious or unconscious loss of a strong will to live. If a reduced will to live is diagnosed using muscle testing, AIT is used to treat the traumas that make someone less enthused about staying alive. In the experience of AIT therapists, after the will to live is restored by treating and removing the traumatic energies, the likelihood of an optimal mental and physical health outcome seems to be greater.

Although people with cancer are often referred to AIT therapists because AIT has specific protocols for adjunctive cancer treatment, AIT therapists also use Multi-Causal Illness Treatment to treat other diseases, such as Hashimoto's thyroiditis, Crohn's disease, diabetes mellitus, fibromyalgia, lupus, multiple sclerosis, heart disease, asthma, chronic or postoperative pain, and bacterial infections, such as sinusitis and bronchitis.

A WANING WILL TO LIVE

If you or someone you love is fighting a dreadful disease such as cancer, you might be wondering, "How could this be?" If you're reading this book, you likely think you have a strong will to live and would try anything to heal. Maybe your will to live is strong, but your disease is meeting another core need or helping to protect you in some way not in your conscious awareness. Maybe not, but what if that's possible? As paradoxical as that might sound, it was a common theme among the healers I interviewed.

AIT therapists are not the only healers I meet who conclude that some people with diseases not responding well to treatment might have a waning will to live that must be reversed before an optimal health outcome is within reach. The good news is that AIT treats those traumas and can bolster the will to live, which can be retested using the muscle test and confirmed.

Many healers also reiterated the idea that people not responding to medical treatment might be getting other core needs met by staying sick, which could sabotage further efforts to heal. If illness is the only way you know how to get core unmet developmental needs met, your body and psyche are going to be understandably reluctant to let go of getting those core human needs met. If being sick helps someone get their fundamental needs met, it would make sense that all efforts to get well might fail unless new strategies for getting those core needs met are put into place. It makes sense that if being sick is helping to protect you, keep you safe, give you financial stability, free you from caregiving or going to a job you hate, grant you a hall pass to get out of something that scares or hurts you, or otherwise help you in some way, some unconscious part of you might be unwilling to let go of this ally, even if it is also causing suffering and potentially putting your life at risk.

I discovered this bewildering phenomenon a decade ago, when my practice shifted from one-on-one integrative medicine, treating sick patients who hadn't responded to conventional medical treatment, to teaching group *Mind Over Medicine* workshops about the Six Steps to Healing Yourself. Unbeknownst to me, I learned from my patients that many of them were horrified to discover during our healing process they were getting core needs met by being sick. Some were getting disability benefits and didn't want to return to the job they hated. Others were getting an excuse not to engage with family members they didn't like. Some were making a living off being sick, writing books about thriving with their disease, for example. How would they make money if they got cured?

Please don't misunderstand this nuance. It can be traumatic for sick patients to discover they might, in some way, be sabotaging their own disease remission. It can feel like blaming the patient and activate "not good enough" traumas, leaving people feeling hopeless rather than empowered. Getting curious about whether you might, in some mysterious way, be blocking your healing can evoke feelings of fear, anger, sadness, guilt, or shame. It's important to be gentle with yourself and remember you're not doing this intentionally—*it's not your fault*. As we discussed with IFS, this is often related to a "protector" part who's trying to help you—and in some way, it is. Usually, there's a good reason. Understanding this helps you love and accept yourself even if you might be unwittingly sabotaging an optimal health outcome.

It's also possible that your traumas or your will to live have nothing to do with the underlying cause of your disease or what is needed for relief. The reason I introduce this idea, often triggering to patients, is because trauma can affect one's will to live, and treating it can reverse that waning will, bolstering life force and potentially bringing disease remission closer. If this insight doesn't feel helpful to you—please, just toss it. If you're curious to consider more, read on.

This idea that our diseases might be helping us meet core needs we don't know how to meet otherwise fit well with what I had observed in my *Mind Over Medicine* workshops. When we reached step five of the Six Steps to Healing Yourself, people would write what I called the Prescription for Healing. This intuitive action plan intended to optimize the body's chance for radical remission often demanded big life changes, such as committing to trauma healing or shadow work, changing the form of a relationship, making a career change, moving to a different location, setting clear boundaries around abusive family members, engaging in a creative project, or fulfilling a lifelong dream. When we got to this part in the workshop, I would ask attendees, "There are no guarantees, but let's say we lived in a magical universe where you would be guaranteed a full cure if you did everything on this list. How many of you would?"

Consistently, about half admitted that, if they were honest, they weren't up to doing what it might take to make such big changes in their lives. They often felt ashamed of this uncomfortable truth. I wanted to understand why, so I asked.

"If I got well, I'd stop getting my disability check and return to that God-awful job."

"If my illness went away, my friends would stop taking care of me, and I'd be all alone again."

"My husband beat me until I got sick. Now he doesn't beat me anymore, but he might start again."

"I write a famous blog about thriving with cancer, and thousands of people follow me. That's how I make my living. If my cancer goes away, what will I write about?"

When I invited people in my workshops to consider other solutions, such as letting go of the disability check and finding another job you love, or asking your friends if they would still come visit even if you weren't sick, or getting out of a violent marriage, or choosing a new topic to write about, I was often met with blank stares and heads shaking. Initially, I figured it must be related to fear, so I started researching it and published *The Fear Cure*. Now, I believe it's more than fear that keeps people stuck; it's unhealed trauma. Fear of change is only one of trauma's many manifestations. Trauma leads to a crisis of imagination, tunneling our worldview, limiting neurological function, and making it difficult for us to imagine other ways to get our needs met. This awareness led me to revise my Six Steps to Healing Yourself based on my new understanding of why we might resist healing. I added AIT as a potential treatment to help those of us who might be unconsciously resistant to treatment so we can learn how to work consciously, compassionately, and energetically with our own resistance, treating the traumas that cause it and plugging the energy leaks caused by having one foot on the gas and one on the brakes.

Muscle testing might come in handy when you're ready to examine the usually unconscious ways in which you might have one foot on the gas of healing and one foot on the brakes of blocking healing. (Before doing any muscle testing, refer to chapter 8 to refresh yourself on the dangers, misuses, and risks of delving into the deep unconscious with muscle testing.)

With the rare exception of floridly suicidal individuals, 99 percent of sick and suffering people consciously desire an end to their suffering and say they are motivated to get well. That said, it's possible that some (but not all) patients might have untreated trauma that interferes with getting optimally healthy—physically and psychologically. This often comes as a shock to patients because many of them have been exhausting themselves traipsing from one practitioner to another; taking one supplement and herb after another; trying every drug, surgery, diet, or alternative remedy they can find. To suggest that in some way they might want to stay sick feels insulting, so it's crucial to reiterate that this unconscious desire to be sick is exactly that—*unconscious*. Nobody is suggesting that sick people are hypochondriacal, malingering, masochistic, or suicidal. Neither are we suggesting that people's illnesses are their fault or they're knowingly blocking their ability to get well.

The AIT Body Alliance

AIT uses muscle testing to screen clients for beliefs that might inadvertently sabotage their healing. Using a protocol Asha calls the AIT Body Alliance as well as 125 other groups of negative core beliefs that might require transformation, AIT therapists use muscle testing to screen for negative core beliefs such as:

> I have nothing to live for.
> I want to get much, much worse.
> It's not safe to be healed.
> I don't deserve to be healed.
> I don't want to be healed.
> I don't want to live in my body.
> I must always be sick.
> I cannot live without illness.
> It's impossible for me to be healed.
> I will never be healed.

I won't do what I need to do to be healed.
I want to die.

If muscle testing is positive for any of these beliefs, it can be used to identify the traumas that might have led to them, which are then systematically identified and treated. The negative core beliefs can be energetically removed using AIT. Then the self-sabotaging belief's "realistic positive opposite" can be installed energetically.

Realistic positive opposites might include:

I have my healing and transformation to live for.
It's safe to be healed.
I deserve to be healed.
I give myself permission to be healed.
I want to live in my body.
I can live without illness.
It's possible for me to be healed.
I'll do what I need to do to be healed.
I want to live.

It's important to note that Asha does not recommend muscle testing the AIT Body Alliance by yourself. Although you might be curious about what your muscle test might uncover if an expert tester screened you for the AIT Body Alliance, it might not behoove you to learn you test positive for "I have nothing to live for" when you have a child you love or a mission you feel called to complete and don't understand what's happening. This isn't as scary with a trained therapist next to you because any traumas causing such a belief will get treated speedily, becoming empowering rather than frightening. But if you don't have a therapist, you might not want to try this *until* you're ready and able to get professional help.

USING AIT TO SELF-TREAT TRAUMA

Because AIT is a complete therapy, just as Jungian analytical psychology is a complete form of psychoanalysis, explaining AIT as a self-help treatment is difficult—but it's possible, within limits. I'll share some relatively simple do-it-yourself healing practices from AIT.

I'll begin with Easy AIT, which I demonstrated in the beginning of the chapter with Philippe blaming himself for his wife, Sophie, dying of cancer. If you've ever tried Emotional Freedom Technique/s (EFT), you'll recognize similarities and differences: AIT uses the chakras, not the meridians; in AIT you touch your body from the top of your head down to your rump, whereas EFT stops at your midsection. Based on the chakra system from Ayurvedic medicine, AIT includes the traditional seven chakras as well as some lesser-known chakras, such as the belly button and the chin.

Easy AIT is a simple self-help version of the more complicated AIT process you would do with the guidance of a therapist. Because AIT depends upon muscle testing—and mastering muscle testing takes practice—Easy AIT skips muscle testing and gives you a straightforward way to remove the emotions, contents, and physical sensations of a trauma without the help of a therapist.

Sometimes when we think about our traumas, our bodies, psyches, and spirits begin to react to what we are remembering and go wonky, making it difficult to treat trauma successfully. We are, among other things, electromagnetic beings whose body polarity can shift when we're stressed. When this happens, our thinking gets muddy, and we're far more likely to trip over our own feet. Also, our bodies can't function normally if we're dehydrated. Remember: We consist mostly of water, our body's electrical conductor, so it's important to hydrate before we do Easy AIT. Finally, we are all resistant to healing sometimes, perhaps when the trauma is too scary or painful for us to bear or when we're afraid to treat what happened because we don't want to look at our part in it. When body polarity, dehydration, or resistance are present, they ruin a treatment opportunity, so we need to correct them before we begin.

Before you start doing any energetic trauma treatment, consider implementing these basic energy hygiene practices for rebalancing body polarity, dehydration, and resistance. Here's how:

Make sure body polarity is working correctly (Modified Cook's Hookup)

1. Cross your left ankle over your right and leave it there.
2. Put your left hand on your right thigh and leave it there.
3. Put your right hand on your left thigh and leave it there.
4. Put your tongue up behind your top front teeth and leave it there.
5. Stay in this position for ninety seconds to two minutes.

Avoid dehydration

1. Drink at least half a glass of water.

Block resistance

1. Find your "sore points": Starting at the concavity below your throat, go down three inches (use both hands), move each hand outward on the side of your chest, left hand moving left, right hand moving right, until each is about three and a half inches out from the center of your chest.
2. Rub the place each hand ends up for ninety seconds to two minutes. These places are usually sore, and that's okay. It's the rubbing that blocks resistance. It doesn't matter if the points stay sore.

Easy AIT Protocol #1

1. **Get ready:** Take a look at the chart on page 278 to see where you're going to be putting your hands. It helps to memorize the energy centers and the order in which you'll be touching them so you can say your phrase nine times in a row without looking back at the chart. But as you're learning, enjoy using the chart like a cheat sheet or a map for removing traumas. To treat traumas, you'll be moving one hand down the chakras the same way each time and leaving the other hand on the same chakra during each round of treatment.

2. **Choose your trauma:** Think of something that's hurting in your life—a simple trauma, something that makes you angry or sad, or a repeating pattern of behavior that unfortunately keeps showing up in your life.

3. **Create your phrase:** A brief one-sentence phrase that describes the trauma you want to treat. You can just state it directly, for example, "My Dad left us and never

came back"; or, if it's a repeating pattern, you can say something like, "All the times and ways the kids on the block teased and humiliated me."

4. **Remember trauma and check its emotional intensity:** Remember the painful event or traumatic pattern; let yourself feel all the emotions that arise from remembering it. On a scale from zero to ten, where zero means you feel no emotions and ten means you feel the greatest possible intensity of emotion, where are the feelings you still have about this memory now? Choose the number from zero to ten that best represents how intense these emotions are.

5. **Stationary hand position:** Sense where in your body you feel these emotions the most. Put one hand there and leave it there.

6. **Go down the chakras:** Keeping one hand stationary on the spot you're now touching, move the other hand from the top of your head to the bottom of your perineum, stopping to touch each of the nine energy centers (chakras) along the way (the ones from the chart). You can use either two fingers or your palm on any of the chakras—your choice. Each time you touch a new chakra, repeat the phrase, reading it off your paper if you don't remember it. Let us guide you through this.

> *Crown Center:* With your stationary hand in place the whole time on the chakra you chose, use your other hand to hold the crown chakra, on the top of your head, and say your phrase out loud or silently until you feel ready to move to the next chakra.
> *Forehead Center:* Move your moving hand to your forehead, and repeat the phrase again.
> *Chin Center:* Move your moving hand to your chin, and repeat the phrase again.

Throat Center: Move your moving hand to your throat, and repeat the phrase again.

Heart Center: Move your moving hand to your heart center, and repeat the phrase again.

Solar Plexus Center: Move your moving hand to your solar plexus, and repeat the phrase again.

Navel Center: Move your moving hand to your navel, and repeat the phrase again.

Pelvic Center: Move your moving hand to the area right above your pubic bone, and repeat the phrase again.

Root Center: Get your giggles out of the way, and move your moving hand to your perineum (for women, this is the area between your vaginal opening and your anus, for men, this the area between the back of your scrotum and your anus), and repeat the phrase one last time.

7. **Deep Breath:** When you're done repeating your phrase while holding each energy center, take a deep breath.

8. **Get emotional intensity level:** Now remember the trauma you're treating again. Check in with your emotions about the trauma, and pick a number from zero to ten that specifies their intensity now. Usually the number has dropped from what it was the first time you checked.

9. **Getting to zero:** If that new number is anything other than zero, start again at the top of your head, and say the phrase over again through all nine energy centers. Do as many rounds as it takes to get to zero.

10. **Hooray!** Once you get to zero, say "Hallelujah!" or some other celebratory phrase with gusto!

Now that you've treated your first trauma, here's your cheat sheet for Easy AIT:

Easy AIT

1. Get Ready

2. Choose Your Trauma

3. Create Your Phrase

4. Remember Trauma and Check Its Emotional Intensity

5. Stationary Hand Position

6. Go Down the Chakras
    Crown Center
    Forehead Center
    Chin Center
    Throat Center
    Heart Center
    Solar Plexus Center
    Navel Center
    Pelvis Center
    Root Center

7. Deep Breath

8. Get Emotional Intensity Level

9. Getting to a Zero

10. Hooray!

That's Easy AIT in a nutshell. Congratulations! You have lightened your trauma burden just the smallest bit, and after you've done many of these, you'll be feeling so much better—mentally, emotionally, physically, and spiritually.

Easy AIT Protocol #2

1. **Find the trauma and create the phrase that you want to treat:** Describe what happened in a short sentence. In Philippe's case, the phrase was "Sophie wasn't willing to get treatment for her trauma, and she died of cancer, and I blame myself and feel like a loser and failure." A few more examples:

   "The lightning hit my car with me in it."

   "They started taunting me, and I ran into my house crying."

   "Shrapnel hit me in both legs before I could find cover."

   If it's a repetitive trauma, it might be a more inclusive phrase:

   "All the times and ways . . ."

   "I get so hurt, ashamed, and angry when I'm criticized that I see red and can't defend myself."

   "I pick partners who betray me with other lovers."

   "I put other people's needs before mine and don't take care of myself."

2. **Discover how intense a reaction you have to this trauma:** Let yourself feel all the feelings and physical sensations arising in you from recalling this trauma. Assess, on a scale from zero to ten—with zero meaning "no emotion or sensation" and ten being the maximum intensity of all the feelings and sensations together—how intense the charge of those emotions and sensations is.

3. **Find where the emotions and sensations constellate in the body:** Because the energetic clearing aspect of AIT is based on the chakra system from Indian Ayurvedic medicine, pick one of the thirteen major and minor chakra points where you feel the majority of this particular trauma lives in your body.

4. **Treatment:** With one hand staying where you feel the trauma in your body, move your other hand over the thirteen chakra points on your body from top to bottom, saying your phrase out loud or in silence upon arrival at each chakra point and staying there until you intuit that it's time to move to the next one. (Refer to page 278 for the thirteen chakra points.) At the end of the round, after you've said your phrase thirteen times, take a deep breath.

5. **Closure:** When you've finished, close your eyes, check back on the intensity of the feelings and sensations, and rate it again on a scale from zero to ten. If you're at a zero, celebrate by saying "Hallelujah!" or another celebratory word or phrase you prefer. If not, do another round or two—it seldom takes more—down the chakras until you get to zero. When you get there, *bam!* The memory of the trauma is still there, but the charge on that particular trauma has been moved out of your body, psyche, and spirit. Most people who've gotten to zero say they feel lighter, and their nervous systems feel more regulated in every way.

THREE-STEP TRANSFORMATION

Although it's possible to use elements of AIT as a quick fix in the way I used it to help Philippe, using Easy AIT alone is more of a bandage than a permanent treatment for trauma. Just as other energy psychology tools, such as Emotional Freedom Technique/s (EFT), can be used in a pinch to improve functioning or reduce suffering, unless the core roots of a traumatic pattern are identified and treated, the problems are likely to keep returning. So how do we treat those deep roots and remove traumatic energies permanently? I'll use my entry into AIT to explain how this works.

When I met Asha, I had just been abandoned by a business partner I thought cared about me personally but later realized was using me. Apparently, I couldn't tell the difference. It wasn't the first time. When I made a list of how often I thought people loved me and later realized they were using me, I felt embarrassed, humiliated, and ashamed. Was I unworthy of being loved on my own merit? Was I somehow sending a message that said, "Take advantage of me?"

I met Asha at the energy psychology conference, and sharing an interest in turning on doctors to AIT as part of a more complete cancer treatment, she suggested we teach some doctors together. But I panicked when I received her detailed proposal, scarred as I was from the business partner who had just abandoned me and not knowing whether Asha would do the same.

Asha seemed sensitive to my hesitation and saw it as an opportunity to demonstrate AIT. She offered to show me how Three-Step Transformation, a unique aspect of AIT that distinguishes it from other energy psychology methods, might help me discover why I was so scared to trust her. I felt hesitant, but I also wanted relief, so I agreed to be treated with AIT, not only for my benefit but also so I could learn more about AIT by becoming the guinea pig myself.

What AIT calls my *Initiating Trauma* was the pain of my abandonment by the business partner. Initiating Trauma is the wound that usually initiates a call to the therapist—something in present time that hurts. In this case, the AIT phrase for my Initiating Trauma was "I thought my business partner loved me, but he was using me instead."

I learned from Asha and other trauma therapists that not always, but often, when something feels excruciating in present time, it's reactivating a traumatic energy from the past. AIT accommodates this as part of its model, recognizing that treating the pain of the present is a stopgap measure unless we treat the pain that makes us hypersensitive to those wounds and perhaps even retraumatizes us. If you've wondered why you keep winding up in the same painful situation, no matter how you try to avoid it, you can probably relate to what I'm talking about. And no—you're not making it happen. Repetitive traumas tend to intensify over time—until we get help and break the cycle.

One fundamental difference between AIT and other energy psychology practices is the intention to treat the Initiating Trauma and ferret out what AIT calls the *Originating Trauma*—the first time a similar wounding affected an individual's energy system. Depending on the belief system of the client, the Originating Trauma might have started in this life, or it might have come from a past life or the trauma of an ancestor. Scientists now have a better understanding of how traumas can literally be passed down from generation to generation.

In my case, Asha found the Originating Trauma (this can be hard to find without a therapist trained in helping you discover it). Essentially, it went all the way back to my mother, who used me rather than loved me and left me confused about the difference between exploitation and love. It wasn't my mother's fault; the same was probably inflicted upon her, and sadly she never sought treatment before she died.

To break the chain of relationships with people who use me rather than love me, the last step of Three-Step Transformation is necessary— the *Connecting Trauma*, a phrase that links the Originating Trauma to the Initiating Trauma, thereby breaking the connection between them.

My Three-Step Transformation went like this:

> **One: Initiating Trauma.** "I thought my business partner loved me, but he was using me instead."

> **Two: Originating Trauma.** "My mother used me rather than loved me."

> **Three: Connecting Trauma.** "Because my mother used me rather than loved me, my business partner used me rather than loved me."

That was several years ago, and so far, my treatment seems to have worked; I'm not repeating that pattern anymore. I can spot someone trying to hook me into that pattern from across a room now, and I'm grateful to have insight and be free of it. Was it fast and easy? *No.* Like sick people who pray for a miracle, I hoped for an instantaneous cure from my lifelong wounding. But that didn't happen. The wounds ran deep, and the process of healing has been slow, laborious, and painful and required discipline, diligence, resilience, and stamina. To tolerate the discomfort, I relied on part one practices to keep me buoyant, but I no longer used them as spiritual bypassing.

My friend Diane was receiving AIT therapy at the same time I was, and she likened the process of weaving in and out of our trauma therapy and our energy transfusion practices to "being like whales." First, we'd fortify ourselves with life force using practices from part one, as if preparing ourselves to go on a solo diving expedition. We'd dive to the bottom of the ocean, making progress on our journey in the depths of the sea of consciousness. Then, we'd return to the surface to breech, smack our tails, play, and catch our breath. When we felt we could handle it again, we'd return to the depths.

What about you? Do you feel fortified enough to take a dive into the depths? If so, try the Three-Step Transformation.

The Basics of Three-Step Transformation

As you begin, try working with simple traumas and short phrases. Don't go straight to the big ones when you're learning, especially if you're doing this yourself. Start with a mild trigger, something less than a five on the zero-to-ten scale of emotional charge.

1. **Identify what's troubling you now.** This would be your Initiating Trauma.

2. **Trace it back to the first time you can remember a similar hurt, your Originating Trauma.** If you're trying this without an AIT therapist, you'll have to rely on your memory and your four Whole Health Intelligences to find the Originating Trauma.

3. **Come up with your Connecting Trauma.** Try this formula: "Because [insert Originating Trauma], then [insert Initiating Trauma].

As an example, let's imagine you get asthma attacks whenever you go see your mother. Your three phrases might be:

>**Initiating Trauma:** I have asthma and have frightening attacks after I visit my mom.

>**Originating Trauma:** All the times and ways that my mother has controlled me, overprotected me, and smothered me.

Connecting Trauma: Because my mother has controlled me, overprotected me, and smothered me, I have asthma and get especially frightening attacks after I visit Mom.

Using the Easy AIT Protocol #1 from page 289, treat your three phrases in the following order:

Step 1. Treat the Originating Trauma first.
Step 2. Treat the Initiating Trauma.
Step 3. Treat the Connecting Trauma.

For extra credit, add a fourth phrase to treat the emotions that might remain after you treat these phrases. For example, "All the rage, sadness, frustration, grief, and regret I feel because I've suffered from asthma attacks my whole life."

Chapter 13

HEALING THE COLLECTIVE

f you've made it this far in this book and in life, you have surely been on a journey. Perhaps you have discovered some fun and delightful tools you're excited to play with. Perhaps others have left you feeling triggered or unsettled. Whatever is arising, try to welcome it without turning away—and take good care of yourself. Be gentle.

You've been through a lot since I first told you about my dog-bite injury, shared with you how to tune in to your Whole Health Intelligences, and taught you about the Six Steps to Healing Yourself. If you've been following along, you might have infused yourself with healing energy and buoyed your life force by journeying with me to Lourdes and learning about the power of pilgrimage, prayer, and group healing. You've indulged your mental intelligence by going to the laboratory and back with me and "the Doc Brown of healing" Bill Bengston. (Yes, I'm dating myself with a *Back to the Future* reference.)

You've educated yourself by going to a different kind of anatomy lab with Donna Eden and learned that what you call *you* might not end at the edge of your skin, something biofield scientists are still trying to validate and understand. You've opened up your somatic intelligence by dancing your prayers, and you might have met your life force–enhancing muse by putting your love into making your art. You've traveled with me to Bali and learned how resacralizing nature and making every tree into a temple can help you attune to your intuitive and emotional intelligence. You've climbed with me to the

Q'eros in the Andes and come back with a greater awareness of our interconnectedness to *Pachamama* (Mother Earth).

You've poured healing light onto your blind spots by learning to understand and love your spiritual bypassing tendencies. You might have had an uncomfortable but illuminating epiphany when you realized these tendencies might lead to personality traits that might put you at risk for disease, such as people pleasing, excessive niceness, anger-phobia, or conflict avoidance. But hopefully you felt inspired when you learned that your personality is not fixed, and you can transform into someone healthier and more authentic to your true nature. You realize this means feeling *all* your feelings and developing more emotional proficiency so you can leverage the healing gifts of your emotional intelligence.

You've recognized that shoring up your physical, emotional, and psychic boundaries could make all the difference, especially if you're an empath. You've learned the potential value and possible risk of Sacred Medicine diagnostics, including medical intuition and muscle testing. You've peered into the startling shadows of Sacred Medicine so you can recognize the sorceresses who still have thorns in their backs, and discern for yourself how to get the most from working with a Sacred Medicine practitioner—*safely*.

I hope an excess of caution and the breaching splashes of energizing transfusions prepared you to dive like a whale to the bottom of the ocean, where you are able to learn about the science linking trauma and disease and get curious about the impact your personal trauma might have on your ability to achieve an optimally healthy body/mind/spirit/energy field. You discovered you are a multiplicity of parts, and those parts are worthy, lovable, and deserving of healing, even the parts who get you in trouble, hurt you or other people, or make your body sick so you'll pay attention and finally get the help you'll need. You learned how to use Internal Family Systems (IFS) and Advanced Integrative Therapy (AIT) so you can heal not only what triggers you in present time but also past traumas that might make your suffering worse.

Take a moment now to check in and celebrate yourself for being so brave! How are you doing? What are you feeling? How does whatever suffering led you to read this book compare now with when you first opened it? What have you learned? What has been helpful? What do you need to toss out because it feels like garbage to your Whole Health Intelligences? What insights have you gained? What traumas have you treated? What, if anything, is different? How have you transformed?

Before I say goodbye, I need to make a confession about a blind spot that came to light during the writing of this book, after much of the travel part of my Sacred Medicine journey was complete. When I set out upon my journey, I admit that I was thinking too small, making the mistake many self-help authors make by trying to help you, dear reader, relieve suffering—*in your individual self.* I wasn't so clueless as to be blind to the undercurrent of trauma permeating American culture. I knew we had an unhealthy obsession with the self and the desire to exert control over it, often with the denial of or blindness to the impact of a sick culture on any individual's mental and physical health. I knew we were a racist, white supremacist culture, a culture that had not reckoned with the impact of colonization and genocide of Indigenous people or with slavery, unfair imprisonment, civil rights violations, and police brutality against people of color. I knew people were starving, capitalism was leading to unrestrained consumerism, and the 1 percent was becoming richer while the most underprivileged were being crushed. I was aware that gun violence was out of control, and addictions, obesity, depression, suicide, and criminal behavior were rising, especially among oppressed, marginalized, and underprivileged people. I knew climate crisis was irreversible, and the planet and her plants and creatures are suffering.

But when I set out on this journey, I hadn't given this awareness enough credence. Although doing what you can to heal your separate self certainly has value, to try to heal the sick self without acknowledging the matrix in which that self is entangled will always be incomplete. This realization had been dawning on me slowly over the course of my Sacred Medicine journey, but it could not have been more obvious than in 2020, when Mother Earth sent us all to timeout. Many of us felt like Mother Earth had to resort to tough love, parenting us by natural consequences because her more subtle cries for help had gone unanswered for decades. Just as the human body tends to whisper its distress before activating the screams of cancer, heart attacks, or strokes, our Earth's body tolerated an inordinate amount of abuse before lashing out with a ferocious "no more."

For a decade I had been studying various ways healers use the breath to facilitate healing. Yet 2020 became the year we collectively could not breathe. This watershed year brought a novel respiratory coronavirus that took away the breath of more than 600,000 Americans and millions worldwide who did not survive it. The year 2020 also took our breath away with out-of-control natural disasters, including devastating wildfires in my home state of California and also across Australia and the rain forests in the Amazon. "I can't breathe" became the chant of the swelling Black Lives Matter movement, echoing, along with repeated pleas for his mother, George Floyd's last words as he was murdered on video by now-convicted police officer Derek Chauvin, who pressed his knee into an unarmed man's windpipe and crushed it for nine minutes and twenty-nine seconds. Some people drew their last breath for mental illness reasons or because of the economic impact of 2020. The fallout was grave as the food supply was interrupted, unemployment soared, immigrants were detained in unlivable circumstances, and more people than usual suffered for a variety of reasons. To become breathless and hypervigilant took on whole different meanings.

I couldn't help reflecting on the synchronicity of the breath-impairing crises that converged in 2020. I started this book by talking about the impact of subtle energies on life force and how many religious traditions spiritualize the breath. The breath is literally *inspiration*—to inspire—from the roots of "in spirit." In many spiritual traditions, the breath is seen as our spiritual essence—as God, if you will. Meditation techniques ask us to focus on the breath. Yoga is about pranayama—breathwork. Even creation myths begin with God breathing life into the world. Human life begins with a baby's first breath outside its mother and ends when we take our last. Breath is life force. Breath animates us. Breath is the difference between life and death, and it became clear in 2020 that way too many of us were being smothered.

In 2020, one of the paradoxes of healing became entirely apparent: We are separate and deserving of self-protection, self-care, self-love, and self-healing—*and* we are intimately woven into the web of life, interconnected to everyone and everything in it. When I embarked upon this book, I had not intended to study healing collective trauma and reckoning with our sick culture as part of my inquiry into Sacred Medicine, yet it became apparent that we cannot separate an individual's body from the planetary body or even from the other human bodies on it. How can anyone have an optimally healthy human body when we are immersed in the poison of a traumatized culture on a brutalized planet, while our fellow humans starve, get gunned down, and lack basic safety and survival resources? My original goal of unraveling the mysteries of healing for any individual's sick body is part of the consciousness that leads to more sickness. We cannot deny that most of us have been swimming in a sea polluted with collective trauma since way before we were born. Before that, our ancestors were hurt, too, passing along their traumas epigenetically.

With a palm smack to my forehead, I realized what many healers outside Western culture (and Indigenous cultures here) never forgot: *The health of your body reflects not only the sum total of your life experiences but all of life and everything you're connected to*—not just your personal history, relational history, and relationship to the planetary body but also the life experiences of your ancestors, your own past-life experiences (if you believe in such things), your kindred earthlings, and the culture in which you were steeped like a complex tea brewing.

Humbled by my ignorance, I couldn't miss the evidence that we humans are all cells in this unified organism of an interconnected planet. Just as you cannot deny the enmeshment between a human heart cell and the heart it pumps or the kidney cell from the kidney that detoxifies, just as the heart and kidney organs in your body rely on each other to keep the whole system functioning, at the most mystical and energetic level you cannot separate the needs and gifts of every sentient being in our planetary body. Whole Health *must acknowledge this.*

SOCIAL JUSTICE AS MEDICINE FOR US ALL

Although each of us would be wise to do what is within our power to use all the medicines at our disposal to relieve suffering when we get sick and make ourselves miracle prone, how can it be possible for any individual human Self to stay optimally healthy when we are all so intimately entangled in a world where access, opportunity, and privilege are so unjustly distributed? Although it took 2020 for me (and many others) to see clearly that optimal health might be more about privilege than personal dedication to a healthy life, I discovered that my previous blind spot had been starkly obvious far earlier to countless BIPOC, LGBTQIA+, financially underprivileged folks, people with disabilities, and other marginalized people. Although spiritual teacher Thomas Hübl has been treating collective trauma as part of his nonbypassing spiritual medicine for many years, the timing could not have been more perfect for his Collective Trauma Summits and his book *Healing Collective Trauma.*[1]

The perception shift was swift—and is still ongoing. Almost overnight, I saw the world as if through new eyes. I had to process my healthy shame and was grateful Karla McLaren had helped me learn how to feel it in a healthy way that motivated me to change my point of view and take a firm stand to do better about making my message about health, spirituality, and wellness inclusive and as actively antiracist as I could, knowing I would continue to mess up, as I'm sure I've done here.

I saw that the spiritual messages I'd been parroting had been helpful to me and to many of my clients, but they didn't always apply to all people. As women such as Layla Saad began calling out "spiritual white women," as she did in her articles "I Need to Talk to Spiritual White Women About White Supremacy—Parts One and Two," I couldn't look away.[2] Because I had done three years of intensive AIT and IFS therapy, I could tolerate the uncomfortable feelings this antiracism work elicited and go public with my apologies, confessions, and desire to be a better ally to the marginalized, oppressed, and underprivileged people I might have been insufficiently sensitive to in my previous work.

The dawning awareness that permeated my consciousness in 2020 and 2021 led me to take a dive not only into my own shadow but also into the shadow of the spiritual self-help, yoga, and wellness industry; conventional medicine; and the integrative and functional medicine world. As a point of inquiry, I allowed myself to grieve, agonize, and wonder. I held my parts compassionately while I examined many of the beliefs I had taken on and parroted, beliefs I now questioned. Although I'm not inclined to succumb to conspiratorial thinking, I considered the actual historical conspiracy of white, cisgender, heterosexual, property-owning men who chose to dominate innocent women, Indigenous and people of color, and those with other gender identities or sexual orientations. Given that these make up the majority of the world's population, how would you get away with something so sinister? If you were to pull off successfully dominating the majority of the population, what kind of psy-op would you have to enact to get them to go along with the domination without rebelling, rising up to make a more powerful majority, and resisting the oppression?

Well . . . as sick as it sounds, if you were interested in getting away with dominating the world, you might use God. After all, God is good, right? If you dress your domination in the Divine, you might sneak your psy-op undercover. This led me to rethink many of the spiritual tropes repeated in religious, New Age, and wellness circles. Everything was up for inquiry, even my most sacredly held beliefs.

What became clear is that we can do better. Waking up means facing the truth, feeling the feels, returning to our bodies, and resolving to love bigger and fiercer—so our love flames into sacred activism and we use our open-hearted, full-throated, gut-intuiting, trauma-informed spiritual awareness to create a more just, equal, passionate, nature-loving, Self-loving, other-loving, and tenderhearted world. This is healing work. It cannot *not* affect the health of our bodies.

We could ignore it no longer in 2020. *The health of the individual is intimately and inextricably linked to the health of our world.* Though people insisted otherwise, you couldn't simply do what you wanted individually when you might poison the air and kill innocent people. Although it behooves us to have good boundaries and treat our traumas so we can establish a sovereign Self and resist collapsing to pressure from others, paradoxically, there's also no such thing as a sovereign Self free to act recklessly during a pandemic. Even the rebellion against public health guidelines during the pandemic revealed evidence of mass developmental trauma. When adults get stuck in a child's regressive rebellion against authority, resisting boundaries meant to keep the collective safe and rejecting limits that could save lives, we know we are in the midst of trauma responses that impede our ability to act collectively so every sovereign being can stay safe.

After the events of 2020 and 2021, one had to *want* to stay intentionally blind not to see how much individual health simply cannot be disentangled from the web of the collective. Denial is a powerful protector part, so many not yet ready to let go of their unearned privileges went off the deep end into mass denial, delusion, spiritual bypassing, gaslighting, lying, and collective psychosis.

Although there's no "silver lining" to 2020 and its aftermath, some of us remembered how much we *needed* one another. It could not be overlooked as those like me, privileged workers sheltering in place and working remotely, were utterly dependent on the essential workers, often BIPOC and people living in poverty, who tended to our needs for food production and distribution, trash collection, grocery store service, and other necessary work. The highest-paid people in modern civilization—sports stars, rock stars, movie stars, and others in the entertainment industry—turned out to be entirely nonessential to the survival of the culture in the face of an emergency.

This greater awareness of how much we rely on each other, especially those with less power and privilege, opened many hearts and evoked gratitude. But we also talked about our guilt, our shame, and our intense discomfort with a growing awareness that our ability to shelter safely at home was built upon the backs of oppressed and marginalized people who didn't have the luxury of sheltering in place. I survived 2020. Many did not, and this weighs on me. In spite of the hall pass given to me by the Balinese healer, I'll admit that I still have world worries on my head.

Touching this pain—without turning away from it, in myself and in the world—fuels my sacred activism and inspires me to leverage my power, privilege, and platform to make yet another offering intended to ease suffering in the world.

HEAL AT LAST: DEMOCRATIZING SACRED MEDICINE

Remember when I mentioned how unfair it is that many Sacred Medicine treatments are luxury goods only readily available to the privileged? Remember how I promised you that my social justice parts were actively seeking to democratize healing so anyone ready to heal can have access to some of the practices shared in this book? Well, I won't leave you hanging.

In 2020, all the world's worries spurred me to start Heal at Last, a nonprofit organization that is my offering to the suffering of the world. Our mission at Heal at Last is to use Sacred Medicine to bring people in recovery from illness, injury, or trauma together in circles of healing, spirituality, writing, art, music, and connection for the purposes of easing loneliness, healing trauma, and improving physical and mental health outcomes, particularly for those conventional medicine has been unable to heal. Using creativity and music as a portal to cutting-edge trauma healing methods, spiritual healing, and energy medicine, we empower individuals and communities of healing ready for the deep dive of treating the root causes of personal and collective suffering. Although cutting-edge healing techniques have become luxury goods in modern cultures, we believe healing and transformation is everyone's birthright and should not be limited to people of privilege. Heal at Last is committed to bringing creative inspiration, soulful intimacy, community connection, and deep healing work to anyone emotionally, psychologically, and spiritually ready for meaningful transformation regardless of socioeconomic status, race, sexual orientation, gender identity, political affiliation, or religion.

By all means, if you can afford to hire one-on-one Sacred Medicine practitioners to support you on your healing journey; if you have access to enough privilege to go on pilgrimages across the globe; if you can go to retreat centers to meditate, dance, make art, or participate in group healings; and if you can hire one-on-one cutting-edge trauma therapists, please do so! But it is my prayer that, God willing, Sacred Medicine be made available to those who might not have such easy access to the kinds of practitioners and experiences I wrote about in this book.

Although self-help tools are great, and I tried to give you everything I found on my own Sacred Medicine quest, delivering what I discovered in the world's medicine bag to you, these tools work better when you can practice them *in community*. Remember one of the paradoxes of healing: You can heal yourself; *and* you can't do it alone.

Although it's a work in progress, Heal at Last is building circles aimed at helping democratize and scale Sacred Medicine for anyone who identifies as being in recovery from illness, injury, or trauma and needs help relieving any suffering that it's possible to relieve, understanding that some suffering cannot be relieved; it can only be carried by a community that cares. If you or someone you love would be interested in participating in Heal at Last, if you're a trauma therapist interested in being trained to lead a group, or if you are in the privileged class and wish to offer philanthropic support to our mission, visit HealAtLast.org.

COMMUNITIES OF HEALING

I am not the only one envisioning a way to democratize healing and bring Sacred Medicine to communities in need. Holistic Health Community in Stone Ridge, New York, is a nonprofit that has offered free healing services to its community for eight years. Gathering in the town's community center, practitioners have been offering acupuncture, reflexology, chiropractic services, massage, Brennan Healing Science, Reiki, OrthoBionomy, NeurOptimal, Biophoton Therapy, One Light Healing Touch, Attunement, Reconnective Healing, Matrix Energetics, Jin Shin Jyutsu, hypnotherapy, the Emotion Code, Spacious Heart Guidance, psychospiritual counseling, craniosacral therapy, holistic medicine—and the desire among healers to participate is outgrowing the space! Clients are invited to give a donation or pay it forward by doing something kind and loving for someone else as a form of sacred reciprocity, but nobody who needs healing is turned away. Practitioners benefit from socializing, sharing a referral network, alleviating the isolation and loneliness Sacred Medicine practitioners sometimes experience, becoming more intimate with their community, enjoying the uplifting emotions that come with selfless service, and trading free treatments with each other.

I was even invited to lead a large community healing session at a local church. I volunteered my services, and everyone who came not only got free admission to the live event but also a free copy of one of my books, paid for by a donor who supports the nonprofit. We sang, danced, meditated, performed a ritual together, shared in group healing, and danced our prayers—together. They even made a documentary film to teach other communities how this model works—and how you might develop a holistic health community in your neck of the woods. Learn more and spearhead an effort to democratize healing in your hometown at holistichealthcommunity.org.

The Trauma Foundation, a philanthropic fund whose mission is to support the healing of unresolved trauma for individuals, families, and communities, also shares this desire to democratize healing. Founder Chris Rutgers, a privileged trauma survivor and philanthropist who spent more than a decade benefiting from cutting-edge trauma therapies, shares this passion to bring the best of what healing has to offer to anyone brave and badass enough to be willing to lean into what hurt. Chris's team and mine are exploring potential collaborations. You can track their progress, learn about their offerings, or donate at thetraumafoundation.org.

BRINGING IT BACK TO YOU

Now, dear reader, we return to where we began, ascending in spirals of consciousness with the paradoxes of healing. I invite you to see if you can loosen any of your tendencies toward one side of a two-sided paradox. Can you see that you can heal yourself, *and* you might need help doing so? Can you acknowledge that we need conventional medicine, *and* it's incomplete? Can you trust your intuition *and* apply critical thinking, science, common sense, emotional intelligence, and body wisdom? Can you cast your vote for healing with laser-sharp intention *and* let go? Can you stay hopeful *and* be realistic? Can you nurture your individual body *and* remember that we are all interdependent and need to look out for each other? Can you participate in activist causes *and* resist the tendency to cast the "other" from the wholeness of humanity? Can you feel yourself as part of this earth—feel your love and care for nature—*and* acknowledge that healing our relationship to nature is indivisible from healing our bodies?

If that seems difficult, maybe you can simply contemplate such things. Let these paradoxes marinate, trusting that within you lives the inner healer you might have been seeking your whole life, always realizing that what you seek has never left you and can rise up to meet you in your heart.

You now have choices, so practice attuning to your Whole Health Intelligences so you can make wise health decisions that allow you to consult all aspects of your being without rejecting others. Will you take in these Sacred Medicine tools you've been exposed to only as an intellectual experiment, an anthropological curiosity, or a cognitive journey? Will you use what you've learned for transformation not just in yourself but also in a world needing your care?

Will you use your Whole Health Intelligences to help you assess which tools might be part of your healing process? Will you heal and treat traumas that might cause you to cling to limiting, trauma-induced beliefs about your health, your worthiness, and your ability to do what it takes to get better? Will you dedicate yourself to learning to cultivate your Whole Health Intelligences, including tuning in and surrendering to the guidance of your Inner Pilot Light or whatever you might call your Self? Will you gather those you might need to support you on your journey, not just doctors, healers, or therapists but also friends, loved ones, and perhaps kindred travelers on the spiritual path? Will you do the hard and deep work of diagnosing the root causes of what might be interfering with the free flow of life force in your energy system and body? Will you employ practices and tools that help bolster your life force when the trauma healing work gets too heavy to tolerate? Will you face your resistance to healing and treat whatever might be inadvertently sabotaging your optimal health?

Will you take one small step right now and take a deeper than usual breath? Will you give yourself a break if some of what affects your health is outside of your control? Because as much as you might treat collective, generational, ancestral, or past-life traumas and as much as you might devote yourself to activist causes, trying to make your body and this world safer, more just, and healthier for all beings, some traumas are built into the culture you swim in, and they are not your fault, and they are not entirely within your power to change overnight.

Will you rest within a final paradox of healing? *Do* everything you can to get better, never forget that one person's impact can move the needle of profound change, *and* relax in knowing that there's only so much you can do?

It really is okay if you're exhausted from fighting for things to be better. Some things cannot be changed, no matter how much effort you exert—and that in *no way* means you're a failure, that you've done something wrong, that you've lost God's favor, that you didn't manifest hard enough, or that you're not worthy of your miracle. I don't know why innocent people who try so hard to be free of suffering sometimes can't get a break, but I do know that you are loved and lovable and worthy of tender care. Perhaps sometimes the greatest healing happens when we finally let go; grieve what we've lost; accept what seems unacceptable; and let others hold, support, and carry us so it's not so lonely.

Thinking back on this whole journey, I can't help shaking my head at myself, remembering how full of hubris I was when I started this book. I thought I might hack healing, cracking the code so I could help save lives, and maybe earn some gold stars along the way. Now, I know healing is a mystery, and perhaps some mysteries need never be solved.

I think about those people at Lourdes, prostrated on the ground in front of the Virgin Mary, praying their hearts out for an unlikely cure, and wonder whether our Creator made us so we might love that which created us *so much* that we would trust it in our most vulnerable moments, dropping to our knees, humbled by great love, and begging for mercy. If we were gods and could grant ourselves a miracle, if we were all-powerful and fully self-reliant, and if miracles could be hacked, what would make us burst into tears of awe, gratitude, and delight when something mysterious happens?

I decided I prefer being down on my knees, my forehead pressed to the earth, flower petals in hand, and maybe even thrumming to the rhythm of whatever strange energy helps us heal. It is from my knees that I say thank you, dear reader. *Thank you.* May we put our knees and foreheads on this same earth together, feeling as we do everyone who will ever read this, everyone who has ever suffered, everyone who has ever transformed and healed, every miracle that did and did not happen.

May we find comfort here—together, alone, together.

I'll close with a poem I wrote for you, dear reader.

Give up trying to perfect yourself.
Root yourself right where you are
And hear the birds sing.
Feel the breeze enliven your skin.
Smell the scent of earth and sea spray.
Fall to your knees, and thank this earth for holding you.
Let your emotions rise and fall like waves.
Allow your sensations to delight or distress you
Knowing this too shall pass.
Notice the life force flowing in you as love itself.
Feel how you are cherished and deserving of belonging
Unblink your eyes and gaze at those who support you on your
   journey.
Touch your deepest longing and your unfettered fear.
Lean in there—and don't turn away.
Open yourself to those places you feel most broken;
Love even that.
Love especially that.
Unguard your vulnerable heart to exactly who you are in this now-
   walking moment.
Give yourself permission to stop efforting so much.
You will never be a saint.
There is no white sofa in the sky that will take away your pain forever.
Thank the stars for this holiness of being human.
Accept what is, and cling to hope.
Dive like whales into the recesses of your being.
Then don't forget to play.
Dance. Sing. Make art. Make love. Rest. Let go.
Love yourself.
Be.

Acknowledgments

Sacred Medicine took me a decade to research and write, so it would be impossible to name every individual who made it possible, though I wish I could. If you were part of my journey in any way, please accept my heartfelt thanks. I am deeply in the debt of countless people whose names I never even learned. This has been a community effort in every way. But let me do my best to name just a few people without which this book would never have been written.

To my mentor and teacher Rachel Naomi Remen, I am forever grateful for the innumerable ways your teachings have become part of my being in such integrated ways that your legacy lives in me and is probably evident in my writing, even when something you taught me has become so much a part of me that I don't remember to credit you. Special thanks for all the lessons in discernment, which helped keep me safe and supported me in separating the wounded charlatans, con artists, and megalomaniacs from the true healers on my journey. I love and appreciate you more than words can say.

To Gabor Maté, thank you for your pioneering work in the field of trauma-informed medicine, and my wholehearted gratitude for writing the foreword to this book.

Many thanks to Michele Martin, the best literary agent anyone could possibly have. Michele, you talked me off the ledge so many times during this book that I am absolutely certain I would not have written it without you.

To my editors at Sounds True, Jennifer Brown and Jade Lascelles, founder Tami Simon, and everyone else at Sounds True who helped out, along with copyeditor Melanie Stafford, thank you! I am in your debt for your patience with my decade-long process, for helping me whittle an unwieldly 250,000-word monster of a manuscript down to something publishable, for tolerating my sometimes fierce 2020 activism, for always making me feel free to be myself and speak my truth, and for making me feel unconditionally supported by the Sounds True team. I feel blessed to have you as my publisher for the hardest book I've ever written.

To all the true Sacred Medicine healers who took me under their wing and were mentioned by name in this book, I am forever in your debt. Thank you especially to Dick Schwartz, Asha Clinton, Bill Bengston, Donna Eden, David Feinstein, Dawson Church, Shiloh Sophia McCloud, Kathy Altman, Lori Saltzman, Del Laverdure, Laurence Heller, Gabor Maté, Thomas Hübl, Jeffrey Rediger, Kelly Turner, Larry Dossey, Sonya Amrita Bibilos, Shamini Jain, Tosha Silver, Karla McLaren, Brandy Gillmore, and the representatives of so many Indigenous people who supported my journey, especially the Q'eros in Peru and the Crows in Montana.

Thank you also to Clardy Malugen, whose energy healing work I studied for many years but whose chapter got cut simply because the manuscript was too long. Thank you also to the healers whose names I didn't name. From these healers, I learned the fine art of discrimination and discernment—and I also still learned a lot about healing. My gratitude is fully in my heart, even if I wound up being unable to use your name. Even the darker lessons made this book what is it—and because we are all human and most of us are wounded healers—I also felt a lot of love, gratitude, and connection with the healers who wound up hurting me or harming other people.

Thank you to Diane Hunter, who traveled to Lourdes with me and who is the best friend a woman could have. Thank you to Casi Zachkariyas for keeping me company, lodging me in her home, and arranging so many beautiful experiences in Bali. Thank you to Emma Harper for joining me in Bali and Thailand—and especially for the Internal Family Systems (IFS) daily parts processing during the whole pandemic. Thank you to Hannah Rae Porst for arranging my trip to the Q'eros and teaching me so much about Q'eros mysticism, history, and culture. Thank you to Suzanne Scurlock-Durana, Maja Rode, Dennis Couwenberg, Christine Gibson, Kira Siebert, Mary Louder, and Rachel Carlton Abrams for countless fascinating conversations about the nature of healing.

Special thanks to Jeffrey Rediger and Edwin Savay not just for your professional contributions to the fields of medicine and healing, but for the boundless emotional and spiritual support you both offered so generously throughout the whole of the pandemic as I rewrote at least half of this book to reflect the greater awareness we all discovered, unpacked, and processed together. I love you both dearly and have been so grateful to have a cocoon of healing with two other doctors within which we could all dissolve, evolve, and pray humbly and mightily for transformation. Thank you also to Rick Loftus for keeping me scientifically current, accurately educated, sane, sensible, and levelheaded amidst a wave of Covid misinformation that left much of the wellness world lost in delusion.

Thank you to Chris Rutgers of the Trauma Foundation for helping educate me about the cutting edge of trauma therapies. Thank you to Tara Carnegie of the Wild Woman Fund for giving Heal at Last our first grant and cheerleading me into the scary next phase of my true calling.

Thank you to April French, Matthew Klein, and Mira Klein for keeping the home fires burning and understanding why I had to keep spiriting away to mystical lands. Thank you to Pearl Macalley and Nicolay Kreidler for running the Lissa Rankin, Inc., business and the Heal at Last nonprofit so beautifully while I was off gallivanting.

Thank you to Asha Clinton, Nancy Morgan, and Dick Schwartz for being great trauma therapists who helped support me through the many traumas of researching and writing this book—and all it brought up in me, especially after my mother died. Thank you to my mother, Trish Rankin, for doing the best she could in light of her own traumas and listening to my Sacred Medicine stories even though they triggered her. I miss you every day, Marme.

Thank you to my pandemic bubble—April French, Mira and Matthew Klein, Steve Sisgold, Dawson and Christine Church, Tiffany Basse, Shiloh Sophia and Jonathan McCloud, and Nicholas Wilton—for helping me survive the collective traumas of 2020. Thank you to the Rankin family for not polarizing and dividing during the tragedies of 2020. Covid is real, science is a lifesaver, climate change is caused by humans, Trump is not a light worker, LGBTQIA+ and immigrants deserve equal rights, Black Lives Matter, and I'm SO grateful we all agreed upon all that when so many families were split by conspiracy theories and political divisiveness. To my daughter, Mira, thank you for all your support, love, sparkle, and understanding about why your crazy mother had to traipse around the world, trying to solve a mystery when parts of me never wanted to leave home without you.

So many others helped me on my journey, and I'm sure I've forgotten to name some important people. So please, if you were part of my Sacred Medicine experience, THANK YOU. I could not have done this without you all! It is with unspeakable joy that I remember what a team effort this book was.

Last but certainly not least, it is with unfathomable gratitude that I bow before the Infinite Divine and say thank you for every miracle, insight, epiphany, breakthrough, illuminated blind spot, synchronicity, and heart-opening intimacy that made this book possible.

Books and Healing Resources

Energy Healing & Shamanism

The Energy Cure, William Bengston, PhD
Energy Medicine, Donna Eden
Hands of Light, Barbara Ann Brennan
How to Heal Yourself When No One Else Can, Amy B. Scher
The Language Your Body Speaks, Ellen Meredith
The Sacred Science, Nick Polizzi
Soul Medicine, Norman Shealy, MD, PhD & Dawson Church, PhD
The Spiritual Medicine of Tibet, Dr. Pema Dorjee, Janet Jones & Terence Moore
Walking in the Sacred Manner, Mark St. Pierre & Tilda Long Soldier

The Science of Sacred Medicine

Energy Medicine, James L. Oschman
Healing Ourselves, Shamini Jain, PhD
Healing Words, Larry Dossey, MD
Science and Spiritual Practices, Rupert Sheldrake
Vibrational Medicine, Richard Gerber, MD

The Shadow of Sacred Medicine & Spirituality

Creating Healing Relationships, Dorothea Hover-Kramer, EdD, RN, DCEP
Ethics Handbook for Energy Healing Practitioners, David Feinstein, PhD
   & Donna Eden
The Ethics of Caring, Kylea Taylor
Eyes Wide Open, Mariana Caplan, PhD
Halfway Up the Mountain, Mariana Caplan, PhD
Spiritual Bypassing, Robert Augustus Masters, PhD
Spiritual Emergency, Stanislav Grof, MD & Christina Grof

Trauma Healing

The Art of Empathy, Karla McLaren, MEd
The Body Keeps the Score, Bessel van der Kolk, MD
The EFT Manual, Dawson Church, PhD

Healing Developmental Trauma, Laurence Heller, PhD & Aline LaPierre, PsyD
Internal Family Systems Skills Training Manual, Frank G. Anderson, MD,
   Martha Sweezy, PhD & Richard C. Schwartz, PhD
The Language of Emotions, Karla McLaren, MEd
No Bad Parts, Richard C. Schwartz, PhD
Nurturing Resilience, Kathy L. Kain & Stephen J. Terrell
The Polyvagal Theory in Therapy, Deb Dana
The Power of Attachment, Diane Poole Heller, PhD
Psychological Trauma, Dawson Church, PhD
Somatic Internal Family Systems Therapy, Susan McConnell
The Tapping Solution, Nick Ortne
Transcending Trauma, Frank G. Anderson, MD
The Trauma of Everyday Life, Mark Epstein, MD
Waking the Tiger, Peter A. Levine & Ann Frederick
When the Body Says No, Gabor Maté, MD
You Are the One You've Been Waiting For, Richard C. Schwartz, PhD

Collective Trauma Healing
Caste, Isabel Wilkerson
Healing Collective Trauma, Thomas Hübl
How to Be an Antiracist, Ibram X. Kendi
Me and White Supremacy, Layla F. Saad
My Grandmother's Hands, Resmaa Menakem

General Health & Healing
The Awakened Brain, Lisa Miller, PhD
The Book of Awakening, Mark Nepo
Brave New Medicine, Cynthia Li, MD
Consciousness & Healing, Marilyn Schlitz, Tina Amorok & Marc S. Micozzi
Cured, Jeffrey Rediger, MD, MDiv
The Cure Within, Anne Harrington
The Daily Flame, Lissa Rankin, MD
Kitchen Table Wisdom, Rachel Naomi Remen, MD
Love, Medicine, and Miracles, Bernie S. Siegel, MD
Mind Over Medicine, Lissa Rankin, MD
My Grandfather's Blessings, Rachel Naomi Remen, MD
Outrageous Openness, Tosha Silver
Radical Remission, Kelly A. Turner, PhD

The Type C Connection, Lydia Temoshok, PhD & Henry Dreher
Unlearn Your Pain, Howard Schubiner, MD & Michael Betzold
The Will to Live, Arnold A. Hutschnecker, MD

Pilgrimage Sites with Healing Waters
Baden-Baden, Germany
Bath, England
Bear Lake, Sovata, Romania
Beitou Hot Springs, Taipei, Taiwan
Esalen Hot Springs, Big Sur, California
Glastonbury, England
God's Acre Healing Springs, Blackville, South Carolina
Liaoning, China
Madron Well, Cornwall, England
Nadana, India
Ojo Caliente, New Mexico
Our Lady of Lourdes Shrine, Lourdes, France
Pamukkale, Turkey
Saratoga Mineral Baths, Saratoga Springs, New York
Yankalilla, Australia

Other Pilgrimage Sites Reputed to Facilitate Healing
Ajmer Sharif, Rajasthan, India
Besakih Temple ("The Mother Temple"), Bali, Indonesia
Bodh Gaya, Bihar, India
Camino de Santiago, Spain
Canterbury Cathedral, Canterbury, England
El Santuario de Chimayó, Chimayó, New Mexico
"Energy vortexes" in Sedona, Arizona
Ganges River, India
Great Mosque of Touba, Senegal
Hazrat Nizamuddin Dargah, Delhi, India
Hazrat Shah Jalal Mazar, Sylhet, Bangladesh
The holy Amarnath cave in the mountains of Kashmir, India
Knock Basilica, Knock, Ireland
Lal Shahbaz Qalandar Shrine, Sindh, Pakistan
Machu Picchu, Peru

Mecca, Saudi Arabia

Mevlâna Museum, Konya, Turkey

Our Lady of Guadalupe Basilica, Mexico City, Mexico

Sainte-Anne-de-Beaupré Shrine, Québec

Shrine of Khoja Ahmed Yasawi, Turkestan, Kazakhstan

St. Mary Magdalene's Shrine & Grotto, Sainte-Baume, France

Stonehenge, Wiltshire, England

Uluru (Ayers Rock), Australia

Vaishno Devi Temple, India

The Western Wall & other Holy Land sites, Jerusalem, Israel

Lissa Rankin's Websites

healatlast.org
lissarankin.com
thesacredmedicinebook.com
wholehealthmedicineinstitute.com

Lissa Rankin's Social Media

Facebook: Lissa Rankin
Instagram: @lissarankin
Twitter: @Lissarankin

Notes

INTRODUCTION

1. Martin A. Makaray and Michael Daniel, "Medical Error—The Third Leading Cause of Death in the US," *British Medical Journal* 353 (2016): i2139, doi.org /10.1136/bmj.i2139.
2. Matthew Remski, Derek Beres, and Julian Marc Walker, *Conspirituality Podcast: Examining the Toxic Ties Between Right-Wing Conspiracism and New Age Utopianism,* May 2020, matthewremski.com/wordpress/what-i-do/conspirituality-podcast/.
3. Marisa Meltzer, "I Refuse to Listen to White Women Cry," *Washington Post Magazine,* September 11, 2019, washingtonpost.com/news/magazine/wp/2019 /09/11/feature/how-activist-rachel-cargle-built-a-business-by-calling-out-racial -injustices-within-feminism/.

CHAPTER 1: GROUP HEALING AS MEDICINE

1. Edward Cody, "Foreign Journal," *Washington Post,* January 27, 1992, washingtonpost.com/archive/politics/1992/01/27/foreign-journal/9b0916e8 -6c35-4470-8c00-562ecd1d2d87/?utm_term=.5341596ea223.
2. Zbigniew Gadek, Takeki Hamasaki, and Sanetaka Shirahata, "'Nordenau Phenomenon'—Application of Natural Reduced Water to Therapy," in *Animal Cell Technology: Basic and Applied Aspects,* vol. 15, edited by Sanetaka Shirahata, Koji Ikura, Masaya Nagao, Akira Ichikawa, and Kiichiro Teruya (Dordrecht, The Netherlands: Springer Science + Business, 2008), 265–271, doi.org/10.1007/978 -1-4020-9646-4_41.
3. Rupert Sheldrake, *Science and Spiritual Practices: Transformative Experiences and Their Effects on Our Bodies, Brains, and Health* (Berkeley, CA: Counterpoint, 2018).
4. American Cancer Society, "Faith Healing," Wikipedia, January 17, 2013, web .archive.org/web/20130427120554/cancer.org/treatment/treatmentsandsideeffects /complementaryandalternativemedicine/herbsvitaminsandminerals/faith-healing.
5. William Franklin Simpson, "Comparative Longevity in a College Cohort of Christian Scientists," *JAMA* 262, no. 12 (September 1989): 1657–1658 (erratum in *JAMA* 262, no. 21 [December 1989]: 3000), doi.org/10.1001/jama.1989 .03430120111031.
6. S. M. Asser and R. Swan, "Child Fatalities from Religion-Motivated Medical Neglect," *Pediatrics* 101, no. 4, pt. 1 (April 1998): 625–629, doi.org/10.1542 /peds.101.4.625.
7. Ted J. Kaptchuk, "Placebo Studies and Ritual Theory: A Comparative Analysis of Navajo, Acupuncture, and Biomedical Healing," *Philosophical Transactions of the Royal Society B: Biological Science* 366, no. 1572 (June 2011): 1849–1858, doi.org /10.1098/rstb.2010.0385.
8. Herbert Benson, Jeffrey A. Dusek, Jane B. Sherwood, Peter Lam, Charles F. Bethea, William Carpenter, Sidney Levitsky, Peter C. Hill, Donald W. Clem

Jr., Manoj K. Jain, David Drumel, Stephen L. Kopecky, Paul S. Mueller, Dean Marek, Sue Rollins, and Patricia L. Hibberd, "Study of the Therapeutic Effects of Intercessory Prayer (STEP) in Cardiac Bypass Patients: A Multicenter Randomized Trial of Uncertainty and Certainty of Receiving Intercessory Prayer," *American Heart Journal* 151, no. 4 (April 2006): 934–942, doi.org/10.1016/j.ahj .2005.05.028.

9.   "Spirituality: Don't Pray for Me! Please!," *Newsweek*, April 9, 2006, newsweek .com/spirituality-dont-pray-me-please-107905.

10. Larry Dossey, "Healing Research: What We Know and Don't Know," *Explore* 4, no. 6 (November–December 2008): 341–352, doi.org/10.1016/j.explore.2008 .09.009.

11. K. B. Thomas, "General Practice Consultations: Is There Any Point in Being Positive?" *British Medical Journal* 294, no. 6581 (May 1987): 1200–1202, doi .org/10.1136/bmj.294.6581.1200.

12. Chittaranjan Andrade and Rajiv Radhakrishnan, "Prayer and Healing: A Medical and Scientific Perspective on Randomized Controlled Trials," *Indian Journal of Psychiatry* 51, no. 4 (October–December 2009), 247–253, doi.org/10.4103/0019 -5545.58288.

13. Andrade and Radhakrishnan, "Prayer and Healing."

CHAPTER 2: THE ENERGY CURE

1.   William F. Bengston, *The Energy Cure: Unraveling the Mystery of Hands-On Healing* (Boulder, CO: Sounds True, 2010), 40–41.

2.   William F. Bengston and David Krinsley, "The Effect of 'Laying on of Hands' in Transplanted Breast Cancer in Mice," *Journal of Scientific Exploration* 14, no. 3 (Fall 2000), 353–364.

3.   Bengston and Krinsley, "The Effect of 'Laying on Hands.'"

4.   Gloria A. Gronowicz, Ankur Jhaveri, Libbe W. Clarke, Michael S. Aronow, and Theresa H. Smith, "Therapeutic Touch Stimulates the Proliferation of Human Cells in Culture," *Journal of Alternative and Complementary Medicine* 14, no. 3 (April 2008): 233–239, doi.org/10.1089/acm.2007.7163.

5.   Gloria Gronowicz, Eric R. Secor Jr., John R. Flynn, Evan R. Jellison, and Liisa T. Kuhn, "Therapeutic Touch Has Significant Effects on Mouse Breast Cancer Metastasis and Immune Responses but Not Primary Tumor Size," *Evidence-Based Complementary and Alternative Medicine* 2015 (May 2015): 926565, doi.org/10 .1155/2015/926565.

6.   Margaret Moga and William F. Bengston, "Anomalous Magnetic Field Activity During a Bioenergy Healing Experiment," *Journal of Scientific Exploration* 24, no. 3 (2010): 397–410.

CHAPTER 3: THE ENERGIES OF LIFE

1.   Ellen Meredith, *The Language Your Body Speaks: Self-Healing with Energy Medicine* (Novato, CA: New World Library, 2020), 22–23.

2. Meredith, *The Language Your Body Speaks*, 23–24.

3. Donna Eden and David Feinstein, "Development of a Healthcare Approach Focusing on Subtle Energies: The Case of Eden Energy Medicine," *Advances in Mind-Body Medicine* 34, no. 3 (Summer 2020): 25–36.

4. Bernard O. Williams, "Exploring Multiple Meanings of Subtle Energy," *Subtle Energies and Energy Medicine Journal* 21, no. 2 (2011): 5.

5. William F. Bengston and Donald G. Murphy, "Can Healing Be Taught?," *Explore* 4, no. 3 (May 2008): 197–200, doi.org/10.1016/j.explore.2008.02.004.

6. Mae-Wan Ho and David P. Knight, "The Acupuncture System and the Liquid Crystalline Collagen Fibers of the Connective Tissues," *American Journal of Chinese Medicine* 26, nos. 3–4 (1998): 251–263, doi.org/10.1142 /S0192415X98000294; Mae-Wan Ho, *The Rainbow and the Worm: The Physics of Organisms* (Singapore: World Scientific, 2008); Petros C. Benias, Rebecca G. Wells, Bridget Sackey-Aboagye, Heather Klavan, Jason Reidy, Darren Buonocore, Markus Miranda, Susan Kornacki, Michael Wayne, David L. Carr-Locke, and Neil D. Theisse, "Structure and Distribution of an Unrecognized Interstitium in Human Tissues," *Scientific Reports* 8 (May 2018): 4947, doi.org/10.1038/s41598 -018-23062-6.

7. Donna Eden and David Feinstein, *Energy Medicine: Balancing Your Body's Energies for Optimal Health, Joy, and Vitality* (New York: Penguin, 2008).

8. Eden and Feinstein, *Energy Medicine*, 245.

9 John Horgan, "Scientific Heretic Rupert Sheldrake on Morphic Fields, Psychic Dogs, and Other Mysteries," *Scientific American*, July 14, 2014, blogs .scientificamerican.com/cross-check/scientific-heretic-rupert-sheldrake-on -morphic-fields-psychic-dogs-and-other-mysteries/.

10. Beverly Rubik, David Muehsam, Richard Hammerschlag, and Shamini Jain, "Biofield Science and Healing: History, Terminology, and Concepts," *Global Advances in Health and Medicine* 4 (January 2015): 8–14, doi.org/10.7453/gahmj .2015.038.suppl.

11. Beverly Rubik, R. Pavek, E. Greene, D. Laurence, and R. Ward, "Manual Healing Methods," in *Alternative Medicine—Expanding Medical Horizons: A Report to the National Institutes of Health on Alternative Medical Systems and Practices in the United States*, edited by Brian Berman and David B. Larson (Washington, DC: US Government Printing Office, 1995), 113–157; Bernard Grad, "The 'Laying on of Hands': Implications for Psychotherapy, Gentling, and the Placebo Effect," *Journal of the American Society for Psychical Research* 61, no. 4 (1967): 286–305; Bernard Grad, "Some Biological Effects of the 'Laying on of Hands': A Review of Experiments with Animals and Plants," *Journal of the American Society for Psychical Research* 59 (April 1965): 95–127; B. Grad, R. J. Cadoret, and G. I. Paul, "The Influence of an Unorthodox Method of Treatment on Wound Healing in Mice," *International Journal of Parapsychology* 3 (Spring 1961): 5–24.

12. William F. Bengston, *The Energy Cure: Unraveling the Mystery of Hands-On Healing* (Boulder, CO: Sounds True, 2010).

13. Shamini Jain, Desiree Pavlik, Janet Distefan, Rosalyn L. Bruyere, Julia Acer, Rosalie Garcia, Ian Coulter, John Ives, Scott C. Roesch, Wayne Jonas, and Paul J. Mills, "Complementary Medicine for Fatigue and Cortisol Variability in Breast

Cancer Survivors," *Cancer* 118, no. 3 (February 2012): 777–787, doi.org/10
.1002/cncr.26345.

14. Susan K. Lutgendorf, Elizabeth Mullen-Houser, Daniel Russell, Koen Degeest, Geraldine Jacobson, Laura Hart, David Bender, Barrie Anderson, Thomas E. Buekers, Michael J. Goodheart, Michael H. Antoni, Anil K. Sood, and David M. Lubaroff, "Preservation of Immune Function in Cervical Cancer Patients During Chemoradiation Using a Novel Integrative Approach," *Brain, Behavior, and Immunity* 24, no. 8 (November 2010): 1231–1240, doi.org/10.1016/j.bbi.2010 .06.014.

15. Shamini Jain and Paul J. Mills, "Biofield Therapies: Helpful or Full of Hype? A Best Evidence Synthesis," *International Journal of Behavioral Medicine* 17, no. 1 (March 2010): 1–16 (erratum in *International Journal of Behavioral Medicine* 18, no. 1 [January 2011]: 79–82), doi.org/10.1007/s12529-009-9062-4.

16. Margaret M. Moga and Dan Zhou, "Distant Healing of Small-Sized Tumors," *Journal of Alternative and Complementary Medicine* 14, no. 5 (2008): 453, doi.org /10.1089/acm.2008.0100; Xin Yan, Feng Li, Igor Dozmorov, Mark Barton Frank, Ming Dao, Michael Centola, Wei Cao, and Dan Hu, "External Qi of Yan Xin Qigong Induces Cell Death and Gene Expression Alterations Promoting Apoptosis and Inhibiting Proliferation, Migration, and Glucose Metabolism in Small-Cell Lung Cancer Cells," *Molecular and Cellular Biochemistry* 363, nos. 1–2 (April 2012): 245–255, doi.org/10.1007/s11010-011-1176-8.

17. Richard Hammerschlag, Shamini Jain, Ann L. Baldwin, Gloria Gronowicz, Susan K. Lutgendorf, James L. Oschman, and Garret L. Yount, "Biofield Research: A Roundtable Discussion of Scientific and Methodological Issues," *Journal of Alternative and Complementary Medicine* 18, no. 12 (December 2012): 1081– 1086, doi.org/10.1089/acm.2012.1502.

18. Shamini Jain, *Healing Ourselves: Biofield Science and the Future of Health* (Boulder, CO: Sounds True, 2021).

19. "Subtle Energy and Biofield Healing: Evidence, Practice, and Future Directions," Consciousness and Healing Initiative, 2021, chi.is/systems-mapping-resources/.

20. Jain, *Healing Ourselves*.

21. Mario Beauregard, Larry Dossey, Lisa Jane Miller, Alexander Moreira-Almeida, Marilyn Schlitz, Gary Schwartz, Rupert Sheldrake, and Charles T. Tart, "Manifesto for a Post-Materialistic Science," Open Sciences (February 2014), opensciences.org/about/manifesto-for-a-post-materialist-science.

22. William F. Bengston and Margaret Moga, "Resonance, Placebo Effects, and Type II Errors: Some Implications from Healing Research for Experimental Methods," *Journal of Alternative and Complementary Medicine* 13, no. 3 (April 2007): 317–327.

CHAPTER 4: PLEASURE PRACTICES AS MEDICINE FOR THE BODY

1. "Subscription," Open Floor Dance, openfloor.discology.me/subscription/.

2. Lissa Rankin, *Sacred Medicine* (Boulder, CO: Sounds True, 2022), thesacredmedicinebook.com.

3. Lissa Rankin, "Lissa Rankin Studio," lissarankinart.com.
4. Lissa Rankin, "Healing with the Muse," courses.lissarankin.com/healing-with-the -muse.

CHAPTER 5: RESACRALIZING NATURE

1. Robert Elphin Smith, *The Fork in the Road: The Divergence and Potential Rejoining of Traditional and Allopathic Medicine* (self pub., 2020).
2. Falk Xué Parra Witte, "Living the Law of Origin: The Cosmological, Ontological, Epistemological, and Ecological Framework of Kogi Environmental Politics," (PhD diss., Downing University, 2017).
3. Robert C. Beck, "Mood Modification with ELF Magnetic Fields: A Preliminary Exploration," *Archaeus* 4 (1986): 48.
4. Luke Hendricks, William F. Bengston, and Jay Gunkelman, "The Healing Connection: EEG Harmonics, Entrainment, and Schumann's Resonances," *Journal of Scientific Exploration* 24, no. 4 (Winter 2010): 655–666.
5. Gib Mathers, "Crow Pipe Ceremony Links Disparate Cultures," *Powell Tribune*, June 14, 2011, powelltribune.com/stories/crow-pipe-ceremony-links-disparate -cultures,7837.

CHAPTER 6: FEELING IS HEALING

1. Robert Augustus Masters, *Spiritual Bypassing: When Spirituality Disconnects Us from What Really Matters* (Berkeley, CA: North Atlantic, 2010), 21–22.
2. The Dalai Lama and Daniel Goleman, *A Force for Good: The Dalai Lama's Vision for Our World* (New York: Random House, 2015).
3. Masters, *Spiritual Bypassing*, 1.
4. Beth R. Crisp, *The Routledge Handbook of Religion, Spirituality, and Social Work* (London: Taylor and Francis, 2017).
5. Tina Forssella, "Human Nature Buddha Nature: On Spiritual Bypassing, Relationship, and the Dharma," interview with John Welwood, *Tricycle*, 2011, johnwelwood.com/articles/TRIC_interview_uncut.pdf.
6. Victoria M. White, Dallas R. English, Hamish Coates, Magdalena Lagerlund, Ron Borland, and Graham G. Giles, "Is Cancer Risk Associated with Anger Control and Negative Affect? Findings from a Prospective Cohort Study," *Psychosomatic Medicine* 69, no. 7 (2007): 667–674, doi.org/10.1097/psy .0b013e31814d4e6a.
7. Black Lives Matter, "HerStory," blacklivesmatter.com/herstory/.
8. Laurence Heller, *Healing Developmental Trauma: How Early Trauma Affects Self-Regulation, Self-Image, and the Capacity for Relationship* (Berkeley, CA: North Atlantic, 2012).
9. Gabor Maté, *When the Body Says No: The Cost of Hidden Stress* (New York: Knopf, 2011), 3.
10. Lydia Temoshok, *The Type C Connection: The Behavioral Links to Cancer and Your Health* (New York: Random House, 1992).

11. Karla McLaren, *The Language of Emotions: What Your Feelings Are Trying to Tell You* (Boulder, CO: Sounds True, 2010).
12. Karla McLaren, *The Art of Empathy: A Complete Guide to Life's Most Essential Skill* (Boulder, CO: Sounds True, 2013).
13. Rachel Naomi Remen, "Helping, Fixing, or Serving," *Lion's Roar*, August 6, 2017, lionsroar.com/helping-fixing-or-serving/.
14. Tania Singer and Olga M. Klimecki, "Empathy and Compassion," *Current Biology* 24, no. 18 (September 2014): R875–R878, doi.org/10.1016/j.cub.2014.06.054.
15. Singer and Klimecki, "Empathy and Compassion."

CHAPTER 7: SHORING UP YOUR BOUNDARIES

1. Brené Brown, *Rising Strong: How the Ability to Reset Transforms the Way We Live, Love, Parent, and Lead* (New York: Random House, 2017).
2. Cindy Starr, "Amy's Story: Severe Spinal Deformity," Mayfield Clinic, mayfieldclinic.com/mc_hope/story_amy.htm.

CHAPTER 8: SACRED MEDICINE DIAGNOSTICS

1. Cynthia Li, "My Personal Health Journey," cynthialimd.com/my-personal-health-journey/.
2. Daniel J. Benor, "Intuitive Diagnosis," *Subtle Energies* 3, no. 2 (1993): 41–64.
3. David E. Young and Steven K. H. Aung, "An Experimental Test of Psychic Diagnosis of Disease," *Journal of Alternative and Complementary Medicine* 3, no. 1 (1997): 39–53, doi.org/10.1089/acm.1997.3.39.
4. David M. Eisenberg, Roger B. Davis, Jeremy Waletzky, Alison Yager, Lewis Landsberg, Mark Aronson, Machelle Seibel, and Thomas L. Delbanco, "Inability of an 'Energy Transfer Diagnostician' to Distinguish Between Fertile and Infertile Women," *MedScape*, medscape.com/viewarticle/408093.
5. Steven Amoils, John R. Kues, Sandi Amoils, Stephen Pomeranz, and Terry Traiforos, "The Diagnostic Validity of Human Electromagnetic Field (Aura) Perception," *Medical Acupuncture* 13, no. 2 (2001).
6. Wendie Colter and Paul J. Mills, "Assessing the Accuracy of Medical Intuition: A Subjective and Exploratory Study," *Journal of Alternative and Complementary Medicine* 26, no. 12 (December 2020): 1130–1135, doi.org/10.1089/acm.2020.0244.
7. Ezequiel Morsella, Christine A. Godwin, Tiffany K. Jantz, Stephen C. Krieger, and Adam Gazzaley, "Homing in on Consciousness in the Nervous System: An Action-Based Synthesis," *Behavioral and Brain Sciences* 39 (2016): E168, doi.org/10.1017/S0140525X15000643.
8. Jeffrey Kluger, "Why You're Pretty Much Unconscious All the Time," *Time*, June 26, 2015, time.com/3937351/consciousness-unconsciousness-brain.

9. Daniel C. Andersson, Matthew J. Betzenhauser, Steven Reiken, Alisa Umanskaya, Takayuki Shiomi, and Andrew R. Marks, "Stress-Induced Increase in Skeletal Muscle Force Requires Protein Kinase A Phosphorylation of the Ryanodine Receptor," *Journal of Physiology* 590, no. 24 (December 2012): 6381–6387, doi .org/10.1113/jphysiol.2012.237925.

10. Silvestro Roatta and Dario Farina, "Stress-Induced Increase in Muscle Force: Truth or Myth?," *Journal of Physiology* 591, no. 12 (June 2013): 3101–3102, doi .org/10.1113/jphysiol.2013.251553.

11. Anne M. Jensen, Richard J. Stevens, and Amanda J. Burls, "Estimating the Accuracy of Muscle Response Testing: Two Randomised-Order Blinded Studies," *BMC Complementary Medicine and Therapies* 16 (November 2016), doi.org/10 .1186/s12906-016-1416-2; Anne M. Jensen, "The Accuracy and Precision of Kinesiology-Style Manual Muscle Testing: Designing and Implementing a Series of Diagnostic Test Accuracy Studies," (PhD thesis, Oxford University, Oxford, UK, 2014).

12. "Dense Breasts," Yale Medicine, yalemedicine.org/conditions/dense-breasts.

13. R. Lüdtke, B. Kunz, N. Seeber, and J. Ring, "Test-Retest: Reliability and Validity of the Kinesiology Muscle Test," *Complementary Therapeutic Medicine* 9, no. 3 (September 2001): 141–145, doi.org/10.1054/ctim.2001.0455.

14. J. J. Kenney, R. Clemens, and K. D. Forsythe, "Applied Kinesiology Unreliable for Assessing Nutrient Status," *Journal of the American Dietetic Association* 88, no. 6 (June 1988): 698–704; J. J. Triano, "Muscle Strength Testing as a Diagnostic Screen for Supplemental Nutrition Therapy: A Blind Study," *Journal of Manipulative and Physiological Therapeutics* 5, no. 4 (December 1982): 179–182.

15. Anne M. Jensen, "Emerging from the Mystical: Rethinking Muscle Response Testing as an Ideomotor Effect," *Energy Psychology* 10, no. 2 (October 2018): 13–27, doi.org/10.9769/EPJ.2018.10.2.AJ.

CHAPTER 9: FIRST, DO NO HARM

1. Martin A. Makary and Michael Daniel, "Medical Error—The Third Leading Cause of Death in the US," *British Medical Journal* 353 (2016): i2139, doi.org /10.1136/bmj.i2139.

2. Brett T. Litz, Nathan Stein, Eileen Delaney, Leslie Lebowitz, William P. Nash, Caroline Silva, and Shira Maguen, "Moral Injury and Moral Repair in War Veterans: A Preliminary Model and Intervention Strategy," *Clinical Psychology Review* 29, no. 8 (December 2009): 695–706, doi.org/10.1016/j.cpr.2009.07.003.

3. Mariana Caplan, *Eyes Wide Open: Cultivating Discernment on the Spiritual Path* (Boulder, CO: Sounds True, 2009), xxii.

4. Paramahansa Yogananda, *Autobiography of a Yogi* (Dakshineswar, India: Yogoda Satsanga Society, 1998), 48.

5. Carole Griggs, iConscious Human Development Model (2018), drcarolegriggs .com/map.

PART THREE: HEALING FROM THE ROOT

1. Daniel J. Siegel, *Mindsight: The New Science of Personal Transformation* (New York: Bantam Books, 2010), 52.

CHAPTER 10: HEALING TRAUMA *IS* SACRED MEDICINE

1. Aditi Nerurkar, Asaf Bitton, Roger B. Davis, Russell S. Phillips, and Gloria Yeh, "When Physicians Counsel About Stress: Results of a National Study," *JAMA Internal Medicine* 173, no. 1 (January 2013): 76–77, doi.org/10.1001/2013 .jamainternmed.480.
2. Nadine Burke Harris, "How Childhood Trauma Affects Health Across a Lifetime," TED Talk, 2014, ted.com/talks/nadine_burke_harris_how_childhood _trauma_affects_health_across_a_lifetime?language=en.
3. "Adverse Childhood Experiences Resources," Centers for Disease Control and Prevention, cdc.gov/violenceprevention/aces/resources.html; Vincent J. Felitti, "The Relation Between Adverse Childhood Experiences and Adult Health: Turning Gold into Lead," *Permanente Journal* 6, no. 1 (Winter 2002): 44–47.
4. "What ACEs/PCEs Do You Have?," ACES Too High News, acestoohigh.com/got -your-ace-score/.
5. "PACEs Science 101," ACES Too High News, acestoohigh.com/aces-101/.
6. Shanta R. Dube, DeLisa Fairweather, William S. Pearson, Vincent J. Felitti, Robert F. Anda, and Janet B. Croft, "Cumulative Childhood Stress and Autoimmune Diseases in Adults," *Psychosomatic Medicine* 71, no. 2 (February 2009): 243–250, doi.org/10.1097/PSY.0b013e3181907888; Katie A. Ports, Dawn M. Holman, Angie S. Guinn, Sanjana Pampati, Karen E. Dyer, Melissa T. Merrick, Natasha D. Buchanan, and Marilyn Metzler, "Adverse Childhood Experiences and the Presence of Cancer Risk Factors in Adulthood: A Scoping Review of the Literature from 2005 to 2015," *Journal of Pediatric Nursing* 44 (January–February 2019): 81–96, doi.org/10.1016/j.pedn.2018.10.009; Dawn M. Holman, Katie A. Ports, Natasha D. Buchanan, Nikki A. Hawkins, Melissa T. Merrick, Marilyn Metzler, and Katrina F. Trivers, "The Association Between Adverse Childhood Experiences and Risk for Cancer in Adulthood: A Systematic Review of the Literature," *Pediatrics* 138 (November 2016): S81–S91, doi.org/10.1542/peds.2015-4268L; Monique J. Brown, Leroy R. Thacker, and Steven A. Cohen, "Association Between Adverse Childhood Experiences and Diagnosis of Cancer," *PLoS One* 8, no. 6 (June 2013): e65524, doi.org/10.1371/journal.pone.0065524; David W. Brown, Robert F. Anda, Vincent J. Felitti, Valerie J. Edwards, Ann Marie Malarcher, Janet B. Croft, and Wayne H. Giles, "Adverse Childhood Experiences Are Associated with the Risk of Lung Cancer: A Prospective Cohort Study," *BMC Public Health* 10 (January 2010), doi.org/10.1186/1471-2458-10-20; Timothy J. Cunningham, Earl S. Ford, Janet B. Croft, Melissa T. Merrick, Italia V. Rolle, and Wayne H. Giles, "Sex-Specific Relationships Between Adverse Childhood Experiences and Chronic Obstructive Pulmonary Disease in Five States," *International Journal of Chronic Obstructive Pulmonary Disease* 9 (September 2014): 1033–1043, doi.org

/10.2147/COPD.S68226; Robert F. Anda, David W. Brown, Shanta R. Dube, J. Douglas Bremner, Vincent J. Felitti, and Wayne H. Giles, "Adverse Childhood Experiences and Chronic Obstructive Pulmonary Disease in Adults," *American Journal of Preventive Medicine* 34, no. 5 (2008): 396–403, doi.org/10.1016/j .amepre.2008.02.002; Robert Anda, Gretchen Tietjen, Elliott Schulman, Vincent Felitti, and Janet Croft, "Adverse Childhood Experiences and Frequent Headaches in Adults," *Headache* 50, no. 9 (October 2010): 1473–1481, doi.org/10.1111/j .1526-4610.2010.01756.x; Maxia Dong, Wayne H. Giles, Vincent J. Felitti, Shanta R. Dube, Janice E. Williams, Daniel P. Chapman, and Robert F. Anda, "Insights into Causal Pathways for Ischemic Heart Disease: Adverse Childhood Experiences Study," *Circulation* 110 (September 2004): 1761–1766, doi.org/10.1161/01.cir .0000143074.54995.7f; Maxia Dong, Robert F. Anda, Shanta R. Dube, Vincent J. Felitti, and W. H. Giles, "Adverse Childhood Experiences and Self-Reported Liver Disease: New Insights into the Causal Pathway," *Archives of Internal Medicine* 163, no. 16 (September 2003): 1949–1956, doi.org/10.1001/archinte.163.16.1949; J. P. Barile, V. J. Edwards, S. S. Dhingra, and W. W. Thompson, "Associations Among County-Level Social Determinants of Health, Child Maltreatment, and Emotional Support on Health-Related Quality of Life in Adulthood," *Psychology of Violence* 5, no. 2 (2015): 183–191, doi.org/10.1037/a0038202; Phaedra S. Corso, Valerie J. Edwards, Xiangming Fang, and James A. Mercy, "Health-Related Quality of Life Among Adults Who Experienced Maltreatment During Childhood," *American Journal of Public Health* 98, no. 6 (June 2008): 1094–1100, doi.org/10.2105/AJPH .2007.119826.

7.   Andrea L. Roberts, Tianyi Huang, Karestan C. Koenen, Yongjoo Kim, Laura D. Kubzansky, and Shelley S. Tworoger, "Posttraumatic Stress Disorder Is Associated with Increased Risk of Ovarian Cancer: A Prospective and Retrospective Longitudinal Cohort Study," *Cancer Research* 79, no. 19 (October 2019), doi.org /10.1158/0008-5472.CAN-19-1222.

8.   "What ACEs/PCEs Do You Have?"

9.   Jessie R. Baldwin, Avshalom Caspi, Alan J. Meehan, Antony Ambler, Louise Arseneault, Helen L. Fisher, HonaLee Harrington, Timothy Matthews, Candice L. Odgers, Richie Poulton, Sandhya Ramrakha, Terrie E. Moffitt, and Andrea Danese, "Population vs Individual Prediction of Poor Health from Results of Adverse Childhood Experiences Screening," *JAMA Pediatrics* 175, no. 4 (2021): 385–393, doi.org/10.1001/jamapediatrics.2020.5602.

10. Deb Dana, *The Polyvagal Theory in Therapy: Engaging the Rhythm of Regulation* (New York: Norton, 2018).

11. David Baumeister, Reece Akhtar, Simone Ciufolini, Carmine M. Pariante, and Valeria Mondelli, "Childhood Trauma and Adulthood Inflammation: A Meta-Analysis of Peripheral C-Reactive Protein, Interleukin-6, and Tumour Necrosis Factor-α," *Molecular Psychiatry* 21, no. 5 (June 2015): 642–649, doi.org/10.1038 /mp.2015.67.

12. "Understanding Acute and Chronic Inflammation," Harvard Medical School, April 1, 2020, health.harvard.edu/staying-healthy/understanding-acute-and -chronic-inflammation.

13. Dawson Church, *Psychological Trauma: Healing Its Roots in Brain, Body, and Memory* (Santa Rosa, CA: Energy Psychology Press, 2016).

14. Oprah Winfrey and Bruce D. Perry, *What Happened to You? Conversations on Trauma, Resilience, and Healing* (New York: Flatiron Books, 2021).

15. Mark Epstein, *The Trauma of Everyday Life* (New York: Penguin, 2013).

16. Laurence Heller and Aline LaPierre, *Healing Developmental Trauma: How Early Trauma Affects Self-Regulation, Self-Image, and the Capacity for Relationship* (Berkeley, CA: North Atlantic, 2012).

17. Pete Walker, *Complex PTSD: From Surviving to Thriving: A Guide and Map for Recovering from Childhood Trauma* (CreateSpace Independent Publishing Platform, 2013).

18. Heller and LaPierre, *Healing Developmental Trauma*, 15.

19. L. G. Russek, S. H. King, S. J. Russek, and H. I. Russek, "The Harvard Mastery of Stress Study 35-Year Follow-Up: Prognostic Significance of Patterns of Psychophysiological Arousal and Adaptation," *Psychosomatic Medicine* 52, no. 3 (1990): 271–285, doi.org/10.1097/00006842-199005000-00002.

20. Vivek H. Murthy, *Together: The Healing Power of Human Connection in a Sometimes Lonely World* (New York: HarperCollins, 2020).

21. Bessel A. van der Kolk, "Developmental Trauma Disorder: A New, Rational Diagnosis for Children with Complex Trauma Histories," *Psychiatric Annals* 35, no. 5 (May 2005): 401–408.

22. Winfrey and Perry, *What Happened to You?*

23. Kathy L. Kain and Stephen J. Terrell, *Nurturing Resilience: Helping Clients Move Forward from Developmental Trauma: An Integrative Somatic Approach* (Berkeley, CA: North Atlantic, 2018).

24. Bruce Ecker, Robin Ticic, and Laurel Hulley, *Unlocking the Emotional Brain: Eliminating Symptoms at Their Roots Using Memory Reconsolidation* (London: Routledge, 2012).

25. Ecker, Ticic, and Hulley, *Unlocking the Emotional Brain*.

CHAPTER 11: ILLNESS AS A TRAILHEAD

1. Mark Nepo, *The Book of Awakening: Having the Life You Want by Being Present to the Life You Have* (Newburyport, MA: Red Wheel Weiser, 2011), 3–4.

2. Laurence Heller and Aline LaPierre, *Healing Developmental Trauma: How Early Trauma Affects Self-Regulation, Self-Image, and the Capacity for Relationship* (Berkeley, CA: North Atlantic, 2012), 41; "Expert Q & A: PTSD," American Psychiatric Association, psychiatry.org/patients-families/ptsd/expert-q-and-a.

3. Frank Anderson, Richard Schwartz, and Martha Sweezy, *Internal Family Systems Skills Training Manual: Trauma-Informed Treatment for Anxiety, Depression, PTSD, and Substance Abuse* (Eau Claire, WI: PESI, 2017).

4. "2014 Membership Survey," Alcoholics Anonymous, 2014, aa.org/assets/en_US/p-48_membershipsurvey.pdf.

5. Anderson, Schwartz, and Sweezy, *Internal Family Systems Skills Training Manual*.

6. Nancy A. Shadick, Nancy F. Sowell, Michelle L. Frits, Suzanne M. Hoffman,

Shelley A. Hartz, Fran D. Booth, Martha Sweezy, Patricia R. Rogers, Rina L. Dubin, Joan C. Atkinson, Amy L. Friedman, Fernando Augusto, Christine K. Iannaccone, Anne H. Fossel, Gillian Quinn, Jing Cui, Elena Losina, and Richard C. Schwartz, "A Randomized Controlled Trial of an Internal Family Systems-Based Psychotherapeutic Intervention on Outcomes in Rheumatoid Arthritis: A Proof-of-Concept Study," *Journal of Rheumatology* 40, no. 11 (November 2013): 1831–1841, doi.org/10.3899/jrheum.121465.

CHAPTER 13: HEALING THE COLLECTIVE

1. Thomas Hübl and Julie Jordan Avritt, *Healing Collective Trauma: A Process for Integrating Our Intergenerational and Cultural Wounds* (Boulder, CO: Sounds True, 2020).
2. Layla F. Saad, "I Need to Talk to Spiritual White Women About White Supremacy (Part One)," August 15, 2017, laylafsaad.com/poetry-prose/white-women-white-supremacy-1; Layla F. Saad, "I Need to Talk to Spiritual White Women About White Supremacy (Part Two)," October 16, 2017, laylafsaad.com/poetry-prose/white-women-white-supremacy-2.

Index

suicide and suicidal thoughts, 230–31,
266, 270

Traditional Chinese Medicine
(TCM)
meridians, 81–82
radiant circuits, 86–87
triple warmers, 87–88
white people practicing, 174–75
trauma, 225–28
backlash, 253, 265–66
childhood trauma/adverse
childhood experiences (ACEs),
229–34, 238–40, 260–61
defining, 235–36
developmental trauma, 236–43
disease, link to, 229–31, 233–34,
279–80
mainstream medicine, 247–48
neuroscience and physiology of,
231–33
Post-traumatic stress disorder
(PTSD) and complex PTSD,
230, 238, 260
stress, 66, 191–92, 228, 231–32
suicide and suicidal thoughts,
230–31, 266, 270
treating, 243–46, 251–53;
Advanced Integrative Therapy
(AIT), 273–98; Internal Family
Systems (IFS), 254–72; somatic
experiencing exercise, 248–50;
Three-Step Transformation
(AIT technique), 294–98
types of, 274
see also Advanced Integrative
Therapy (AIT); Internal Family
Systems (IFS)

triple warmers, 87–88
trustworthiness of Sacred Medicine
practitioners, 201–23
finding and discerning an ethical
healer, 220, 223
harmlessness ("first, do no
harm"), 209–11
Kirikou and the Sorceress (film),
206–7
virtuosity and spiritual
enlightenment, 202
The Type C Connection (Temoshok
and Dreher), 145–46

vulnerability, 2

Welwood, John, 133, 141
Whole Health Cairn, 18–20
Whole Health Intelligences, 15–17
see also healing
Whole Health Medicine Institute
(WHMI), 7, 162
wholehearted, 161
wholeness, 3–4

About the Author

issa Rankin, MD, is the *New York Times* bestselling author of *Mind Over Medicine*, the prequel to *Sacred Medicine*, as well as six other books. She is a former OB/GYN physician, founder of the Whole Health Medicine Institute certification program for doctors and therapists, a radical remission researcher, and founder of the nonprofit Heal at Last. Dr. Rankin is a passionate ambassador for trauma-informed medicine, integrative approaches to treating chronic and life-threatening illnesses, and bridging science and spirituality. Her four TEDx Talks have been viewed more than five million times, and her television specials *Heal Yourself: Mind Over Medicine* and *The Fear Cure* were widely viewed on the Public Broadcasting Service (PBS).

Dr. Rankin is also a social justice activist advocating for health equity, antiracism in medicine and spiritual teaching, and health-care reform. Her desire to democratize Sacred Medicine healing modalities and ensure health equity for oppressed and marginalized people inspired her to spearhead her latest project, Heal at Last, a 501(c)3 nonprofit organization modeled after 12-step programs that aims to help treat the public health epidemic of loneliness and bring cutting-edge trauma healing methods and other Sacred Medicines out of their current status as luxury goods, making these healing modalities available and accessible to anyone who needs them regardless of socioeconomic status, race, or gender orientation.

Dr. Rankin lives in Marin County, California, with her daughter, Mira, and housemate, April. She is an avid hiker, nature ritualist, dancer, singer, painter, chef, raw chocolate maker, and amateur DJ. To learn more about her, visit lissarankin.com. To learn more about the Whole Health Medicine Institute, visit wholehealthmedicineinstitute.com. To learn more about Heal at Last, visit healatlast.org.

About Sounds True

Sounds True is a multimedia publisher whose mission is to inspire and support personal transformation and spiritual awakening. Founded in 1985 and located in Boulder, Colorado, we work with many of the leading spiritual teachers, thinkers, healers, and visionary artists of our time. We strive with every title to preserve the essential "living wisdom" of the author or artist. It is our goal to create products that not only provide information to a reader or listener but also embody the quality of a wisdom transmission.

For those seeking genuine transformation, Sounds True is your trusted partner. At SoundsTrue.com you will find a wealth of free resources to support your journey, including exclusive weekly audio interviews, free downloads, interactive learning tools, and other special savings on all our titles.

To learn more, please visit SoundsTrue.com/freegifts or call us toll-free at 800.333.9185.